I0838910

A FITFUL

LIFE

A story about Epilepsy, Depression, Anxiety and so much more...

TIM BONE

Copyright 2021 Tim Bone

The right of Tim Bone to be identified as the author of this work has been asserted by him in accordance with the Copyright, Designs and Patents Act 1988

All rights reserved. No part of this publication may be reproduced, stored in a retrieval system, or transmitted, in any form or by any means, electronic, mechanical, photocopying, recording or otherwise, without the prior permission of the copyright owner.

A WORD FOR THE STIGMATISERS AND PSYCHIATRISTS

For those of you who see those with disability, of any type of description, as being a member of a population of people who are deserving of less preferential treatment, as well as, deserving of less human rights, due to possessing what one would call a feature that compromises one's potential to satisfy societal expectations, I would strongly recommend you read the following before commencing the reading of this book as come the end of this book you will either be of the opinion that I am a member of an underclass whose life has been made complicated by issues that would fill you with shame and less deserving of human rights; or you will see me as belonging to an admirable group of people who have endured and survived storms and turbulent, confrontational living conditions in an inhospitable world that takes up to 1 in 7 lives where the only way in surviving has been to learn life skills and knowledge, that they don't teach you at any educational establishment; as well as, develop personality traits that enable you to bounce back from every traumatic experience a stronger and much more mature person.

We live in a society where if you belong to a minority, where the minority feature is one that is associated with wealth, status and power; you are admired and adored by others where others all wish to be like you to the point where some will even go as far as go out and pay for the same hair cut as you, in their attempts to be like you, however, if you are a member of a minority where the minority feature is associated with disadvantage and social injustice; you are made unemployable, bullied, raped, beaten up etc, where some people will even go as far as set you on fire. You may ask "why is this?". The answer to this question is quite simply because civilians are from a very young age raised by society to want to be like the "ideal person". The authorities that make up society create this image of the "ideal person" who everybody is encouraged to be like for the purpose of getting everyone walking, talking, wearing, spending etc the same things for the purpose of making huge fortunes, as well as, raising everyone to have the same set of beliefs and values so that the authorities can get away with giving us minimal human rights.

Society promotes this image of the ideal person through the use of media, codes of conduct, rules and regulations, family values, marketing etc. People are encouraged to be like this ideal person from a very young age. Everybody grows up trying to be like this ideal person which causes people to naturally evolve towards just trying to be like everyone else, and this is where conformity comes from. For some, the wearing of school uniform was the beginning of this, where if we wore the wrong shade of blue to school we got hounded by the teachers in front of our peers, which taught us to believe that it was forbidden to be different to the rest, and it was okay to treat someone with hostility for being different. For others, they will have learned this same message in some other setting that promoted the same principle.

The "Self" is by nature the most different thing to "the rest", therefore, due to everybody's aversion toward anything seen as different, most people have an aversion towards the self, causing them to grow up with a self-loathing. This has made people grow up with a love for the "one of the crowd" identities and a love for majorities. It is this love for majorities that has everyone disapprove of anyone who is seen as belonging to a minority or different, unless the minority feature is seen as being one that makes the person "more ideal, than ideal" which is a feature that gives one wealth, status or power.

People measure how well they are fitting in by how much acceptance and approval they are getting from others; where how well they fit in determines how much moral and self-esteem they have due to society convincing them that you need to be like this ideal person i.e. like everyone else, to be taken seriously and to be worthy of being treated with respect. People, therefore, know what the consequences of not fitting in are, which would be very low moral, self-esteem and no confidence. There is, therefore, this assumption that if someone does not fit in; as they belong to a minority, they will be someone with very low moral and self-esteem, therefore, as people also have a sadistic streak in them, they tend to get a gratification out of victimising those who belong to a minority believing that they are reducing that persons moral/self-esteem and confidence to intolerably low levels causing them to feel lots of pain. Victimising these minority members also gives people a feeling of gratification, as it makes them feel more secure about what they see as their shortcomings of being this ideal person. Victimising others remedies their own insecurities.

People in general are relatively very life inexperienced. There is too much stagnation in our society. People find roles that they fit into in society that are better known as jobs, that create comfort zones, resulting in far too many people choosing to just play the one role all their lives, thus, learning no new knowledge, new skills nor new experiences; causing them to mix with, as well as, get to know very few people; and have very little exposure to the world, meaning, that they rely on media to inform them of things like being black in America or sharing a home with someone who has schizophrenia, giving them a naïve understanding and very inaccurate images of people who belong to certain minority groups.

It can, therefore, be said that the stigmatising of others as a result of them belonging to a minority group evidences one to be insecure, needy, naïve, easily taken advantage of, inexperienced, ignorant, cynical, pretentious, vain and very likely someone who gets jealous. I would say that these traits of personality sound very much like the symptoms of a psychiatric condition worthy of being listed in the Diagnostic Statistic Manual Version 5 (soon to become Version 6, at time of publishing) under a name such as **"Insecure Attitude Disorder"**. Therefore, if come the end of this book you have become more judgemental or remain just as judgemental of people with disability; especially those with conditions that involve psycho-sensory hallucinations, then remember this unlisted mental health complaint that you as a stigmatiser could be described as ticking every box of; which I remind you, would be called **"Insecure Attitude Disorder"**

About the Author

Tim Bone, the author of this book is a 45 year old gentleman who graduated from the University of Glasgow with a BSc (Hons) in Molecular Biology in 1997. The author has been an advocate for people with neurological disability as well as a symptom management trainer for those living with long term disabilities. As well as having these credentials, the author has lived with lifelong epilepsy, symptoms of obsessive- compulsive disorder, social anxiety disorder and major depressive disorder; resulting in social exclusion as a result of the complete breakdown of education, employment, social and family functioning. The author has coped with these mental health conditions that have been both organic and psycho-social in origin using mental health symptom self-management techniques discovered through his own self-directed learning. It is through the learning of these techniques that the author has managed to avoid using anti-depressant and tranquiliser medication in the controlling of some mental health conditions and the conquering of others. As a result of the successful use of these symptom self-management techniques, the author has a passion for teaching these techniques to others with anxiety and depressive disorders. This passion has enabled the author to acquire years of experience of teaching these techniques to others affected by anxiety and depression as well as inspire him into starting his own mental health symptom self-management service; teaching in groups as well as one- to- one sessions, these symptom self-management techniques that are better known as "Cognitive Techniques".

A story about Epilepsy, Depression, Anxiety, self-empowerment and the links between politics, industry and psychiatric scientific theory.

INTRODUCTION

My name is Tim Bone and I was diagnosed with 'Complex Partial Epilepsy' at the age of ten. I have chosen to write this book as a result of the many social injustices I have had to live with, and continue living with to this day; that have been created by living in a society that could only be described as judgemental and penalising of those it sees as belonging to a vulnerable group. My experience of society, combined with being a meditator, has made the world transparent enough for me to realise what a "reckless blindfolded bull in a china shop" people can be as they have no knowledge of the collateral damage their everyday decisions have on the lives of others. I write this book with the hope that readers will become more aware of the collateral damage their decisions have on others' lives, with the aim of preventing others from becoming future casualties. I also write this book to make others who manage and make up the infrastructure of society aware of the needs of those with hidden disabilities, that to date get very little attention and tend to be treated as low priority by those in positions of power and authority. This book hopes to educate and inform with the aim of bringing about positive cultural and political change for those with disability in education, employment, social circles, law, family life, and other areas of a person's life.

The reader at the end of this book will either think that many of the things mentioned do not apply to them. If this is so then that means you are one of the ones' who is of high worth and what chapter 29 of the book would describe as 'high functioning'. You may however notice that there are many things that apply to yourself and your reaction will be to recognise that there are some things about the nature of yourself that you need to change. Well done, it means you are now a smarter, wiser, more informed and life educated person. You may however also recognise many things in this book that apply to yourself and get defensive by getting offended. The latter of these three people that one will find themselves being at the end of this book is the very type of person who is the driving force behind the troubles that this book is about, and therefore, it might make sense that a book that is a critical reflection of a society that such people make up a significant fraction of, would get defensive and possibly go on the attack after reading this book.

Happy Reading!

CHAPTER 1

You've bought this book because you are interested in epilepsy, you may be a sociology/medical/psychology etc, student wanting to gain a greater insight into the psychosocial impact that epilepsy has on one's life, you may have learned of a family member or a friend who has been diagnosed with epilepsy and wish to know what the future looks like for them, you may have been diagnosed as having epilepsy; and wish to learn about how your disability will affect you and what precautions you may wish to take to minimise the possible disabling effects that epilepsy can have on your life; you may have noticed that this book also concerns the self- management of anxiety and depression which you may have been diagnosed as having and would rather self -manage than be on psychotropic medication, or you may have another of the many reasons for buying this book.

As this book is primarily about the life of someone living with epilepsy co-existing with anxiety and depression, the first thing you will wish to know is: "What is that condition that makes someone go unconscious, collapse and suddenly start shaking very violently?". One question you most likely won't be asking is: "What neurological disorder is making that man look very drunk and behave in a very bizarre way?", nor will you be asking: "What neurological disorder caused that man on the same train as me to suddenly start screaming out loud, shouting all types of offensive statements/ words, terrifying everyone around him, resulting in the British Transport Police placing him under arrest upon arriving at our destination?". One thing I could be confident with is that you would know the word 'epilepsy' to be part of the answer to one of these three questioned scenarios. I could also be confident that if you are a layman reading, you would most likely not know nor even consider the word 'epilepsy' to be part of the answer to the other two questioned scenarios. I could also be confident that when those that can identify epilepsy as being behind the cause of each of these three questioned scenarios are asked what epilepsy is, those asked would either not be able to explain at all; or would at best give a very unsure, unclear and most likely very inaccurate definition.

So what is epilepsy? The first thing that one must clarify is that it is not a mental health condition. Many people struggle to either tell the difference between, or appreciate the difference between a condition of 'brain'; and one of 'mind'. Epilepsy is a condition that affects the brain and not the mind. Epilepsy is what we call a 'neurological disability'. A doctor called a 'neurologist' treats this condition where as a doctor called a 'psychiatrist' treats a person with a 'mind condition' such as: schizophrenia, depression, anxiety etc. Many do question whether schizophrenia is a mind condition or a brain condition. Many conditions that affect state of consciousness were at one time believed to be conditions of mind in the days where little, if any, of the biology of these conditions was understood. This is why many conditions that were once treated by psychiatrists are now treated by neurologists. Such an example of a condition that was first believed to be a mind condition but has proven to be a brain condition as we have learned more about the biology of the condition is epilepsy. Many expect depressive disorders such as 'bipolar disorder', and other conditions that are still treated by mental health professionals e.g. schizophrenia, will eventually prove to be conditions of the nervous system as more is discovered about the biology of these conditions. There are already theories, such as bipolar depressive disorder being caused by fluctuations in levels of different neurotransmitters in the central nervous system; that are chemical messengers that are responsible for the creation of electrical energy in the brain. Such theories would evidence that bipolar depressive disorder is caused by an imbalance in one's brain chemistry, making it a condition of brain and not of mind. Therefore, those who are being treated by psychiatrists today for having a condition such as bipolar depressive disorder, could find themselves being treated by neurologists tomorrow. In other words, bipolar depressive disorder, obsessive compulsive disorder and other, could end up following the same route that epilepsy took; which began in the field of psychiatry, ending up in the field of neurology; as doctors and scientists became more informed.

Epilepsy is a complicated condition, but a simple condition at the same time. Epilepsy is biologically simple, but politically and culturally very complicated. As someone who has lived with epilepsy since the age of three, I have compared notes of what living with epilepsy is like with people living with other neurological conditions such as multiple sclerosis. One thing I am told consistently by those affected by multiple sclerosis, Parkinson's disease, stroke, motor neurone disease, spinal injury etc is that living with epilepsy is much more of a political/socio-cultural battle than it is a medical battle. It's more society's reception towards our disability that disables us more than it is the actual impairments in our biology. I would say that society is the enemy more than it is the actual disability. If I were to split the issues faced by a person with a disability as belonging to one of two types i.e. medical and political/socio-cultural, in the case of someone living with my type of epilepsy the percentage of issues faced that have been medical in nature have been around the 15% mark and the issues that are political/socio-cultural in nature have made up 85% of all issues faced.

It can therefore be said that living with epilepsy, like other conditions, creates issues borne from a mixture of biology, politics and culture. First of all, let's look at its biology and then the rest of the book will look at the political, sociological and cultural side to living with epilepsy from the perspective of someone who lives with the condition. That person being myself, who is the author of this book.

SO, WHAT IS EPILEPSY?

Everything we think, how we behave, what we say, our perception of time and place, memory, our emotions, our personality etc, is controlled by the electrical activity in our brains. Our brains are made up of brain cells like a brick wall is made of bricks. These brain cells generate the electrical activity responsible for brain function, in the form of electrical waves that repeat themselves. This electrical activity is generated by a simple physiological process involving changes in electrochemical gradients brought on by changes in concentrations of sodium and potassium both inside and outside the brain cells. Let's look at how the brain cell creates the electrical activity that controls your nervous system.

Like a battery each brain cell has a voltage. This voltage is -70mV. In part 1 of the graph below, a substance called sodium enters the brain cells. Sodium has a positive charge and therefore the voltage of the cell increases. At part 2 of the graph, the brain cells' voltage has reached +30mV and the channels in the brain cell walls that were allowing sodium to enter close; preventing further increases in voltage. Once the sodium channels close, a substance called potassium, which has a positive charge; leaves the cell through potassium ion channels, causing the charge of the brain cell to start to drop. This decrease in voltage is further assisted by a sodium/potassium pump, where three sodium ions (positively charged) are pumped out and two potassium ions (positively charged) are pumped in, resulting in a further net loss of positive charge (Part

3 of graph). This results in the charge of the cell decreasing to below -70mV, to -90mV (Part 4). It is during part 5 of the graph that the sodium/potassium pump, pumps three sodium ions in and two potassium ions out, until the brain cell's charge increases from -90mV back to -70mV where the whole process starts again at part 6 of the graph.

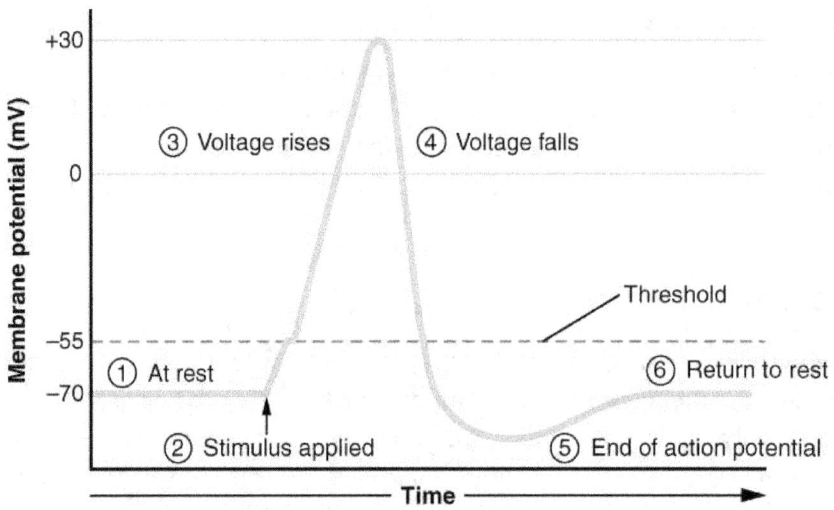

The brain waves that make up the brain's electrical activity are always of the same frequency i.e. number of waves per millisecond, and wavelength i.e. distance between the peaks of each wave; just like a radio station's radio waves are.

What controls the opening and closing of the sodium channels (part 2 to part 3 of graph) are structures called "receptors" that sit to the side of the entrance to the sodium ion channels, opening the channels for sodium to enter at -70mV; and then closing the channels to sodium at +30 mV.

In some people, these sodium channels can from time to time suddenly start opening and shutting much more frequently and for different durations of time than they usually do. This results in the generation of disorganised electrical activity made up of electrical waves of different wavelengths and frequencies. This disorganised electrical activity is what is referred to as a 'seizure', and can last between a few seconds and a few minutes; before returning back to normal. The symptoms one experiences during a seizure is determined by what part of the brain is affected by the distorted electrical activity.

A person who has a "tendency to have recurrent seizures" is diagnosed as having epilepsy. Anyone can have a seizure at any time without having epilepsy. For example, a person in the gym can have a seizure if they lose too much sodium in their sweat, are withdrawing from the effects of alcohol intoxication, sleep deprived, hypoglycaemic (especially in the case of diabetes) or had a stroke.   These are just a few examples. These types of seizures are one off seizures, and do not tend to be reoccurring seizures, that can happen at anytime and anyplace; thus meaning that these seizures do not mean that the person affected has epilepsy.

Medications for seizures are called 'anti-convulsants'. Some anti-convulsants act by blocking the sodium channels when they are supposed to close. Other anti-convulsants act on the receptor, thus helping the receptor control the closing and shutting of the sodium channels; preventing them from becoming "disobedient".

It requires a lot of trial and error with many different medications before a combination of medications can be found that control the seizures; however, with perseverance 85% of people with epilepsy do eventually find a combination of anti-convulsants that get the epilepsy under control without having to endure intolerable side effects.

If most people were to be asked about epilepsy it would be a safe assumption to make that all would have a knowledge of the seizure type that causes one to lose consciousness, collapse and undergo violent shaking of head and all four limbs, and experience urinary or faecal incontinence. This seizure is referred to as a "Tonic-Clonic Epileptic seizure". It would also be a safe assumption to make that the odds of lay people having heard of any of the other seizure types other than "Petit-Mal" are very low. It is unfortunately an ignorance that not only the vast majority of the public possess but also a large number of our public sector workers, and those who work in other service industries where they could come across someone with epilepsy having a seizure on any given day also possess; and this book will highlight the consequences of such ignorance amongst these public sector workers e.g. police, teachers, social workers, public transport workers and other service industry employees such as doormen.

Seizures can be split into one of two categories. One of these categories is called 'Generalised Seizures' and the other is called 'Partial Seizures'. As the names would suggest with 'Generalised Seizures', the seizure involves the whole brain; however, with 'Partial Seizures', the seizure activity only affects a part of the brain.

There are a number of different types of 'Generalised Seizure' as well as there being a number of different types of 'Partial Seizure'. Let's have a look at the different types:

Generalised Seizures are: **Tonic-Clonic Seizures, Atonic Seizures, Tonic Seizures, Myoclonic Seizures, Absences.**

Tonic Clonic seizures have already been described and are the stereotypical epileptic seizure. This is the seizure that everyone thinks of when you mention the word "Epilepsy". It is also referred to as "Grand Mal Epilepsy".

Atonic seizures are also known as "Drop Attacks" and these are seizures where a person suddenly loses muscle tone and will collapse like a puppet whose strings have been cut. These attacks are only momentary. There is no period of unconsciousness. The person will get back up on their feet but unfortunately because of the nature of the seizure and the environment, injuries to the head and face are very common. These people can often have eye injuries as a consequence of hitting themselves of corners of tables and work surfaces as well as burn injuries. I witnessed a man have one of these seizures on Argyll Street in Glasgow while I was walking to a stationary shop to get some whiteboard pens. This man was crossing a road and suddenly collapsed and got straight back up and kept walking. This man had hit the side of his face off the tarmac while he was crossing a road. You knew it was a seizure as there was no attempt made to break his fall. People affected by this type of seizure should always use the pedestrian lights and would be seriously unwise to ever run across a road giving themselves just enough time to get to the other side.

Tonic Seizures are the opposite of Atonic seizures and they result in a person's muscles suddenly going stiff causing them to fall backwards. These seizures are also momentary. Injuries to the back of the head are common.

Myoclonic Seizures are seizures that cause the person to suddenly undergo many uncontrollable muscular contractions of their arms and legs. This can also cause them to have falls and injuries. With this seizure there is no loss of consciousness.

Absences are seizures that cause someone to become unresponsive, still and stare blankly with no facial expression for around twenty seconds.

There are also a number of partial seizures. The most common partial seizures types can be categorised as '**Complex Partial Seizures' and 'Simple Partial Seizures'.**

Complex Partial Seizures are seizures where consciousness is not lost, but consciousness is affected; and the person can behave in a very bizarre way and say very bizarre things. The person is overcome by an overwhelming feeling of anxiety and fear. The person loses awareness and may appear drugged and may start shouting out loud uncontrollably or they may go up to people in the street and start speaking nonsense that does not make any sense. They may also experience loss of familiarity with surroundings as well as anyone they are with, and believe themselves to be elsewhere. There is a period of blackout, that they have no memory of after the seizure, which is the period of the seizure where they say bizarre things and behave in a bizarre way. The blackout is usually followed by a period of confusion that can last for several minutes where they have no knowledge of date, day of week, time of day, anything about themselves e.g. occupation, their plans for today, no memory of yesterday etc. This loss of information can be very distressing and cause a lot of anxiety, as they have no knowledge that they have just had a seizure, nor have any memory of having had previous seizures; therefore, there is no previous experience that they can recollect that will inform them that memory will recover. Gradually over a period of several minutes this essential information that makes up identity, time and place comes back to them. This period of confusion is referred to as the "Post-Ictal State".

Simple Partial Seizures are like complex partial seizures, but as the name would suggest, there is no impairment in consciousness i.e. blackout, nor is there any post-ictal state. In other words, the person will experience the onset of symptoms such as immense fear and anxiety, loss of familiarity with surroundings and those around them, feeling of being elsewhere and then sudden wearing off of the seizure. They could maintain a conversation with you throughout the seizure in theory, but the anxiety and fear may be incredibly difficult to hide from someone they are speaking to. I have had these sitting in coffee shops and pubs and there is no better feeling in the world than the feeling you get when the seizure wears off and you learn that for this time you are not going to have a complex partial seizure. You feel a tremendous feeling of getting away without getting caught.

Complex partial seizures, which is the seizure type that I have, occur in a part of the brain called the 'Temporal Lobe'. There is a temporal lobe on both sides of the brain, and with simple partial seizures only one of the temporal lobes are affected; but with complex partial seizures the seizure activity starts off affecting just one of the temporal lobes, but then spreads into the other temporal lobe, thus affecting both temporal lobes. This is why in complex partial seizures there is an impairment in consciousness but in simple partial seizures there is no impairment in consciousness i.e. no period of loss of awareness, nor period of post-ictal confusion. It is often the case that medication does not have any effect on complex partial seizures, and as a consequence of this; surgery is seen as the only option, which involves the removal of the temporal lobe where the seizure activity begins in. Just like a kidney, a person can live with just one temporal lobe, but removal of a temporal lobe can leave the person with significant memory impairments.

Complex partial seizures can also take place in a part of the brain called the 'Frontal Lobes'. The frontal lobes are responsible for inhibiting your behaviour. It is the part of the brain that stops you from acting out intrusive thoughts, such as jumping when you are looking down from a very high height or punching the bride; or groom at a wedding when making your vows, or shouting out loud "I have a bomb" when walking through airport security in a country where there are armed guards who will shoot on site. This type of seizure can result in someone behaving in an extremely anti-social way, which can get them arrested or injured, and in worst case scenarios even killed as a result of getting themselves into confrontational situations. This type of complex partial seizure is referred to as 'Frontal Lobe Epilepsy'.

The seizures listed here are the most common ones, and only make up a fraction of the number of the different epileptic seizure types. There would be too many to list here as there are over forty different seizure types, but they can all be categorised as partial seizures or generalised seizures.

Epilepsy is diagnosed using medical apparatus called an MRI scanner which looks for abnormal brain anatomy that could be behind the cause of someone's seizures such as previously undiagnosed brain damage, damage left behind after stroke, brain tumour or scar tissue. A person who is suspected of having epilepsy is also attached to an 'ambulatory electro-encephalogram', also referred to as an 'EEG', which measures brain wave activity so that doctors can see what happens to the electrical activity in the brain when someone experiences the seizure like symptoms that they have previously reported to their neurologist. It is from this EEG trace of brain electrical activity that doctors can both diagnose epilepsy as well as diagnose what part of the brain the seizure affects and thus what type of epilepsy a person has.

You may be asking: "What is different about the brains of people with epilepsy and those without?". I would first of all like to say that everyone is at risk of having a seizure. No person's brain is not capable of having a seizure at any one time. Every person's brain has what is called a 'Seizure Threshold', and the difference between those with epilepsy, and those without is that those with epilepsy have a lower seizure threshold than those without epilepsy; therefore, it does not take much to antagonise the brain enough to bring on a seizure in these people with epilepsy i.e. those with a low seizure threshold. In fact, the brain can be antagonised into having a seizure so easily in those with a low seizure threshold that seizures are a common occurrence and this is called 'Epilepsy' i.e. a tendency to have recurrent seizures. What causes a person's brain to have a lower seizure threshold at rest than the average person's can be the presence of scar tissue, brain damage at birth, stroke, brain tumour, genetics, head injury, alcohol and drug abuse as well as unknown cause. Someone who has a tendency to have recurrent seizures where no cause behind their low seizure threshold can be identified is referred to as having "Idiopathic Epilepsy".

What can trigger seizures in those with a low seizure threshold are triggers such as: sleep deprivation, wakening from sleep, depression, anxiety, food additives such as aspartame and mono-sodium glutamate, alcohol and drug withdrawal, over exertion, stress, acute emotional reactions, strobe lightening and others.

It is important to communicate to others that epileptic seizures brought on by strobe lightening is symptomatic of a type of epilepsy called 'Photosensitive Epilepsy', and only affects 5% of people with epilepsy. In 95% of cases of epilepsy it is perfectly safe to engage in activities that result in exposure to strobe lightening; however, there is this widespread belief that strobe lightening affects all people with epilepsy, and anyone found with anti-convulsants on them by a doorman at a nightclub is going to have a hard time convincing him that they are one of the 95%, as even they believe all people with epilepsy to be affected by photosensitivity. This can unfortunately result in a lot of discrimination, prejudice and denial of luxuries that the mainstream are not denied.

Many people with epilepsy report that the most disabling part of living with epilepsy is not the symptoms of epilepsy, but the reception these people get from society, after society learning about their epilepsy. There have been statements such as: "My epilepsy does not disable me, but people's attitudes do", spread around that have gone from being personal statements made by individuals to widely held findings amongst the population of people living with epilepsy. We do unfortunately live in a society that penalises those living with epilepsy, and this can be evidenced by many bits of factual information that highlight the disadvantages living with epilepsy in British society invites into one's life. For example, the suicide rate amongst the mainstream population is **1 in 200,** but the suicide rate amongst those with complex partial seizures is **32 fold** this rate; which equates to **1 in 7** according to a University of Western Ontario, Department of Psychiatry study carried out in 2012 . This figure is determined by the fact that the prevalence of major depressive disorder amongst those with complex partial seizures is 37% (Oliveira et al 2010) .The prevalence of people with epilepsy in society is **1 in 130,** whereas the prevalence of people living with epilepsy in the prison population is   **1 in 50** if you are a man, and **1 in 20** if you are a women (Sulfolk Cluster 2015). In fact, if you have epilepsy and are a man, you are just under three times more likely to end up in prison. If you have epilepsy you are far more likely to remain single or get divorced. Only 27% of people with epilepsy get married, whereas 90% of the mainstream get married by the age of 45 (Ghaemi et al 2014). There has been a widespread belief that up until 1970 there was a law in Britain which forbid people with epilepsy from getting married. The World Health Organisation was also under the belief that such a law existed; however, this belief has been nothing more than a myth. It is however the case that back in 1937 there was a law called the 'Matrimonial Causes Act', that allowed for a marriage to be declared invalid if one of the partners of that marriage were to suffer from recurrent seizures. This meant that a marriage could be broken up without there being any need for divorce proceedings if husband or wife were to have recurrent seizures. The Archbishop of Canterbury did speak out against the Matrimonial Causes Act, but unfortunately it would take another thirty four years before parliament shared the same view as the archbishop.

The unemployment rate of people with epilepsy has been reported to be between 25% and 69% (Epilepsy Toronto 2013), and 20% have to retire early (Boer, Science Direct 2010). Those with epilepsy also experience a lot of discrimination in the workplace. In fact, as many as 54% of those with epilepsy have experienced discrimination in the workplace; and as many as 67% of those with epilepsy believe that their careers have been adversely affected by their condition. As many as 75% of those with epilepsy feel that their colleagues are not understanding enough, and that the stress caused by this can cause them to have seizures at work. (Epilepsy: Everything you need to know, Closer online, March 2016)

Childhood is a very vulnerable period in a person's life as it is the time where a person is undergoing their formative years, and therefore it is the time where the most damage can be done to a person's confidence, morale, self- esteem and future mental health thus affecting future achievement and happiness. In fact, 50% of all mental health problems amongst the mainstream adult population can be attributed to incidents that happened during childhood, according to 'Anxiety UK'. Children with epilepsy are therefore especially vulnerable, and therefore more prone to future underachievement, unhappiness, low life satisfaction and diagnosable mental health problems. It has been recognised that children with epilepsy face discrimination, hostility, exclusion and taunting on a regular basis. It has been found from a report, released by the organisation 'Young Epilepsy', questioning adults' and childrens' attitudes towards epilepsy, that as many as 79% of those with epilepsy across all age groups have been the victims of discrimination and that there is particular concern for young people with regards towards their ability to cope with the negative reactions they receive from others. According to the same report, it has also been found in research carried out that almost 50% of children with epilepsy are on the receiving end of hostility or ill feeling as a consequence of their condition and that almost 20% experience such negative reactions at least once daily. It has been reported in the same report, published by 'Young Epilepsy', that as many as 40% have experienced discrimination or exclusion from members of their peer group, and that around 33% feel that they have received discrimination from their teachers. After experiencing a seizure as many as 41% have been told by their peers that they are sick, 43% have been told that they are crazy, 29% accused of having something contagious, 20% have been told that they are possessed, 18% have been asked if they speak to spirits and 16% have been told that they should be locked up. It is most likely because of these bad childhood experiences that adults with epilepsy do not tell people they have just met that they have epilepsy due to fears of negative reactions.

All of these figures demonstrate that there is a negative attitude towards epilepsy in our society that seriously disadvantages an individual to what is often an even greater extent than the actual medical condition itself. There are other settings where people with epilepsy are disadvantaged because of public attitude as well as attitude amongst those in professional roles working with people with epilepsy; however, this chapter would probably be the length of a book if all of these were to be covered. The rest of the book will be looking at these settings mentioned in this chapter, and some other settings from the perspective of an individual living with epilepsy. That individual is myself and what you will learn from my experiences in the settings I have encountered difficulties in, should provide you with an insight into the difficulties one with epilepsy would encounter in settings not discussed, and your learning from my experiences; combined with your own intuition, will enable you to see the collateral damage that the difficulties in these undiscussed settings creates. In other words, this book will make you a much more holistic thinker which is a life skill that has kept many people alive, which sadly too many people do not have.

I must emphasise that this book is no attempt of one person living with epilepsy to capture the sympathy of those who have bought this book. This book is instead wanting to draw to the attention of the reader the failings of our society in terms of the behaviours and reception people with epilepsy are on the receiving end of from its people; with the intention of changing these through the spreading of the word by the reader to those they come into contact with every day. Some of these will be people who need their behaviour towards, and perceptions of people with epilepsy changed for the better, whereas others will not; but will know of people who do need such behaviours and perceptions changed. I would hope that through this book the attitude and perceptions of others towards those with epilepsy, other physical disability, learning disability as well as mental health problems will change in the same way that "friendship" and "people you may Know" spread on social media, such as Facebook. These attitudes and perceptions of other people will not change painting a pretty picture of living with epilepsy; co-existing with depression and anxiety, nor would this book be read if it were to be about what a wonderful life living with epilepsy accompanied by depression and anxiety is when it doesn't make you a millionaire, a celebrity or a person of influence and high social position.

As the person writing about the negative experiences found in this book is the person who was affected by these experiences, the tone may sound sympathy seeking in parts, but it is instead the tone of someone communicating a dissatisfaction with experiences and treatments; with the intention of opening the mainstream's eyes and bringing about cultural change for future generations of those struggling with a disability. Despite these two tones sounding very similar they are not to be confused if the book is to fulfil its purpose by taking society steps closer towards the desired cultural change required for social justice to prevail. To label the dialogue of someone with epilepsy communicating their bad experiences with the world as "sympathy seeking" would be detracting from the message this book has been written to communicate. This labelling the communicating of bad experience of living with epilepsy as "sympathy seeking" would also be an example of the very cynicism that creates many of the issues that people with epilepsy have to live with as well as an attempt to run away from the real issue. This book is written to bring about an improvement in society as opposed to obtaining sympathy from society. Sympathy is just 'talk' and what this book wants is 'action'. It is for this reason that this book has been sent to First Minister Nicola Sturgeon, Scottish Labour Leader Richard Leonard, Scottish Liberal Democrat Leader Willie Rennie, Scottish Conservative Leader Jackson Carlaw and the Scottish Charity Regulator as the charities serve no purpose whatsoever for mainstream people like me. This is not only evidenced by the lack of any difference the charities make to the lives of those with neurological disability, such as epilepsy; but also from the discrimination towards people with neurological disability that they themselves are guilty of, such as constructive dismissal that you will read about later on in this book. If the Charity Regulator put this book down now then it evidences the very accusations that I make and let's not get hung up over strong words like "Accusation". This politically correct climate has made me very ill, where the word "ill" is a word I would now probably be slapped on the wrist for using as it sounds too strong.

This book can also serve as a guide for those with depression, anxiety disorders including panic as well as other mood disorders e.g. anger, low confidence etc; as it introduces you to the cognitive and other self- help techniques that can be used to control these mental health conditions as an alternative to anti-depressants and tranquilliser medication. The effectiveness of these cognitive and self-help techniques is put into context through this storytelling of an individual living with epilepsy co-existing with anxiety and depression. These techniques aren't just taught as theory, but taught as 'applied theory'; as you will read about these techniques being used in real life scenarios. Too many mindfulness courses available in our society, that just teach theory. It is 'Applied Theory' that people relate with, and are inspired by, as opposed to text book theory. You will be a fly on the wall in the life of someone who has used these techniques to fight the everyday mental health battle of living in an intolerant society towards anyone living with a disability; giving every reader with a mood disorder confidence in the using of these cognitive techniques as an alternative to anti-depressant and/or tranquiliser medication.

This book, as well as being a symptom management guide for those suffering from mental health problems, can also be used as a guide for personal development for the average member of the mainstream population as a number of cognitive techniques introduced to the reader in this book to boost confidence, morale and self- esteem can also be used as strategies that can help someone work towards successful outcomes with any present and future goals they find themselves wishing to achieve. Finally, the book also provides the reader with advice on how to prepare for a universal credit medical assessment, exampled by my own application, which I managed to put together using the skills developed from my experience as a disability advocate.

CHAPTER 2 - MY EPILEPSY

I chose to write this book as I am too aware of the lack of education and ignorance that surrounds the subject of epilepsy in our society. There is no source that educates and informs those who will come across those with epilepsy as part of their roles within society, other than a few hours of in-house training every few years for people working in caring and certain teaching roles that lasts a half day, which in my own opinion is taught more for the sake of ticking a box and getting funding for charities than it is the improvement in services for people with epilepsy. This is especially concerning when those in such roles, play roles that give them responsibilities and decision- making powers that will have a huge influence on the quality of lives of those living with epilepsy, which if compromised can also have a huge influence on the quantity of life of those living with epilepsy, and cause an explosive amount of collateral damage such as years of social isolation resulting in drug and alcohol addiction, a career on the benefits system, jumping from a tall bridge; resulting in a mother experiencing a reliance on community mental health services, to then be made unemployable as a result of having a history of mental health problems, to then acquire a condition like angina resulting in early grave. This sounds very depressing, but it is; and it's a reality going on right now, and you may need a thick skin to read this book, but if we avoid talking about the realities of living in such an intolerant society then I'm afraid that is showing an intolerance in itself.

It is not just those in roles with decision making powers, that have a big impact on the lives of those with epilepsy, who need educating on epilepsy; but anyone who could, and will most certainly at some time in their life come into contact with someone with epilepsy; such as lay people, educators and employers etc.

I am only too aware of this great need for public education on epilepsy as a consequence of myself being on the receiving end of such discrimination and ignorance in education, employment and social settings; as a consequence of having complex partial epilepsy, which I was officially diagnosed with at the age of ten, despite remembering my first seizure at the age of three, when I was running around the lounge with my toy hoover and suddenly experienced the onset symptoms of a simple partial seizure. These simple partial seizures only occurred once or twice per year up until the age of ten, and as a consequence of this, remained unnoticed until seizures started to become much more frequent; where they were starting to occur at a frequency of two every three days and were now complex partial seizures. It was at the age of ten that I was referred to a neurologist and was given a diagnosis of 'Complex Partial Epilepsy'. These seizures occurred mostly upon awakening in the middle of the night, as well as within the first couple of hours of being out of my bed in the morning. Despite morning seizures happening within the first couple of hours after awakening, they mostly occurred within the first twenty minutes of being out of my bed, the vast majority of the time. It was the case that maybe there would be three events a year, where I would take my morning seizure on the train going to school or upon arriving at school. Although these seizures occurred upon awakening in middle of night or within first couple of hours of being awake, I could still have two or three events a year during the day such as during class at school, watching the television in the evening or out with my friends having lunch.

These complex partial seizures, as has already been mentioned in chapter one, do not involve any loss of consciousness; however, they do involve impaired consciousness, where during the seizure you lose all alertness and orientation and start saying bizarre things and behave in a bizarre way which you are not aware of doing at the time of being in this bizarre state. These seizures are not the stereotypical epileptic seizure that everyone thinks of when you mention the word "epilepsy". It is a seizure type that next to no one has heard of who does not work in the field of epilepsy/medicine/life sciences, and as a consequence of this, the first thing members of the public believe when they witness such a seizure is that the affected person is either drunk or is intoxicated on some illegal recreational drug. If someone is with you at the time of taking the seizure and doesn't know you have epilepsy, they will think you have become deranged, as onset of symptoms is so sudden. As a consequence of this ignorance, neither the public nor people in service provision roles e.g. police, public transport workers, doormen etc, take a sympathetic approach to managing the person affected by the seizure. It will be discussed in further chapters what kind of issues such seizures have created for myself when out in the public and the inappropriate treatment I have received from others during the seizure such as police and gym staff.

Up until 1998 my seizure frequency remained what it was since the age of ten. Up until 1995 I was having seizures immediately upon awakening, within the first couple of hours of being awake and anytime during the day. In 1995 seizures that were had during the day were eliminated but seizures within first two hours of being awake or upon awakening in middle of night, were still continuing at a high frequency of one every 36hrs. Seizures during the day were still possible if there were a trigger such as sleep deprivation, excessive alcohol consumption and missed doses up until 1998, when my medication was changed and I was put on two types of anticonvulsant drug. One of the anticonvulsants types prevented seizures, and the other type acted when you were about to take a seizure. Two of the anticonvulsants that I was put on in 1998 acted on the sodium ion channel receptors 24/7, and the other drug blocked the sodium ion channels when they started to misbehave. Since being on this drug combination I have had no seizures during the day, still have seizures upon awakening in the middle of the night, but these are only once every ten days, and I have not had any seizures within the first couple of hours of awakening in the morning over the last 5 years.

The seizures that I have had to live with have been seizures that are not dramatic for the observer to watch, unless the person having the seizure seriously injures themselves or gets themselves into an incident that could result in seriously regrettable lifelong outcomes. If the seizure takes place in a quiet place with privacy and no environmental hazards, they are not dramatic to watch but very dramatic to experience. The rest of the chapter describes the experiences that I experience during a complex partial seizure.

WHAT IS IT LIKE TO EXPERIENCE A COMPLEX PARTIAL SEIZURE?

The following descriptions make reference to the different pictures that describe the onset of a complex partial seizure originating from the left temporal lobe, causing a psycho-hallucination, right through to loss of awareness and orientation, followed by amnesia to full recovery. I have put links beside each picture that take you to a website with these same images, where the images are in colour. The reason for this is because colour is required to truly communicate to the reader what the atmosphere of the world feels like around me at the time of having a seizure. Just like some people think "red" when you say the number "three", or "green" when you say the number "four"; when you have a seizure, the world is "experienced" in the colours found in these images. A better explanation of this can be found in the appropriate part of the seizure description that you are about to read. The book shows these images in black and white as a result of the extra costs that publishing in colour would have put on the price of the book.

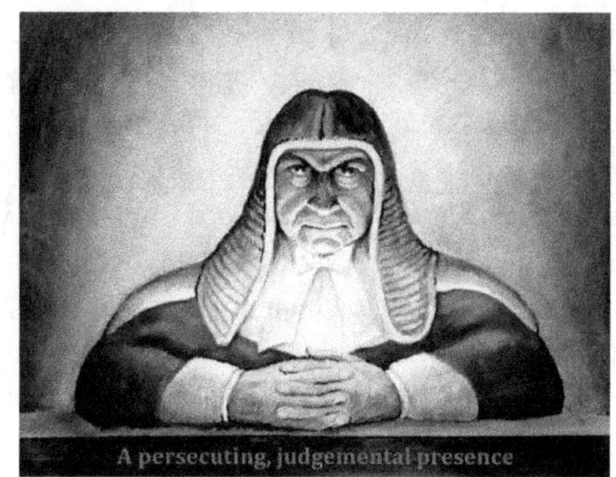

Picture 1

View colour version: http://www.afitfullife.com/index.asp?pageid=717241

Picture 1 describes the emotional experience that tells you that you are about to have a complex partial seizure. Just before the onset of a complex partial seizure I feel a strong nervousness in my gut and the presence of a great threat. It is a similar feeling to what you would feel standing in front of a judge before you, awaiting persecution from a persecuting; intensely authoritative authority, combined with the unknown consequences of such persecution, other than that you are going to become majorly compromised. This feeling of nervousness can be described as being accompanied with the paralysing feeling of helplessness that one feels when uncontrollably heading towards the "edge of a cliff", where going over the edge will result in very compromising consequences. You feel that there are three consequences if this warning develops into a seizure. One consequence that fills you with overwhelming dread is the thought that you are on the brink of experiencing a mentally distressing experience which is strong enough to leave you traumatised; another consequence is a traumatic experience that could also be accompanied by irreparable damage caused by self-humiliation, where you might not feel able to show your face again. A final consequence that terrifies you is the judgementalism of other people causing you to become seriously compromised in the long term e.g. assaulted, arrested, made redundant etc.

This brings on a feeling of panic and loss of control; and has you want to just stand up from whatever conversation you are having with someone or setting you are in, such as a meeting at work, and "run- away"; but you can't "run" as there is no place to run to. You could say, "Help me! I'm about to have a seizure!" but you are having thoughts about how asking for help could in itself majorly compromise you; as it could probably result in loss of job, future bullying in the workplace or simply the negativity of others towards you; causing you to lose roles and responsibilities from your job description as well as loss of promotional prospects, without good reason. The asking for help could also have you thrown out of a night club, as doormen think "once he's out the door, he's no longer our problem". The asking for help of a stranger on the street could also result in you being without your jacket, wallet and watch etc once you are fully recovered from the seizure. You also don't wish to ask for help, as to hear yourself ask for help is confirming in your mind that you are going to have a seizure which you don't concede to as these seizures are just too frightening to even contemplate having. You are effectively gagged from asking for help as you are in a state of fear induced denial during the warning stage.

The picture gives the judge, the same amount of presence as what you feel the fear of the majorly compromising outcomes of a seizure have during the warning to a seizure. The threat of the negative outcomes that result from a seizure have an incomparably greater amount of presence than anyone I am with or anyplace I am in. Time and place have become irrelevant. You feel you are going to be abducted from the world around you and "taken away" as you are aware of what symptoms are to come, which you will learn about very soon. You feel overwhelming isolation as this experience is one that only you are having, and the experience comes entirely from within yourself; which is the mind and brain, which combined are as large as the universe; giving you an overwhelming feeling of vulnerability that makes you feel the size of an atom that's about to lose all its electron shells. An overwhelming feeling of "you came into this world on your own, and you will leave on your own" overcomes you, which you feel couldn't apply more to the present moment.

At this stage of the seizure experience the beginning of the warning is slow in progressing towards seizure. If "1" is beginning of warning and "10" is seizure, then up until "6" the warning is travelling towards the "edge", which in the case of epilepsy is the 'seizure threshold' i.e. the score which if the warning progresses beyond you are definitely going to have a seizure. On average, up until "6" the warning is travelling at a slow speed, and it lasts for around ninety seconds. Once the warning gets to "6", it accelerates rapidly to "10" in a period of around ten seconds. The ninety seconds is full of anxiety over "will it happen?", and the next ten seconds is full of panic as "it is going to happen!!". The seizure warning can be prevented from progressing beyond "6" by using techniques such as mental arithmetic, using the self- talk that a boxing coach would give his boxer, or thinking about scenes in your mind of places that make up a large part of your identity and thinking to yourself as much as you can "What's going on there now?". The likelihood of the seizure happening can be increased by having opposite thoughts about places you've never been before, places you have only been once or twice; such as a hotel room you were in over the summer holidays five thousand miles away, or places you've been but have not visited over the last twenty years; and think to yourself "What is going on there now?". These thoughts of unfamiliar places that ally with the odds of having a seizure can come on in the form of intrusive thoughts. My theory for why thoughts about places far removed from my identity bring on seizures, is that loss of familiarity of myself and whereabouts is such a strong feature of the complex partial seizure.

If you can defuse the warning through these symptom management methods mentioned i.e. positive self-talk, mental arithmetic, thoughts of familiar places; you suddenly feel the relief of all the fear, anxiety, nervousness in the gut and blood returning to your face; and a massive relief, where you want to shout out loud, "Thank fuck for that!!!!". If you're a child you will start crying with relief, which I did when I was fourteen on a French exchange, where I had a warning at the family table during dinner and had to be comforted by an English lady afterwards. I just used my boxing coach self- talk to defuse it, which is why I have probably grown up a very bold person, as I relied on this positive self-talk to fend off seizures up until the age of twenty which was when I discovered the strategy of mental arithmetic to defuse warnings that had a much greater success rate. Positive self-talk defused around 1 in 3 seizures from developing, and mental arithmetic defused about 8 out of 10 seizures from happening. I discovered the technique of mental arithmetic when I was at university sitting in a double lecture, where for a full two hours I was having lots of onsets of warnings trapped amongst 200 people. The arithmetic has to be very complex. The kind of arithmetic that you get lost trying to calculate, and can just about do if you really put your mind to it. What I would call "Brain Blowing Arithmetic".

The warning to a seizure progresses gradually from "1" to "10". It is at "10", when you experience the onset of 'psycho-hallucination'. Once the warning has progressed to a "6" there is what is called "the point of no return", which means you are going to have a seizure. Once "10" is reached, you experience onset of seizure that involves you having a full blown psycho-hallucination where you feel the world around you become a world with an overwhelming church hall like atmosphere. You believe that there is sun shining in from windows to your left, where the rays are beaming down on the front of the church hall like place. The feeling of being judged that was experienced during the warning remains, and it feels like this judgement is coming towards you from the front of the hall, giving you an overwhelming feeling of fear, self-consciousness and vulnerability. You also feel the presence of a congregation of people to your right, and this foreign world that you believe yourself to be in exists both inside the church hall as well as outside it. The world around you feels overwhelmingly eerie and gothic-like and totally unrecognisable from the place you are having your seizure in. The world you believe yourself to be in feels the same place wherever you are having your seizure e.g. train station, class room, bedroom, café, gym, bar, walking up a street, sitting in an airplane etc

This world that you believe yourself to be in is so overwhelmingly convincing that you are never at any time under the belief that it is an illusion, and are 100% convinced that this world is real. During this powerful illusion you believe this world you are in to be everything that there is to existence. It is not just the entire world but also the entire universe, giving the world you believe yourself to be in so much credibility as well as feel so real. There is no visual component to this psycho-hallucination. Psycho-hallucinations involve disturbed sensory perception and interpretation of your environment.

During this psycho-hallucination stage of the seizure, you have no knowledge of what happened before, nor have you any idea as to where you are; and your mind is so fixated in the present moment that there is no knowledge of past nor future, therefore no recollection from memory of previous seizures as to what happens next; therefore you cannot tell yourself that the world you believe yourself to be in will subside and things will be back to normal. You believe the world you are in is normality, and there has never been any other normality experienced before now, and nor will there be any alternative to this "new normality" in the future. As the mind can only be in one time zone at any one time i.e. Past, Present or Future, and as the present moment is so frightening; your mind being fixated in the present moment makes reflection on past experience impossible, resulting in me having no knowledge of any previous seizures, therefore every seizure is experienced like it is your first seizure, making you terrified by the unknown, as well as the atmosphere of the world around you; and the overactivity of the part of the brain responsible for emotions i.e. temporal lobe

The going into this seizure world is something that happens gradually once the warning gets to "10". What happens beyond the warning stage is that the real world you are in goes from 100% present to 80% present, to 60% present, to 40% present, to 20% present, to 0% present; and at the same time as this happening the seizure world goes from being 0% present, to 20% present, to 40% present, to 60% to 80% to 100% present. During this transition from real world into seizure world, it is as if the real world is superimposed on top of a very faint seizure world, that becomes increasingly present while the real world becomes increasingly fainter until 40% real world/**60% seizure world.** The real world continues to get fainter while the seizure world continues to become more present. When the world around you becomes 40% real world/**60% seizure world** it is now as though the seizure world is superimposed on top of the real world. This transition from **60%real world**/40% seizure world to 40% real world/**60% seizure world** brings on a very strong feeling of depersonalisation i.e. a strong ying-yang feeling, resulting in an "out of body" sensation as the world around you continues to progress towards 0% real world/**100% seizure world**. Essentially, throughout the transition, the seizure world; that has been drawn in picture two overleaf, becomes more and more present until fully present, and the real world around you becomes less and less present until the real world is 0% present; and as far as you are aware, there never was a previous world to the one you find yourself in now. This nature of this transition can be demonstrated in the small boxes to the right of picture two, that depicts the seizure world; where the diagonal cross is the real world, and the seizure world is the vertical cross.

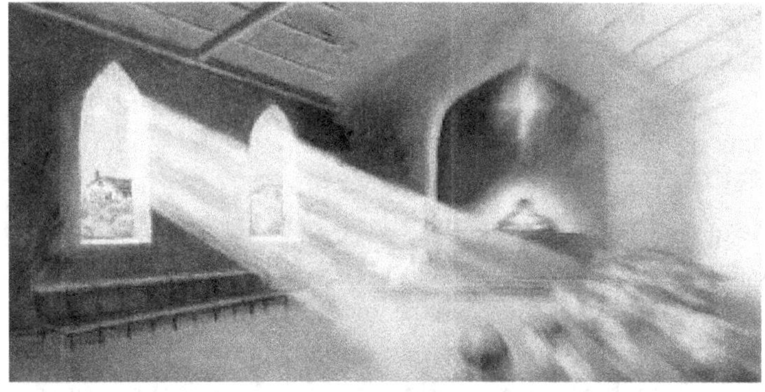

Picture 2

View colour version: http://www.afitfullife.com/index.asp?pageid=717242

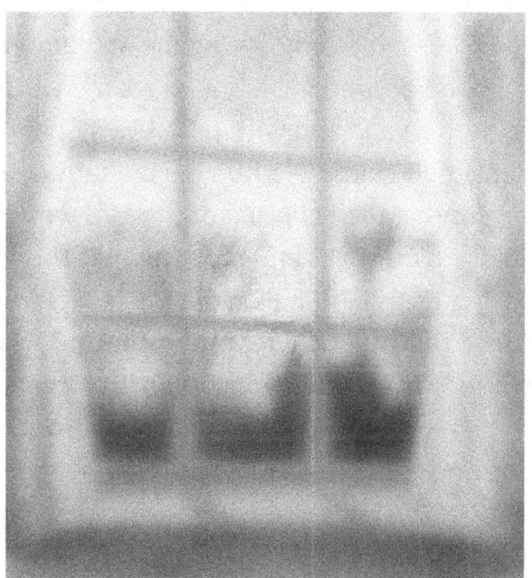

Picture 3

View colour version: http://www.afitfullife.com/index.asp?pageid=717243

Above is a picture that depicts the place I believe myself to be once full blown seizure comes to fruition. As can be seen from the picture, the seizure world feels overwhelmingly eerie and gothic, and has no similarity with the real world in terms of atmosphere, and where you feel and believe yourself to be.

During seizures upon immediately awakening in the middle of the night, the onset of the seizure world comes on in a different way to the onset described for awake seizures taken within first two hours of awakening, and the daytime seizures. It is not the gradual onset and fruition of being in a haunted like church hall in another world, that you feel gradually replacing the world around you but in fact a sudden, convincing, overwhelming belief and feeling of being in a farm- house like room looking out on a sunset sky with another farmhouse in the distance that freaks me out, that is depicted in picture 3 below. I feel myself being pushed by overwhelming feelings of helplessness into a tighter, and tighter mental corner; where instead of one world disappearing and another   appearing at the same time, I instead feel a strong eclipsing of the real world by the seizure world, where the closer the seizure world comes to fully eclipsing the real world, the tighter and tighter   that mental corner starts to feel in that eerie farm house like room I believe myself to be in, where I find myself being suffocated by increasing panic. Once the seizure world has totally eclipsed the real world I experience a feeling of me becoming mentally detached from something, giving me an out of body sensation, and then find the world around me being the same world that comes to full fruition during both awake and within first two hours of awakening attacks that is depicted in picture 2 above. The farmhouse like room I believe myself to be in during the eclipsing of the real world by the seizure world can be depicted in picture 3, remembering that this is not a visual hallucination and is instead a psycho-hallucination i.e. you're not 100% deceived into seeing something that's not there, but instead 100% deceived into feeling and believing yourself to be somewhere you are not. Psycho-hallucinations are not visual hallucinations; but instead, atmospheric and perceptual hallucinations convincing you into believing yourself to be elsewhere.

Some of you reading will understand what I mean by associating numbers with colours, as well as in some cases; words as well. For example, I think the colour "red" when you mention the number "three". I think the colour "green" when you mention the number "four". I think the colour "yellow" when you mention the number "seven". I think the colour "black" when you mention the number "nine". You may associate these numbers with different colours to the ones I associate them with. They call this association of words and numbers with colours, "Graphemic Synesthesia". Just like I associate numbers with colours, I very strongly associate the atmosphere of the seizure world with a colour; and that colour, is the colour of the background in "picture 1" with the judge, that was made reference to during the warning of the seizure. During the warning to a seizure, I am anticipating being abducted by a world with an atmosphere that is that colour i.e. dark green/yellow, and during the seizure I am experiencing the world in that colour, with the world feeling ancient and church like. This colour that I experience the seizure world in, plays a big part in making the seizure world feel terrifying.

Once the seizure world becomes fully developed, where I feel the presence of a large crowd of people to my right, I then feel the presence of a large number of people move across from the right immersing me amongst a crowd. I don't know who these people are, and have no idea what my relationship with them is. The feeling the presence of other people that are not there, can make my flat where I am on my own during my seizure feel as busy as the concourse in a busy airport terminal building. The seizure world does not feel any particular size. The seizure world feels the same size standing in Glasgow Central Station, being aboard the Waverley boat sailing up the Firth of Clyde, in my bedroom etc. These people, therefore, are not a set amount, but just people; and its busy and you are just elsewhere. The word "feel" has been used in this paragraph a lot reinforcing the point I make that there is no visual hallucination. When I am experiencing this fully developed seizure world as well as presence of other people around me, I am not thinking "I feel the presence of other people, but it is a symptom of a seizure that will wear off". I am instead thinking "I feel the presence of other people because there are other people". This being convinced of there being other people being around you then fills you with paranoia, as you feel that these peoples' presence is going to seriously compromise you in some way. This part of the seizure also gives you a strong feeling of "stage fright". You feel that the world has changed around you, and you would associate the experienced changes with disturbed electrical activity, as much as you would associate a window cleaner with mashed potato. There is a belief, once you get to this stage of the seizure, that you are about to experience massive exposure, that will be followed by massive accountability due to the feeling of the presence of many people around you. You feel that same massive feeling of "going to be held to account" that a person would feel after they had accidentally left the gas on, and came to realise this while standing outside their tenement house and had just witnessed someone go back in to get something, that would result in the light being switched on, where that person knows they have no way in preventing the explosion.

During this period of the seizure you feel like the sky has opened up above you, giving you a feeling that you are going to be held to massive account. It feels like a bomb has exploded above your head, giving you a massive stage fright feeling akin to the feeling you get when a fast train goes through a train station, where the tannoy tells you to, "stand back, fast train approaching" and you get that intrusive thought of jumping in front of the train that gives you the jitters as it passes through at very fast loud speed. The difference is though, to the person standing on the platform their mind knows that the intrusive thought of being hit by the train is just imagination and the jitters are irrational, whereas I have been brain washed into believing that this feeling of the jitters comes from a very real threat with guaranteed worst outcomes, therefore, greatly increasing the significance of the jitters, which in turn greatly increases the strength of the fear.

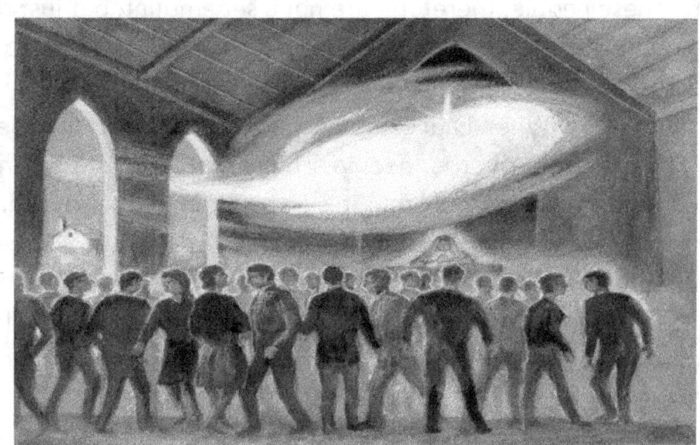

Picture 4

View colour version: http://www.afitfullife.com/index.asp?pageid=717244

It is after this part of the seizure that where I believe myself to be starts to disappear with me in it. It is at this part of the seizure that I experience blackout. The blackout does not involve unconsciousness but instead involves loss of awareness and orientation as well as bizarre behaviour in terms of the things you say and do.

The next stage of the seizure after the blackout is the amnesiac episode, that has me walking around confused about time, place, day, where I am, what has happened, what was I doing yesterday, what do I do for a living, what I have got on today etc. The world around me feels very eerie but not church like eerie. It is now the eeriness that I associate with the noise that comes from the inside of a seashell. It's no longer gothic, but still very alien. There is a feeling of isolation, with no one around for miles. It's like a bleak beach atmosphere, with tide out a long way. This alien ghost town feeling brought on by an impaired interpretation of the world around me remains throughout the amnesia, but at the very beginning of the amnesia the world is mentally very foggy, where the fog starts to lift gradually with the amnesia. The beginning of the amnesia has me feel and believe that I am in a world of corridors, where the trying to answer key questions about me, time and place has me feeling lost; as though I am just going down corridors, wanting them to lead to answers but instead they lead to dead ends. Trying to work out the initial answers to the key questions about time, place and self are like walking around a maze trying to get to each answer. Trying to work these things out is like trying to work out what you had for dinner two weeks ago to this day. You find yourself having to try and answer about seven or eight different questions about you and your whereabouts, to bring you back to full orientation. It is a period that can last up to twenty minutes, where fortunately the answering of some questions answers others. You do also tend to stumble across answers. For example, you may be wandering around your home thinking "What do I do for a living, and what day is it today?". You're emotionally experiencing that same feeling you get when you forgot to set your alarm clock and slept in late, or you gave yourself ten more minutes in bed at 7am and you waken up to see its 8.20am. The difference is, the distress during the amnesia is much greater as you do not know that you have had a seizure, as having epilepsy is one of the things you do not know about yourself, and if you can't remember something as simple as what you did yesterday, you will not know what the prognosis of someone experiencing amnesia after a seizure is i.e. does it ever lift? The amnesia is very like the seizure in that you remain in the present moment, where it is the distress of not knowing essential information that keeps you present, thus further disabling your ability to recollect past and anticipate future e.g. "Where was I yesterday?" and "What do I have on today?".

Answers to some questions do however answer others. For example, if I pick up a pair of trousers and put them on thinking "Let's get changed at least", I might have change fall out my pockets with a train ticket from yesterday, where I pick it up and I have a flash memory of being on a train yesterday which immediately reminds me of where I was yesterday, which then reminds me of what day of the week yesterday was and therefore what day today is. I then realise that I am not due anywhere because yesterday was a Saturday and therefore the odds are, whatever I do for a living I do not need to be anywhere today as it is a Sunday. Answers to questions probe answers to other questions until I am fully back

The world around me during the amnesia part of the seizure feels like the world in the following picture:

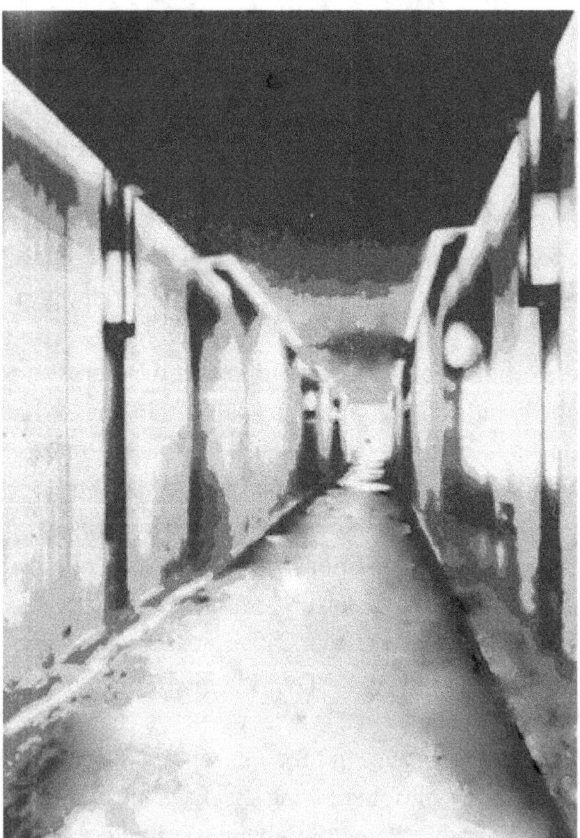

Picture 5

View colour version: http://www.afitfullife.com/index.asp?pageid=717245

Once everything comes back to you, the seizure has been and gone, and you are back to normality. Back to knowing who you are, where you are and who you are with. People around you asking you if you are okay, and explaining to you that you had gone and sat on a table that had coffee mugs on it, where you had spilt the cups and the coffee all over the floor, plus fell off the table during the blackout. It is during the blackout that your behaviour becomes impaired, and you start behaving in a bizarre way, saying the most bizarre things; that can too often result in injury, trouble with the judiciary or just plain humiliation to live with; and face the consequences of the next day.

The fear during the warning to a complex partial seizure is a mixture of biological induced fear and psychosocial induced fear. The "thunder and lightning" going off in your temporal lobe, combined with the fear induced by thoughts about how members of the public will treat you, the judiciary, the impact it will have on career etc makes the onset a torturous experience that you are just expected to cope with living with. Anticipating your next seizure can cause for you to live a very disturbing life. During upon awakening seizures in the middle of the night you don't have these psycho-social fears but that does not provide you with any comfort at all at the time of onset of warning just before middle of night seizure.

Complex partial seizures can lead you astray to the most unexpected places. I did on one occasion fall asleep during the day when I was a nursing student back in 2003, where I woke up at around 7pm in the evening and had a seizure. As I was coming round from my seizure I looked at my clock and again fell victim to the confusion between AM and PM. I unfortunately believed I was due on placement, and got in a taxi asking the driver to drive me out to a hospital in Greenock, which is 25 miles away from Glasgow, despite my nursing placement at the time being at the Western Infirmary in Glasgow, which was literally just across the road from my house.

The taxi driver, who drove me to Greenock, took the M8 motorway heading west, and by the time I was recovered from the amnesia I asked the taxi driver where we were going and he said, "Greenock like you asked for". I panicked and asked him where we were, and he said that we were on the M8 approaching the exit for Paisley on route to Greenock, which I responded to by telling him to instantly bring the taxi to a stop, which he did by pulling the taxi aside after coming off the next exit, where he told me that I owed him a black cab price, which is not cheap, of twenty pounds. I told him that I had had a seizure and had been suffering from amnesia, but he told me that I was still to cough up. I was furious as I knew that it would have been obvious to this taxi driver that I was confused and disorientated at the time of recovering from the amnesia, and I feel that he just took advantage of a situation where he could make a quick fortune out of someone who was temporarily cognitively incapacitated therefore, a seizure that started in a lounge on a couch in a flat on Byres Road in Glasgow's West end came to a close in a taxi approaching Paisley, which was a good eight miles from my flat in a straight line, and around ten miles road journey away. This seizure also found me at a bank machine having to withdraw twenty pounds for a taxi driver.

Don't ask me why I asked the taxi driver to drive me to Greenock. One theory is I could have had a seizure when the news was on, and during the amnesia there may have been a story on the news concerning the town of Greenock, as I always fell asleep in front of the television. I don't know if maybe it had something to do with my dream while asleep, or if it was some kind of spontaneous memory about Greenock from childhood that jumped into my mind during the amnesia, as it was a town me and my family drove through every Sunday between the years 1980-1989 on route to Largs, where my Grandad lived.

Another example of a time where the seizure experience can invite trouble, is the time when I worked at a challenging behaviour home in Nottingham in 2003 and had come home from work after completing my early shift that began at 7.30am that morning. What had happened was I fell asleep after returning from work at 5pm. When I woke up at around 7.30pm I had an upon awakening seizure, and next thing I knew, I was suffering from amnesia and saw the clock display 8.00. I panicked when it came to me recollecting what I did for a living and where I worked, and was immediately on the phone asking to speak to the shift leader, who turned out to be Martin, who was also my team leader. I told him how sorry I was for being late and I would be in on the next bus. Martin told me to calm down. He asked me why I was talking about being late. Fortunately it was a rhetorical question and instead of waiting for an answer he told me that I had come of shift earlier that day at 4pm. I looked at my clock and the little red dot was at the "pm" sign. I felt a hybrid of relief over not being late, and anxiety over what Martin would think of this phone call. I suddenly responded by saying, "Sorry" and just put the phone down. The next day I said nothing about the evening before phone call, and neither did Martin. No questions asked, and I thought to myself how glad I was that I practiced my right under, what was at the time, the Disability Discrimination Act, where I did not tell my employer about my "within first two hours upon awakening seizures" and instead described myself as having "controlled epilepsy", which in practice could be described as "controlled", when these seizures were controlled to only being experienced within the first two hours of awakening. This was at a time where I had to be daytime free of seizures to be a support worker, which I was, but in this risk averse society would anyone have taken my word for it that I had been sleeping prior to this seizure taken at 7.30pm. My previous experiences would certainly provide supportive evidence that one should expect the answer to that question to be a resounding "NO".

My Complex Partial Seizures last maybe five minutes i.e. onset to end of blackout, followed by around ten to twenty minutes of amnesia. The total amount of time from onset to full recovery is on average around twenty minutes, however, during a seizure you have no perception of time and therefore, a twenty minute seizure experience i.e. onset to full recovery, feels around forty five minutes in duration. A five minute experience of losing awareness and orientation is a very long time in terms of what can happen to you during that period of time and what trouble you can get yourself into. To put into perspective how long five minutes is, just think about a car in motion, where for five minutes it is without its brakes and steering, and the driver hopes to God that he will come across no lights, dead ends, turns in road, roundabouts, absent minded drivers as well as pedestrians etc

CHAPTER 3

We live in a very complex world. This world, as you will go onto read about, is a world that could be described as a big "University", that has its own teaching staff, where all those playing an educational role at this "university" are teaching PhD level subjects, where the majority of those teaching don't have as much as a standard grade, GCSE etc in the subjects they teach. It is why we have recessions, wars, punch-ups, thefts, professional negligence and so many more illnesses in our society. It is also true that most students at this university called 'society' will learn nothing and skive most of their lectures. Most people reading chapter 2 would say, "I didn't know epilepsy was like that? I thought you fell to the floor, became unconscious and started shaking". It probably wouldn't be instinctive, for the vast majority of the population, to think the words "they might even injure themselves" if the only thing I had described about the complex partial seizure were to be warning, transition, blackout, amnesia, recovery. If you would have thought these words then well done! You probably have an IQ above 125, and a high ability to apply intellect to practice.

I wanted to do medicine when I left university back in 1997. I was told I could not get in as I had only got a third class honours degree in Molecular Biology and I needed at least an upper second class honours degree. I had written in support of my application, that I had lived with epilepsy, and that I wished to do medicine because of this. I wanted to treat people with epilepsy as I had an empathy with them. I knew how difficult people find living with this condition, and as an NHS patient I only saw my doctor once every three months, and between these months I had no one to share my experiences with who played a professional role as I needed that to cope with the psycho-hallucinations. You go back to that diagram about the brain wave and I can tell you that with that explanation I could still not cope as I thought "How can a disruption in brainwave frequency and wavelength cause you to believe yourself to be in a church far removed from here and walking around a deserted beech like feeling world of corridors." When I went to my doctor's and smelt the corridors of the hospital, I got a sense of security. I felt that I was in a place that understood me and was on my side and it was the only time I believed the brainwave diagram, but when I was back out on to Dumbarton Road, I was back to believing myself to be possessed, and when I had my next warning that got to the "point of no return", just after the 6 on the 1 through to 10 journey towards the edge of the cliff, I thought to myself "How much I wish to be in the Western Infirmary with Professor Brodie" and then the symptoms of the transition into seizure totally discredited any appointment that I had had with Professor Brodie and any theories on what epilepsy is. It was for this reason that I needed more professional contact, and I never got this. My father, believe it or not, was a Professor of Neurology, and life is full of coincidence. Despite my father being a neurologist, I didn't get the sense of security that I would have got off a professional, as he was my father. I didn't see my Dad as a neurologist. I instead saw my Dad, as just "Dad". It didn't have the same effect seeing Professor Brodie in the hospital had.

 I decided I wanted to give the knowledge and experience of living with epilepsy, to epilepsy patients, as I knew what those with temporal lobe seizures were experiencing, in some cases on a daily basis, and therefore applied to do medicine for these reasons; and received a letter informing me that Glasgow University medical faculty could can make no exception to those applicants who fell short of the entry criteria of 6A's in their Highers, or at least a 2:1 Honours Degree in a life science". I feel that this was a gross mistake, especially when I had discovered ways in defusing seizures with techniques such as mental arithmetic, and was not given the opportunity to share this with patients, and could have improved services for people with epilepsy, considering I had the personality to run an advocacy charity for those with neurological disability, evidenced by the creation of a charity advocating for those with neurological disability called 'Fairway Advocacy' between the years 2014-2017. The person who did get my place was very likely someone wanting to do medicine for the salary and the status, and I am not afraid to appear arrogant, but that person most likely did not have as much to offer as I. There have probably been epilepsy patients that I would have seen, if I had been allowed to study medicine, who have probably taken their lives; as 1 in 7 people with my type of epilepsy will attempt to take their life, as evidenced in a study on depression in temporal lobe epilepsy by a Neurologist called Garcia back in 2012. Garcia comments that the chances of suicide in those with tonic-clonic epilepsy is 5-fold that of the general population, and those with complex partial epilepsy is 32 fold, which equates to 1 in 7. My teaching of arithmetic to defuse seizures could have saved lives, both in terms of preventing suicide by enabling those with complex partial seizures to defuse the seizure simply by telling them to do in their mind a sum like "42x63x15…….." that would have an 80% success rate, thus allowing these people to work, get married and have families, as well as making life much more mentally endurable with an 80% reduction or more in seizure frequency.

Medicine must stop saying, "You need to be academically gifted", and instead look at the whole person, looking at what life knowledge and experience they bring to the job. They did those with epilepsy in the Greater Glasgow Health Board Area a great disservice. Assessing a person's suitability to do a job like medicine done correctly prevents doctors qualifying and shooting off on a plane to America where the money is even greater or staying here but just doing private practice. The two things medicine should look for in people when determining suitability to become a doctor is evidence of living and coping with disability or evidence of believing and having been involved in achieving social justice for those with disability.

Come on, medicine, think outside the box!! And please could everyone else from other relevant backgrounds think outside the box as well!! We live in a world where people are judged by the type of car they drive, the size of their house, their wealth, their accent, their looks, the clothes they wear and the grades they get in their exams. Judging a person's suitability for a vocational course on the basis of grades is as cheap as judging someone by the type of car they drive when the grades being asked for are not a reflection of the ability required to successfully complete the vocational course and make a competent professional.

WHY WE DON'T THINK OUTSIDE THE BOX:

It's time for society to become more qualified in their knowledge of this complex world. Society is simplistic and has a simplistic knowledge of a very complicated thing called "living". There's so much to be said about the "University of Life". Most of us are guilty of skiving, not attending our lectures, not going to tutorials, not doing our research, failing our exams etc yet still getting into the next year.

People just like to learn what they need to know to get through today and tomorrow. This is sad, especially when new interests, passions, discovery of talents etc come from learning new knowledge, and doing these things makes you a much more interesting person who doesn't rely on "small talk" to have a conversation, as you can talk about intelligent things. "Small talk" I do not do!

Part of the reason why we are guilty of these things is because we only speak to a small clique of people in this world. The fewer people you know the less you will learn from others. You learned about complex partial epilepsy from meeting me in the form of this book. Throughout this book you are with me and you will learn a lot. I am not the only person in the world with knowledge and experience and there are so many others, but I would say they are sadly too few at the same time. When I go out for a drink I stand at the bar. I stand there and I talk to people, and you will find that the people at the bar have life experience. They are very often alone people who are disappointed in what simple minds they have found the human race to be in terms of its ignorance and its lack of knowledge about anything. Many who like "large talk", and have not been able to remain in contact with like- minded friends from their school years and university years due to emigration, have found themselves very short of like- minded people to form new relationships with, resulting in many people standing alone in bars being "large talkers". We don't want to be in a bar talking football, weather and coronation street. We want to be talking politics, science, social justice and everything else intelligent.

I was in a bar the other night in Glasgow where I got talking to two former military men. One had been thrown out the army for being homosexual and had been blinded as well; and the other had hydrocephalus as well as peripheral blindness, and had; had a huge number of operations, telling me that his mother kissed the doctor after his successful operation, and told me that he could speak Turkish and Russian as he loved learning. He was hilarious to be with, and the three of us stood there and drank together for around three and a half hours only having three pints as we were so busy exchanging life experiences and knowledge thus distracting us from our drink. Pubs can be great places to meet new people and come out your comfort zone at the bar (not the dance floor) as well as introduce yourself to people you don't know; instead of congregating in your clique of seven friends, in a world of seven billion people, gossiping at a table about football, the prices in shops and what's going on in the soap operas. You learn new knowledge at the bar that encourages you to try out new experiences and allows you to develop a wealth of views, opinions, beliefs; encouraging you to learn new things, making you more open minded and more of an outside of the box thinker as well as giving you such a wealth of information that you will never fear running out of things to talk about when you meet a complete stranger.

Too often you get speaking to strangers at the bar, and you get a bar member of staff growling at you, as you and the people you are speaking to have this instinctive ability to just start talking to strangers, and find so much common ground as well as share lots of new ground; and I think to myself "Well come out, and join us!", "Instead of hate us, come out and grow and develop, then you won't have to hate us!". If they did this instead, their confidence would grow, and every day would start with the question: "I wonder what interesting person I will meet today, what interesting things will I learn and what new experiences will I have?". Now that's a much better definition of the term "You need to get out more!".

We only learn what we were taught at school, further education and through personal development in our jobs. We let our jobs and wealth define who we are, which shapes us into a very limited person and sadly where you have "limited", you have "ignorant", that leads to the very types of behaviours that come from others in this book. It annoys me that those people who have been given the autonomy to make decisions about my life don't have any of the knowledge required to be able to do so. They don't see how their decisions on housing policies cross paths with performance at work and symptom management of disability. They are a "reckless bull in a china shop with a blind fold on". They are an "airport with no air traffic control". They just say to the plane landing from New York, "Yup, the run way is clear all permission given to land" without even thinking about that plane crossing paths with the plane from Paris, as they've never heard of a radar and have no respect for first come first served; and the colleague who has heard of the radar, with respect towards first come first served, is on the plane flying back from Paris, guaranteeing a collision. Lives are quite literally lost every day in this world purely because of those in position of authority being blind to 99.99% of the knowledge of this very complicated thing called "LIFE & LIVING".

Unfortunately for people with complex partial seizures, society's lack of outside the box thinking is an everyday reality. A good example is the person who has a complex partial seizure when standing in the pub at the bar that has doormen wandering around inside and manning the entrance. In such circumstances, the man in the pub whose overcome by a seizure can end up going up to a table and sitting himself amongst a group of people he is not with and not budging when asked to do so. This is especially a problem if he is fifteen stone and sits himself down on the lap of an eight stone woman out with her partner. In response to this he could be seriously assaulted by the customers sitting at that table. The doorman may witness the incident and see that the man is confused and disorientated and immediately assume that he is on recreational drugs or heavily intoxicated on alcohol and immediately grab him and throw him out. The doorman may even assault the man if the man demonstrates any attempts to resist the doorman. Both incidents could result in hospitalisation or imprisonment. You will remember from chapter one, that 1 in 50 people in prison have epilepsy, and this is one of the reasons that explains this. In fact, as I write this chapter of the book on the 16th of September 2017, I have just learned from the BBC website that there has been a bombing on a London Tube train at Parsons Green tube station. It has resulted in many people having to be treated in hospital for burns as well as resulted in three members of the public being left in a critical condition. The news story informs me that the terror threat in the United Kingdom is now at critical and that the Scottish Government will now have a presence of armed police at train stations where they will be on guard protecting the public from anything suspicious. As I read this story I think to myself that there was a time when I used to have seizures in train stations where the public were sympathetic towards me because I was wearing a school uniform, but had I been a middle aged adult dressed in plain clothes I would have ticked the box of acting suspiciously, and I don't want to think how armed police would react if I were having day time seizures today, or seizures within the first couple of hours of awakening and were to have one in a London station when the country is on high alert. I think it is particularly concerning for a person with my type of epilepsy who is of asian origin. It is even worse for someone whose complex partial seizure originates in the frontal lobe as they will lose their inhibitions and might start screaming out loud, that could result in armed police opening fire during high alert. I have to ask this question: Will the police and other security who will be bearing an arm get any lectures on conditions that affect state of consciousness e.g. stroke, hypoglycaemia, seizure etc before they are given a gun where they will be allowed to shoot someone who gives an officer reasons to believe they pose a threat. No, they won't! This is what I mean by not thinking outside the box! Our society can not link poorly controlled seizures with country being on high alert with armed officers. They call this "not being able to join up the dots". People with learning disability are accused of not being able to do this but you will learn later on in the book that the majority in our society are very poor at doing this.

CHAPTER 4

With my type of epilepsy, the consequences of having a seizure in certain environments can be very great causing you to avoid certain settings; hindering your education, your employment, prospects for personal development, social life, development of relationships; and with poorly controlled seizures you can become socially isolated. I have had anxieties about having seizures in particular settings. Anxiety can in itself bring on a seizure, and as a consequence of that, you can find yourself becoming trapped in a vicious symptom cycle where environment causes anxiety, that causes seizure, that causes more anxiety in environment, that causes seizure..... etc; where you feel the only way to defuse that symptom cycle is to avoid the environment that brings on that anxiety. I could have found myself becoming phobic of going into lectures when I was at university as well as sitting in exams, which if I had become, would have crippled my higher education.

There have been a number of triggers that I have identified over the years that bring on seizures. Very often society is a trigger to seizures. Due to bad experiences created by other peoples' attitudes towards your epilepsy, that are both traumatic and cause you to have to live without closure, you can find yourself living with anger and rage, which develops into depression, which in itself anger and rage is a symptom of. This is another one of the vicious symptom cycles that a person with epilepsy can find themselves having to live with as well as the environment-seizure vicious symptom cycle. This anger-rage-depression-anger-rage-depression etc vicious symptom cycle, created by discriminative experiences, then has psychiatrists make claims like: "Those with temporal lobe epilepsy, tend to have anti-social personality disorder; as they are always angry, full of rage and fallout with everyone". There are many campaign groups in America that are trying to have psychiatry scrapped as an area of medicine, as there is a consensus amongst many that it is just a massive "front". These psychiatrists know that their discipline is being found out, and are now trying to involve themselves in neurotransmitter research, which is neurology, which is just an attempt to try and make their discipline look like a legitimate discipline in my opinion. I was told that many people do psychiatry as it is the area of medicine where you cannot be sued. Someone kills themselves the attitude is: "Well he had mental health issues". There's no such thing as killing a patient in psychiatry, unlike disciplines such as cardiology or neurology.

This anger/rage/depression/anger/rage/depression etc vicious symptom cycle, as well as depression alone; can cause mood swings, poor sleep, impaired memory; resulting in missed doses of drug treatment and sleep deprivation, thus resulting in seizures. The increased anger and rage can result in anxiety, as you feel yourself being pushed into a tight mental corner; as you get closer and closer to your "freak out threshold", which then brings on seizures, resulting in more anger and rage, leading to further anxiety and increases in seizure frequency, so you are now in an increased anger and rage/increased anxiety/increased anger and rage/increased anxiety etc vicious symptom cycle that also increases seizure frequency which causes that 1 in 7 person to have a nervous breakdown and attempt to end their life in the case of someone living with complex partial epilepsy originating from the temporal lobe.

Another trigger to my seizures has been food additives that despite me bringing to the attention of my doctor, it has never been given the recognition or interest that it should have been given. One food substance that you are most likely familiar with is a substance called Monosodium Glutamate better known as 'MSG'. This compound is used as both an emulsifier and a flavour enhancer. It is also said to be a compound that gives people food cravings thus making them spend. It is very often used in Chinese food which I must avoid like the plague. You will remember in Chapter one that receptors control the opening and closing of sodium ion channels; and that it is rapid, frequent, irregular opening and closing of sodium ion channels that bring on seizures. What was not mentioned was that you get substances called" Neurotransmitters", that bind to the receptor, causing the receptor to instruct the ion channel to open. One of these neurotransmitters is called 'Glutamate', and MSG mimics glutamate, thus effectively flooding a person with epilepsy's brain with excess glutamate, bringing on excessive as well as irregular opening and shutting of sodium channels, thus bringing on seizures. It used to be the case that when I ate Chinese food, the MSG got into my brain across the blood brain barrier so quickly that I would have a seizure while eating my King Prawn Curry. My brain became so excitable that I did not get a warning i.e. a climb from 1-10. The first thing I experienced was a sudden onset of full blown psycho-hallucination followed by the remainder of seizure. Obviously, Chinese meals had an amount of MSG that could bring on a full blown seizure, whereas other meals with MSG did not contain enough to bring on a full complex partial seizure, but enough to bring on a very brief simple partial seizure. This response to MSG in people with epilepsy would explain why other people experience migraine after eating Chinese food or complain about being restless and not being able to sleep, as migraine and restlessness are also symptoms of an antagonised central nervous system. It is worth noting that if this compound can cross the blood brain barrier so quickly as to have myself have a seizure while I'm half way through my Chinese king prawn curry, then it is feasible that you could take your child out for a meal in a restaurant, and by the time they are home they are swinging from the lights if they suffer from Attention Deficit Hyperactivity Disorder which is another condition that is related to a restless Central Nervous System .

I have also experienced seizures in response to consuming 'Aspartame', which is found in low calorie soft drinks. Aspartame is an artificial sweetener. As well as there being a neurotransmitter called 'Glutamate', there is also a neurotransmitter called 'Aspartic Acid' that is found in the synapses that are the gaps between the nerve cells. Aspartic acid transmits the electrical activity from one brain cell to another by binding to receptors on the brain cell wall causing sodium ion channels to open and close, generating new electrical activity. Aspartame is very similar in molecular structure to aspartic acid, and when consumed it travels to the brain and mimics aspartic acid thus binding to receptors causing excessive opening and closing of sodium ion channels, thus bringing on seizures. Not all low- calorie soft drinks with aspartame in them have caused me to have seizures in the past. The low- calorie drinks that have caused seizures are those where the aspartame is used in amounts where the aspartame creates an artificial sweetener taste. There are other low- calorie soft drinks with aspartame in them that have not caused seizures. These have been low calorie soft drinks that have no artificial sweetener taste, evidencing that not all low- calorie soft drinks use aspartame in large enough quantities capable of bringing on seizures.

Even though my seizures do not involve collapsing there is an element of risk of injury during one of my complex partial seizures. One thing I must do at night is ensure that there are no shoes lying around the floor space in my room as well as ensuring there are no bags or anything else I can trip over. I did back in 2015 waken up at 7am in the morning feeling absolutely fine to find my bedroom door open and got out of bed to go to the toilet. After my visit to the toilet, I washed my hands in the dark feeling fine. When I switched the light on to shave I looked in the mirror and was overcome by the disturbing shock of seeing several semi- dried streams of blood that had been running down my face and that my hair line was covered in blood. This was one of the most disturbing sites I have ever been exposed to. In response to this view in the mirror, I walked into my bedroom and discovered that my bedroom wall attached mirror behind my opened door had been smashed and that there was broken glass all over the carpet. I now have a scar about two inches long above my right temple where it is evident that this was the site of injury when I made contact with the mirror which backs up the theory that I fell into this mirror. I don't lose my balance during a seizure therefore the only thing that could have caused me to fall was something lying in my way that tripped me up. As a consequence of this, never do I go to sleep without ensuring that there is nothing that I can trip over during the blackout phase of a night time seizure. I also have to ensure that my laptop cable is not lying across the lounge carpet at the door before going to bed so there is no chance of me tripping over in the lounge if I have a seizure that night and go into the lounge during the blackout or the recovery phase when I am suffering from amnesia. If I were to trip over the laptop cable I would most likely give myself a bad head injury as my head would hit the lounge table. When I go to visit my friend Alan who lives in Sheringham I find myself sleeping in a room that has mirrors covering the perimeter of the room in the form of mirrored wardrobe doors and just enough room between the edge of the bed and the mirrored wardrobe doors to accommodate the length of your foot. It is when I stay in this room that my friend has to put duvets and blankets over the wardrobe doors so that there is no chance of me hurting myself during a seizure. My room back in my home has a built in wardrobe with mirrored doors. With this I just ensure that there is nothing in the vincinity of the wardrobe that I could trip over. It just requires one moment during a period of confusion to go over, cut yourself badly leaving yourself with a bad scar and destroy your future employment prospects, meeting a partner, getting into bars and pubs, being refused membership of anything that requires a meeting such as a golf club etc This is an example of how society's attitude towards the casualties of a condition like epilepsy can result in the social exclusion of those with epilepsy. This is how a person with epilepsy could find themselves on job seekers allowance for the majority of their working life, and then called a "scrounger" by society. Too often, those who persecute others because of the predicaments these others find themselves living with, are the very creators of these predicaments. Another one of the many things that causes someone like myself to live with a rage.

CHAPTER 5

The previous chapters have looked at the symptoms of my seizures, as well as the secondary mental health problems that are created by living with epilepsy in an intolerant society, and how so many of these mental health problems are dressed up as being clinical complaints when in fact they are normal human emotions caused by a cultural attitude towards people with disability. What now needs to be covered is the side effects of the medications.

Believe it or not, but the side effects of some of the medications I have been on have been worse to live with than the prospect of having a seizure every day. Many of the medications I have taken have caused as side effects a combination of blurred vision, double vision, running vision, dizziness, loss of balance, loss of appetite, tremor, irritability, excessive hunger etc. When I was on a drug called 'Tegretol'; I had running vision, double vision, blurred vision and dizziness for two hours every day. When you take these medications, there is what is called a 'Peak Dose', which is when the medications have got into your system and are present at their highest levels. The liver will start to metabolise the drugs, and clear it from your system over a period of around seventeen hours; but for the first two hours of being in your system, the drug levels are at their highest and this is when the side effects are at their strongest. After these two hours the side effects get less, and after three hours the double vision, running vision, blurred vision and dizziness have subsided; however, side effects like irritability, increased appetite, loss of appetite, tremor etc tend to remain. I found that during the period of time that I was experiencing the visual disturbances, as well as dizziness, I was at increased risk of injuries. You can imagine having running and blurred vision, and going onto an escalator with an impatient commuter behind you, pressurising you to walk fast down the moving stairs, when you cannot see the edge of the steps due to the running and blurred vision. This is when you can land on the edge of a step believing you are landing your foot on the centre of a step, and combined with the dizziness, fall down the stairs. This is just as much the case on a stair case as it is on an escalator. Falling down these structures can result in head, back and neck injuries which can possibly result in a spinal injury. It is possible for a person to take their anti-convulsant medication, experience peak dose side effects, fall down a steep stair case, have a spinal injury and find themselves wheelchair bound for the rest of their life. As for the other side effects that don't lift such as increased appetite, it is possible to put on so much weight that you end up developing circulatory problems, resulting in heart problems and possibly resulting in a condition such as stroke. It is a bit ironic that the treatment for your epilepsy could be the cause behind a stroke, which can cause epilepsy. I have also experienced serious weight gain due to increased appetite as a side effect, where I went from twelve stone up to fifteen stone as I could not stop eating. I never felt full and always felt hungry. It was physically dangerous but also mentally harmful as it can become mentally distressing always feeling hungry. Constant hunger can become a real "thorn in the side" that can mentally antagonise you. It was the case that when I attended my doctor's epilepsy outpatient clinic and told him about my weight gain and how concerned I was, his reply was, "Well what would you rather be, fat or epileptic? I know that I would rather be fat". I expected this attitude from this doctor, as he was not a neurologist, and was instead a 'clinical pharmacologist' who had too cosy a relationship with the drug companies, who he carried out clinical trials for. This man was a money man, and this especially showed in July 1997 when I bumped into him in Glasgow's west end after I got my honours degree in molecular biology and I told him that I got a third class honours degree, where all he could do was put an expression on his face like he had just sucked a lemon and responded by saying, "let's be honest, there's few jobs out there and for someone like you it could be a life on benefits". I was very upset and found that having a bad doctor could be classified as a bad side effect especially when your doctor is a clinical pharmacologist i.e. a drugs man and not a neurologist, thus putting you at risk of being treated by a doctor who has very little understanding or concern for people living with epilepsy. I always felt that this doctor was just a statistician for the drug companies who had a vested interest in prescribing you certain anti-convulsants and choosing to treat epilepsy, as according to a neurologist that I know, this clinical pharmacologist had said that he was going to specialise in epilepsy as it was the field of epilepsy care where the money was to be made doing clinical trials for the drug companies. My father who was in Seville in Spain attending a drug conference, witnessed this doctor being ridden through the streets with his wife by a horse and carriage while every other professional attending the conference was mobilising by foot. This was probably a privilege granted to him by a drug company. Just in case there are any neurologists reading this book, let's just say he was Glasgow based, treated me in the 90's and he was a clinical pharmacologist and not a neurologist!

It was the case that the drug that put on a lot of weight had controlled my seizures; however, at the same time I had put on three stone and was most likely going to continue piling on the pounds as I continued to eat to excess and my stomach continued to stretch. Fortunately for 80% of patients with epilepsy, perseverance will eventually allow for them and their doctors to find a combination of anti-convulsant medication that will control their seizures with minimum side effects, but this does require a lot of trial and error.

This clinical pharmacologist that I was treated by did not have a good relationship with my father. My father was a neurologist at what was called at the time the 'Southern General Hospital' in Glasgow, and he was well known in his field. My father always said that he believed my seizures originated in the temporal lobe of my brain, and he told the clinical pharmacologist this but my father's opinion was met with insults such as: "Your Dad's an amateur in the field of epilepsy. Tell your father to stick with stroke. That is what he's good at!". My father started coming to my appointments and the clinical pharmacologist just said to my Dad, "Ian, this is frontal lobe epilepsy and not temporal lobe epilepsy". It was because of this dispute that I was sent to the National Society for Epilepsy just outside London in 1998 by my G.P. to be investigated.

As already previously mentioned, in the year 1998 I was seen by a very good neurologist called Professor John Duncan who saw me at the National Society for Epilepsy down in Chalfont St Peter. I spent a week at their centre where I wore an ambulatory electroencephalogram (EEG) which recorded seizure activity. I had a seizure upon awakening one evening and the next day I was seen by Professor Duncan who told me that I had epilepsy where complex partial seizures occurred in the left temporal lobe. My father had been correct and that the clinical pharmacologist, the money man, had been wrong in saying that it was frontal lobe epilepsy. Making reference to my father as an amateur who should stick at stroke and not interfere with the doctor patient relationship had very likely been defensiveness. My diagnosis was "complex partial epilepsy originating from the left temporal lobe". My doctor in Glasgow could have been diagnosed with "defensiveness originating from an inferiority complex".

 I was put on a good cocktail of drug therapy made up of three different medications i.e. Diamox, Lamictal and Gabapentin; with no side effects, that has had my seizures controlled while awake since 1998, and reduced my awakening seizures during the night to one every ten nights, which I continue to have to this day; and since five years ago, has totally eliminated the seizures that I could have within the first two hours of being out of my bed in the morning. I also have no seizures upon awakening if I fall asleep during the day. In the past there had been Saturdays where I had fallen asleep during the day and then gone out with friends to pubs and clubs and had seizures. I can now have confidence that seizures upon awakening during the day; or even a couple of hours later, no longer happen. I don't know why daytime sleep doesn't bring on seizures, but night time sleep continues to bring them on.

As my epilepsy starts in the left temporal lobe, I am by nature vulnerable to the development of anxiety disorders that are clinical in nature, but these are because of the neurophysiology of my brain and not because of anything psychiatric. Unfortunately, I have therefore had to live with anxiety that has required medical attention. As a child and adolescent, I was constantly anxious about the world coming to an end, and also had 'Obsessive Compulsive Disorder' like symptoms concerning the fear of cross infections. I also suffered from 'Hypochondriasis' which caused for me a lot of distress. I had also developed a subtype of 'Social Anxiety Disorder' called 'Performance Anxiety', which is a condition where you fear negative evaluation by others in performance settings. I developed 'Performance Anxiety' as a consequence of a combination of being educated by an education system that had been way too overly critical towards me, being put through bad humiliating performance related experiences that I had with my peer group that are typical of childhood because of the nature of horrible children, and the vicious symptom cycle effect in adulthood that is a result of all the trauma of childhood i.e. trauma from past, impairing performance in the present, causing more trauma, causing further impaired performance in the present etc; resulting in avoidance, withdrawal and isolation; which has played a large part of why I can't work for people and need to work for myself, as I have a zero tolerance for the workplace culture as it has a zero tolerance for me, and I see so many parallels between it and the school culture, both in terms of people attitude and infantile behaviour. This society has an addiction for criticising people and putting people down. It uses people as punch bags the moment an achilles heel becomes evident that makes someone not the 'ideal student' or 'ideal employee'. It's a shame we can't help people overcome achilles heels and instead choose to attack them. It is the case though that I see so much learned helplessness amongst the mainstream population and think to myself: "Well if they can't help themselves, then they certainly can't help me!". A major criteria for helping others is the ability to help yourself, which my observations of the world would support the conclusion that most people can't do, evidenced by their love for the comfort zone and their fear of turning weaknesses into strengths, as well as their over reliance on others to confront life's challenges.

CHAPTER 6

I have since 2008 had what I would call "Blue Moon Days", where maybe once every six months; for the whole day, the world feels very unreal. The atmosphere of the world is of the same atmosphere that you associate with the sound of the inside of a sea shell, just like the amnesia after a seizure. That kind of past tense feeling. That "been and gone" feeling. That "once was, but no longer is" feeling. You wonder if it is some sort of epileptiform activity, as it is essentially an impairment in your interpretation of the world around you. You also feel that today's version of the world is a blend of the real world around you, and "another world" that you have been in before that is very alien, but you can't quite place, and you are spending the whole day in the "overlap" of these two worlds. For most of the day the real world component of the blend of both worlds is the predominant world; however, throughout the day there are many frequent moments i.e. one every ten minutes, lasting up to twenty seconds, where you feel the other world component of this blend of two worlds become the predominant world that has feelings of familiarity and unfamiliarity, where you can't quite place the familiarities. All day it feels as though the world around you is a blend of a world from a past life and the world of this life, where you feel from time to time that you are on the verge of identifying memories of being in this other world and what experiences you had there as it becomes the predominant component of this blend of two worlds. It feels like it belongs to the same family of illusionary experiences that déjà vu belongs to. Déjà vu is a one- off experience lasting seconds, where as, these "blue moon days" last all day, where the feeling of the world around you being a blend of a 'past world' and a 'present world' never wears off. Déjà vu is like, "You have lived this before"; but this feeling is like, "You have been in this other place before, but where, when and what were you doing?", where throughout the day there are many frequent moments where you feel you are only seconds away from being able to answer these questions as the past life world becomes the predominant of the two worlds to then suddenly find yourself no closer to being able to answer them as the real world goes back to becoming the predominant world in this blend of two worlds.

What the world around you has become on these "Blue Moon Days" shares traits with the seizure experience i.e. very alien and unfamiliar, but unlike seizures, there is no feeling of fear or anxiety, but instead a feeling of euphoria and a "buzz" from the curiosity combined with a feeling of escapism that accompanies experiencing the whole day in the overlap between the alien feeling familiar world and the impossible to recollect other world. This feeling of euphoria is even more greatly enhanced as the other world momentarily becomes the predominant world in this blend of two worlds. Star Trek fans would buy this illusionary type all day experience if they could. It won't be long until they put neuro-transmitters into these e-cigarettes! I used to know someone who was studying Genetics at Glasgow University who smoked every bit of weed under the sun, took ecstasy and LSD. Your superficial character found him funny, but your principled underneath character i.e. your beliefs and values, thought he was an idiot; and when I told him the symptoms of my seizures, his reply was, "Wow, You're Lucky!"

I don't know if these blue moon days are seizure related, if they are an effect that the gym has on my neurotransmitter levels, if it's a type of pleasurable migraine or if it's my diet. Some foods can increase your 'Serotonin' levels, which is the good mood neurotransmitter; as well as your 'Dopamine' levels, which is the feelings of reward and motivation neurotransmitter. Since 2008 I do eat a lot of garlic, whole wheat/wholegrain, oily fish and many other dopamine/serotonin producing foods and think that it may have something to do with this. There is so much to learn about the brain and the mind. I can't remember what I did the day before these blue moon days as they are so few, and therefore wonder if I might have been to the gym the day before them, where I might have had a lower seizure threshold due to a poor previous night's sleep the night before the workout, where I had been lucky not to have a seizure but continued to have a low seizure threshold; which when combined with the effects of increased Dopamine, Endorphins and Serotonin levels from the workout done at the gym, caused the following day to be a blue moon day.

I have just recently over the last year started making a point of buying lots of apples, red bell peppers, tomatoes, onion, garlic, oily fish, olive oil which are all dopamine producing foods and I have found myself on a number of occasions having a couple of days where for 36-48 hrs I experience a really strong "feel good factor" accompanied by a very strong feeling of confidence, optimism and self- esteem; and life becomes something that gives you a high. I believe that this is a combination effect of the diet, the exercise as well as the two lots of forty five minute meditation sessions that I have been doing every day since September 2017. I find myself once every ten nights having a seizure but I also waken up probably one every four nights feeling strong euphoria brought on by feelings of self- belief and feeling really optimistic about the world being a garden of opportunity, and it's up to you to get out your bed tomorrow early and grab the opportunities and bring to fruition achievements; and make life a really rewarding experience. I put these awakenings accompanied by very strong feelings of optimism and motivation down to burning two lots of 1500 calories per week on the cross-trainer and the stationary bike, as I started having these awakenings back in 2009. As you will learn later on in the book, I took up cardiovascular exercise to combat my OCD symptom like anxiety back in July 1999. I also took up consistent meditation in 2017 to fully combat my 'Major Depressive Disorder', on top of the cardiovascular exercise. If my attendance at the gym drops though I still continue to have these awakenings and I attribute that to the consistent meditation that I am also doing. Meditation and exercise both increase your dopamine and serotonin levels in the brain. These feel good awakenings can very often cause me to have feel good factor for the entire day. All I will say is that never would I have made this progress under the influence of tranquillisers and anti-depressants. Meditation and cardiovascular exercise have saved my life, and without them I would have been one of the 1 in 7 people with epilepsy who attempt self harm, who would have taken his life back in March 2015 when my entire family abandoned me but for my father.

As I am seizure free during my awake hours, I learned to drive towards the end of 2011 and have held a driving license since June 2012. As it is not unusual to have a missed night sleep, and as I have had a history in the past of having seizures during the day after missed night's sleep, I never drive my car if I have not had a minimum of 5 hours sleep per night. I also do not drive within the first two hours of being awake, to ensure that my morning dose is in my system, and that there is no chance of having one of those freak attacks that used to happen two to three times per year during my childhood and adolescence upon travelling to school. If there is as much as a suspicion that I might have not had my medication I do not go anywhere near a car for that entire day unless I am the passenger. Even though blue moon days are not seizure experiences nor are they warnings to seizures they still could be described as noticeable changes in neuro-cognition and I therefore do not drive a car on these days either, yet I have not had a seizure on any of these days and they do go back to 2009.

CHAPTER 7

Up until diagnosis at the age of ten, I had been having seizures since the age of three. These seizures, between the ages of three; and ten, were different to the ones between the age of ten, right up to the date of writing this book, as there was no blackout phase. I can remember being in my primary school classes, being round at friends' homes, playing in my back garden; where I would suddenly find myself experiencing a transition, where the world would go from a place of feeling very familiar, to feeling very unfamiliar and foreign. During this transition, as well as throughout the experience of the world becoming very alien, I would be thinking to myself, "I am having one of these really, really weird things that I get very rarely and do not know what it is". After thinking this thought to myself, I would then feel the subsiding of the unfamiliar world, so that the world felt like it was back to normal again. As opposed to feeling anxiety, I instead felt a very disturbing feeling of not trusting my environment, as it had become very alien to me, but the alienation just passed; unlike seizures from the age of ten onwards, that had all the features previously described in the seizure description chapter. I was suffering from no blackout phase; simply because only one of the two temporal lobes of the brain were affected by the seizure activity. It is possibly the case that only a small part of the affected temporal lobe was affected; however, from the age of ten onwards, seizure activity started in the left temporal lobe, and then spread into the right temporal lobe, causing me to experience a blackout. As has been mentioned in a previous chapter, it was at the age of ten that my seizures became noticeable to onlookers, and this was because the seizures now involved a period of blackout where behaviour became bizarre.

My parents never used the word 'epilepsy' in front of me, and nor did my paediatrician neurologist. What I was having was always referred to by myself as "feelings", and so this was the word everyone else used, as opposed to using the word "seizure" or "epilepsy". It was only around the age of fifteen that I was made aware that these "feelings" were in fact seizures and that I had epilepsy.

Childhood from the age of ten onwards was very difficult as every morning was a battle not to have a seizure. Every morning I woke up, I felt vulnerable and found myself having to concentrate on not having a seizure. Every morning was about getting out of the woods unscathed by epilepsy. It was the same case with awakening in the middle of the night. It was hoping sleep would capture you before epilepsy did, when you were trying to get back to sleep after your night time awakening. These middle of night awakenings, and morning rises, were especially stressful when I was staying the night at friends' houses, away on scout camps or foreign French exchanges with the school.

Once the seizures became complex partial seizures, this was when the seizures brought with them a number of risks that compromised my health and safety, when I was out and about in public or using public services. The first time the reality of having seizures with impaired consciousness, when out in public, came to surface, was back in 1986, when I took a train to school one morning. My usual commute was from Maxwell Park Station, on Glasgow's southside, to Glasgow Central Station. I can remember being with a friend on the train going to school at 8.00am, and as we were pulling into Glasgow Central Station, I could feel a rising feeling of fear in my stomach that felt like going over a hill in a car. This rising feeling of fear was telling me that I was about to have a seizure, and I suddenly felt a feeling of panic and an overwhelming feeling of helplessness, as I knew a seizure was going to be had, while looking around the train that was pack filled with commuters. I thought to myself that there was going to be some audience to this seizure and that after today I would not be able to take this train again due to humiliating myself in front of others. I was overcome by that feeling a child gets when they want their Mum & Dad. I tried fighting the warning with self- talk, telling myself I would not have a seizure, as well as focussing on thoughts of places and events that I was very familiar with; that played a big part in the making of my identity, which had managed to prevent the seizure on some occasions in the past from occurring. What I felt was the feeling of fear in my stomach subsiding, like you do when you get that sudden relief feeling, and the blood returning back to my face when we were around 5 minutes from pulling into Glasgow Central. For that 5 minute period I thought to myself how lucky I was not to have had a seizure and that I was at present skating on incredibly thin ice as I saw everyone around me just talking to one another and thought to myself "You don't know that you nearly saw a seizure", as I looked out the train window seeing cars going over the Kingston Bridge, feeling very vulnerable. When the train stopped at the platform, everyone stood up, some giving way to others, and others just selfishly, as well as assertively, budging forwards. When the doors of the train opened, another warning came on which I tried to fight, but the transition came on as I stepped down onto the platform and started walking towards the concourse. I can remember feeling myself going into another world, as I looked up at the dark grey walls of the interior of Glasgow Central and saw the dark grey morning sky through its glass roof. This made the transition even more chilling, especially when I was surrounded by commuters at the same time as starting to feel the presence of people who are not there. To take a seizure in such a place was incredibly traumatising, as the two traits of the world that I go into i.e. gothic and busy, are traits that Glasgow Central possesses, being an old Victorian building in the centre of Europe's fifteenth biggest financial centre at rush hour. A train station that has one thousand passengers, customers; and people taking short cuts, pass through it every six minutes. My friend at the time did not know what was happening to me as the blackout phase developed, and he just left me there on my own, as he continued to the underground to do the last stretch of the journey to school. The next thing I remember is a man, and his wife, escorting me away from the concourse. All I remember is saying, "Where am I?", "Who are you?", "Where are you taking me?"; but still very cloudy with no recollection of what had been, nor what was still to come. It was then that I next remember sitting on a bench in a reception area until I was fully recovered. Once I was recovered, I noticed a police man standing behind a counter looking at me asking me how I was feeling. The policeman said, "You don't remember much do you?". I said, "All I know is that I had a funny turn coming off the train". The policeman said that a man and his wife had noticed my attack, and had brought me to the British Transport Police Station. The policeman was kind and offered to phone my Dad, but I said to the policeman that I would be fine as the attack had now been and gone, and I never took more than one in the morning. I also informed the policeman that my medication would now cover me for the rest of the day. The policeman said that if I felt comfortable going to school then he would just let me go. I said thanks, and left. I then arrived at school still on time for my first class but had missed my morning assembly. I look back now, and think to myself at the age of forty three how different the outcome might have been if the incident had happened today, where instead of being a ten year old in a school uniform, I was instead a middle aged man in jeans and a leather jacket. I especially wonder how different the incident could have been if it were to happen at the age of forty three, in a station that has armed guards due to recent terrorist threats. As already mentioned, a person of asian origin having a frontal lobe seizure could get shot during high security alert moments in a train station if they suddenly started to experience uncontrollable screaming. I wrote to the 'Scottish Police Force Personal Development Department' back in 2001 to ask them if they would wish me to come along and give a presentation on living with epilepsy in an uneducated community, but their response was to tell me that their curriculum was too full, and that they did not wish to be given such a presentation. Ego costs lives, and this is especially the case when addressing the needs of those with any type of seizure disorder. I have to ask what is the biggest enemy of those with epilepsy. Is it the seizures and all the other clinical symptoms that accompany it, or is it the inadequate as well as penalising legislation that is passed by law; as well as the egoistic attitudes of people who think you are telling them how to do their jobs by giving them a first person account of living with a condition that makes up a large proportion of a neurologist's medical-legal work due to wrongful arrests. I will touch on epilepsy and the law later on in the book.

CHAPTER 8

The side effects of the anti-convulsant medication had been as crippling as the epilepsy, throughout both childhood and adolescence. The side effects of the anti-convulsants hindered learning in the classroom, and also hindered my ability to enjoy my hobbies and interests. These hinderances led to a frustration that could affect mood for the worse, which in itself led to risk of other complications arising that are too great to list here.

These drugs prevented me from having bad things happen to me, such as being robbed during a seizure. They also prevented me from becoming housebound through fear of having a psychologically disturbing experience when out in public, where I could have ridiculed/humiliated myself and invited all sorts of unwanted trouble. Despite these drugs preventing an endless list of possible medical, social, economic, educational, legal, political complications etc, they could create their own endless list of possible complications as a consequence of introducing into your life, side effects that could be as worse as the actual condition these medications are prescribed to treat.

These drugs on one occasion, in 1994, had me fall when walking along a pavement, where during my fall; I hit my head off a wall and ended up in hospital as an inpatient due to their decision to keep me in overnight for observations. Another example would be when I was at school, back in 1993, and I was playing golf with my father, teeing my ball up on the fourth tee of our local golf course. The first three holes I had played badly as a consequence of having double vision. To overcome this double vision, I had to close one eye to put my vision back into single vision. The only problem with doing this is that when you close one eye when addressing the ball, you swing your club at an angle that doesn't make good contact with the ball. You need the combined information from both left and right eye to swing the club on a plane that makes sweet contact with the golf ball. With one eye closed and the other open, the plane you swing your club on hits the ball above its equator, and as a consequence of this you mishit the shot, producing a notoriously bad shot. This playing with one eye closed was ruining my game and I was so frustrated; as these were side effects that I had been living with for years. While I was losing my temper on the fourth tee, a group of youths walked past me and my father, and they were all looking at us. I out of sheer rage shouted, "What the hell are you all looking at!!"; gripping my club like it was a baseball bat. These guys suddenly started shouting a whole load of abuse at me and my father, and one of them started running towards us. Once this member of the pack showed some leadership by running towards me and my father, all the others started running with him, and both me and my father found ourselves being chased and having to run for our lives. Me and my father were chased the combined lengths of a par 4, par 3 and par 5, back to the clubhouse with our hearts in our mouths. If we had been caught, we could have been beaten up or stabbed. This happened during an era in Glasgow where it was common practice for young guys to go through a phase of carrying a knife. It was an era when it wasn't unusual to see a private school boy carrying a knife around with him on a day off school. Whether he would use it or not does raise a question, but it's a question where you would rather not hang around for the answer. It is evident that people did use them from the deaths that you read about in the newspapers at the time. The area of Glasgow that these young men were from was an area of deprivation, where those residing feel there is less consequence for them to carry a knife and use it, than a middle class private school boy does, who most likely has a better quality of life and much more promising future prospects. These are young men who come from deprivation, and have had upbringings that give them lots to be angry with society about, and like myself, do not feel they owe society a good civilian, simply because they do not see such a society as deserving of one. There comes a time where you no longer let morality navigate your behaviour as the preaching of morality has come from people who have done nothing but treat you with immorality in their own subtle way, thus, discrediting any lessons on morality that you were taught by these people. If you were to ask someone from my background or theirs, what the difference between morality and immorality is, their answer would be "subtlety". Is other peoples' morality just a front for "Immorality"? I will let your life experiences answer that question for you.

I have therefore demonstrated, using two examples of events that had happened to me, that the side effects of anticonvulsants can result in more harm happening; than harm brought on by a seizure. With one of these examples, I could have had a head injury to live with; and with the other example, I could have been beaten up, scarred or murdered. This could have been the case with my father as well. I might not have just lost my father but I would have had to have lived with his murder on my conscience for the rest of my life. I am glad to say that side effects of medication have not caused many dangerous events to happen in my life, but it only takes one dangerous event to cause your life's fortunes to become majorly compromised. It would not be beyond the side effects of these medications to be the cause of you living with a head injury as well as spinal injury, leaving you paralysed from the waist down, with no mobility in the legs, having to mobilise in wheelchair, being pushed by carer and having no sexual function. Such a head injury could leave you housebound or living in a nursing home for the rest of your days. One peak dose of anticonvulsants could be the end of career plans, prospects of marriage, loss of independence; and even accidental death. The side effects of anticonvulsants can also cause you to underperform in both exams and courses, or training that requires the using of skills such as manual dexterity. These medications can also get in the way of you learning new manual skills as well as being able to safely carry out manual tasks, thus majorly hindering educational and employment prospects. The side effects can therefore be as detrimental, or even more detrimental than the epilepsy can.

CHAPTER 9

Childhood was also a period of great trauma in my life. Most days at school were days where I mixed with peers like any other child in the country did. I was accepted and had a group of friends. They still to this day are the best friendships that I have ever held in my life. Unfortunately, the days that I have a clear memory of are the ones that have given me reason to remember for the wrong reasons, and that what is to be remembered are experiences that could only be described as traumatic. These traumatic days cast a shadow over all the other days spent at school, despite the traumatic days being heavily outnumbered by the good days; because of the scars they left me with and the crippling effects this has had on earning and further skill development. I have already mentioned that people with my type of epilepsy are prone to developing anxiety disorders because of the part of the brain that epilepsy is present in. This part of the brain being the 'temporal lobe'. As a consequence of this, I have been more vulnerable to mental scarring from anxiety provoking incidents in childhood than my peers have been. There is a long record of anxiety provoking incidents that happened in my childhood and adolescence years that have left their scars affecting me vocationally and academically.

I would hope in this part of the book those reading will learn the importance of raising children to be more considerate of the feelings of their peers, and to not see slagging off and calling others names as something they can do for a bit of entertainment and joy, which will be short lived for those satisfying their sadistic streak; and instead appreciate and be in the knowledge that the damaging effects on those attacked by such slaggings and name calling can last a lifetime. The after effects of such ridicule or humiliation of others can last from hours right through to lasting a lifetime even though the event itself only lasts from seconds to minutes. Very like a seizure! It is also the case that if events like this repeat themselves then they start to have an accumulative effect, which can last for years beyond the slaggings, and require intense therapy from mental health professionals to conquer. The long term after effects of childhood torment from, I sadly say, both child and adult, can surface as academic underachievement, vocational misery, family strain, strained social relationships and social isolation; leaving those in old age to the vulnerability of exploitation and inhuman treatment by establishment, due to having no one to fend for them; it can even lead to suicide. This is especially the case in a person experiencing torment in childhood or adulthood with a medical condition, where the incidence of suicide is much greater amongst those living with that medical condition e.g. Asperger's Syndrome. This is a reality of childhood trauma, in the form of slaggings and ridicule, that most people are not even aware of. Many people who would call themselves nice people have made their contribution during childhood towards the scarring of someone, causing them to be without friends nor family throughout life, right through to old age; meaning they have no one to fend for them, leaving them vulnerable. Not having anyone to fend for you in later life could allow someone like social work to deem you incapacitated as a cost cutting exercise, when you are more than fit enough to make financial and welfare decisions for yourself; allowing social work to make decisions on your behalf, such as choosing to put you in a residential home thus freeing up a housing association home for a couple with family and friends to move into. I have seen these kinds of situations arise for people during my time in advocacy, and know how vulnerable someone becomes when they tell a social worker they have no next of kin nor any family or social connections; and how strongly related, experiences at school are with being in such a situation in later life. Ridicule in the playground or the classroom in childhood can result in denial of a house in middle age, or placing someone against their will in a residential home in old age. Bullying and mistreatment at school can also result in the police mishandling you in later life as a result of having no friends, nor family and having no earnings to pay for a lawyer due to being without a job for the same reasons; at a time when it is impossible for you to find a lawyer in this country who provides legal aid representation.

When I look at the people that surround me every day, I see so much human insecurity that goes back to our school days. Meditation has made me very much a human psychologist, and I realise that insecurity is society's biggest plague; not money (but this would come a very close second), and that this insecurity is something that is acquired at school, and installed in us by the children we grew up amongst. When I see a child, while everyone else is saying, "Oh, how cute, what's his name?", "Isn't he so nice"; I am thinking "He is of that age when they are the most evil and cause the most lasting damage to others". I also recognise that he is at that age where he is most vulnerable. That child is at that age where he is either contributing towards the developing of future scars of others the same age, or is one of these others whose acquiring these future scars. In 50% of mental health cases, the damage is done at this age, by those of this age. They, at this age, are anything but cute. The words "vulnerable" or "evil" would be more accurate at describing a child's true nature. This is when they are most damaging. I recognise that there are good children, but just like the bad days at school overshadow the outnumbering good days, unfortunately in those with damaged confidence from their childhood, the bad children overshadow the good children in terms of the lasting effects their company has had on the lives of others' and future personal development.

In my experience, teaching staff were evidence of how people don't grow out of this love of ridicule or humiliation and nor do they ever learn of the potentially devastating effects such ridicule and humiliation can have in the long term. I went to an all boys School in the 1980's and I had a large number of these experiences with both my peers and my teachers over the thirteen years that I attended school i.e. 1980-1993.

The first traumatic experience I had was back in primary 1 when we were given a list of arithmetic sums to do and I was very stuck as I found arithmetic a difficult subject. Did I really, or was I just taught badly? I sat there anxious all day and had only managed one sum. At the end of the day my teacher went around the class asking to see every pupil's work. When the teacher saw that I had only done one sum her immediate response was to get very angry. My teacher's first response was to get red faced, throw a fit of rage and shout out loud, "Guess what everyone! How many sums do you think Tim Bone has done today!!!!". Without giving the class an opportunity to make a guess she put her index finger up to the class and shouted, "One!!!!!!!" in both an aggressive volume and in a disgusted as well as aggressive tone of voice and facial expression. My teacher was full of so much rage that I thought she was going to smash the classroom up. My teacher marched towards me and took me by the hand and pulled me out of my seat, dragged me out of the classroom by one arm into the empty cloakroom, where I was smacked hard a number of times. I was told by the teacher that I was lazy and that I was a little skiver as I had lied to my mother about being unwell and having to take a day of school a few days before. My mother wrote in her letter to the teacher explaining my absence that I was skiving and was in fact not unwell. In truth I kidded on to be unwell as I was insecure about going to school. I wonder why? And I also wonder if this reaction of the teacher was helping. I remain scarred by that experience which has in itself had major disabling effects on me worse than the epilepsy.

Arithmetic was a subject that I had great difficulties with at school and it was the reason behind my mother constantly being invited down to the school to meet with teachers to discuss my lack of progress, and was also the reason behind me having to listen to my mother threatening to go down to the school and murder teachers. I remember my mother shouting at me at the fireplace going over fractions, where one night she said that she would go down to the school tomorrow and choke my teacher Mrs Tindsell and then go up to Mrs Ferguson's office and tell this headmistress that her school was "crap!". My mother was displaying the motions of choking someone with her hands as she was shouting this out in absolute psychotic rage. I was so scared as I was only eight at the time and I believe that this played a huge factor in the development of my performance anxiety in later life which is the original reason as to why I turned to meditation practice in 2014 which took me three years to eventually become consistent with. Becoming consistent with meditation was difficult for me but when I started losing my literacy skills as well as my ability to follow conversation, due to years of living with major depressive disorder, I was so overcome by anxiety that I managed to start doing it consistently twice per day for 40 minutes. When you've had a health scare you just pull your act together as you worry you are going to dement if you don't, especially when you hear stories about social isolation and cognitive decline as well as the effects major depression has on cognitive function.

If it were not for arithmetic being an essential life skill, I would have the subject banned, as I believe that the teaching of arithmetic is for many the beginning of the destroying of existing confidence, at a time in one's life where confidence is only just starting to develop. The same is true for literacy as well. It is a skill that is more difficult for some to acquire than others, and is probably the first time when people in authority start comparing us with others i.e. A-D streams/mixed ability; and we start comparing ourselves with others, as we begin for the first time to see ourselves being categorised on our ability. It is, at the end of the day, how good your literacy and numeracy is, that determines whether your school career gets off to a good start, which more often than not determines whether you will be in the A-stream or D-stream for the rest of your school days; which shapes your self-belief for your adult years. Low self-belief can be remedied, but it often requires a therapist.

It's like golf; if the first hole goes "pear shaped", then the rest of your round, much more often than not, goes pear shaped. A good round of golf always starts off with a good tee off on the first hole, with the exception of the odd "freak round". This couldn't be more true for education. Governments have scrapped 'streaming' in favour of 'mixed ability', but this doesn't stop the confidence damaging 'comparing and contrasting' that starts in early childhood. The only difference between streaming and mixed ability is, with streaming; the comparisons are made between students within different streams, whereas with mixed ability, the same comparisons are made between different students within the same class. The class is "closer to home" than the stream, therefore ironically, mixed ability classes might be more confident bashing, and cause you to be more likely of having a bad "first tee shot".

As a consequence of this damaged confidence, I did not trust my own initiative nor intuition when I was a kid. If my initiative was telling me to do something in a particular way, I did not listen to it, as I had little faith in it due to my low confidence. An example of this lack of faith in intuition was when I was told by my form teacher, in primary seven, to take a book down to another teacher's class, which I did; where upon my arrival the teacher said, "Just put it down there". My initiative told me he meant his desk, but I had such little faith in my initiative that I ended up putting it down on the floor. In response to this, the class just started to roar with laughter, which was a belittlement further encouraged by the teacher who dropped his jaw and just twisted his head right to left like one of these model clown heads at the carnival that you throw balls into the mouth of. I remember this humiliation, to this day, confirming it had a scarring effect on me. It is a massive failing of the teacher, as he had just watched someone with complex partial seizures behave in a bizarre way and never thought to question that I might have had a seizure. It just shows you though that low confidence can make you behave like you are having a seizure. If a scar on the brain can cause symptoms of seizure, then I suppose a scar on the mind could bring on behaviours that could be mistaken for seizures. It could also be said that if depression can cognitively impair you, then it's possible that anxiety can make you behave as though you are cognitively impaired.

I was at one time shown up by Mr Robertson; who was my geography teacher, in front of the whole class when I was in first year secondary school. It was over a problem that was arithmetic in nature, and he caught me out as being someone who was weak in this area. He noticed that I had difficulties understanding the logic behind the solution to the problem, and he started coming up with examples of similar problems, asking me in front of the whole class to solve these problems. I was struggling with this, and he was giggling at me with a red amused face like a child, and he had the whole class laughing at me as well. This ridicule went on for around half an hour, in a lesson that lasted forty minutes. My teacher would not let it go. I could not think when trying to solve the problem because I was suffering from mental block as a result of being so anxious, which just gave the teacher more reason to keep showing me up in front of my peers. My teacher made me look like a fool in front of everyone, and when he eventually let it go and moved on, we were given a class activity to do from the text book. It was then that I hoped that the bell would never ring, as once it did, I would have to stand up and look every class mate in the eye after my humiliation.

There was another time, in primary seven, when I was in French: which we started at my school a year earlier than in the other schools, where we were doing the times on the clock face which I had great difficulties doing in English, never mind French. I used a digital watch right up to the age of fifteen, as it took me to this age to be able to tell the time on a clock face. I could not get my head round how "9" could also be "Quarter to" and "45", or "6" could be "30" and "half past"; and had great difficulties combining the information from the minute hand with the hour hand. I wondered if it were a type of dyslexia with numbers, or if it were just confidence. It turned out to be confidence. It was a symptom of being taught how to tell the time on a clock face at a one size fits all pace in the primary years, and getting left behind. It was also a belief that anything that involved the teaching of numbers was not going to be a good experience when previous numeracy skill teaching had involved physical assault by the teacher and the belief that I was going to be responsible for the murders of my teachers by my mother.

During this French class; my teacher, whose name was Mr Johnstone, quoted times in French, and called out a name of someone who was to come down to the front of the class and put up the times on the clock; or he would put up the times on the clock and nominate someone to say them in French. The teacher mentioned the name of the first boy, where I found myself thinking "please, don't choose me, you will make a fool of me"; and then thinking "maybe someone else in the class will have the same problem". The first boy put his time up on the clock face and got a clap. This boy walked away with a smile back to his seat. I looked at my digital watch to see if there was the possibility of being saved by the bell. My watch told me that I still had thirty minutes before the end of class. This just made me feel even more nervous, as well as helpless. The name of another boy was mentioned, which provided me with no relief as I watched him stroll up, put a time up on the clock face and get an applaud. I was starting to have images in my mind of being humiliated in front of the class. This made me look at my digital watch for the second time, which provided me with no relief to learn that only a couple of minutes had elapsed since I last looked at it. The teacher then called out another four boys to the front of the class giving them exactly the same task, which each did with no problems before strolling back to their seats. The teacher then looked at the class register to determine who he would next call out to the front of the class to have their fluency in French tested; and if you were me, your inability to tell the time on a clockface exposed. This pause the teacher took to have a look at the class register caused me to have an intrusive thought of the teacher shouting out, "Bone". In the midst of this intrusive thought, my teacher shouted out, "Bone". I got a shock and remembered standing up and walking down to the front of the classroom, with a class size of thirty looking at me. I remember his face staring at me, and making eye contact with me, as I approached the front and did my right turn towards the centre front of the classroom, with him looking me right in the eyes. I could feel the adrenaline and apprehensiveness. I knew that this man would turn nasty in a matter of seconds from now, and I would be reduced in front of everyone, and that this was going to be entertainment for them; and a scarring humiliation for me. It was at a time like this that you would have thought of a seizure as a morale and self-esteem saving experience. I don't know what is worst, a seizure resulting in a lifelong implication, such as a physical scar; or a classroom humiliation that can go on to haunt you in future years, whenever you are taught any new skill, which to have difficulties with; will inevitably affect your future educational and vocational opportunities.

When I was out at the front, the teacher quoted a time, which I could translate into English; but I thought to myself, "how the hell do you put that time up on a clock face". I was full of anxiety, the palms of my hands were sweating, and I could feel blood draining from my face. I also felt my legs starting to go weak. I ended up putting up a random time with the two hands of the clock face. In

response to this time that I had put up the teacher looked at me and then the clockface and said that the time I had put up bared no resemblance to the time that he had given. He said this in a demanding, impatient tone of voice nodding his head towards the clock face. I felt panic, and felt like I had taken a stride further towards the edge of the cliff where there was only enough space for one more stride before my moral and self-esteem went over the edge. The teacher gave me another time to put up on the clockface, and history repeated itself, in terms of putting up a time that did not resemble in the slightest the time the teacher quoted. The teacher quoted another time in French, and then in a patronising "here's a test for you" tone of voice, asked me what the time was in
English that he had just given to me before giving me the opportunity to attempt putting the time given in French up on the clockface.

The teacher had a smile on his face, and some of the class were starting to snigger. I thought, "Fucking Bastard. I will show you I at least know the time you are quoting", but this just backfired on me as I told the teacher the time in English, and he then told me to put the time up on the clockface in a way that evidenced this difficulty of mine to be annoying him and entertaining him. I didn't attempt to put up a time as I knew it would just give him more ammunition to use against me in front of my class peers. The teacher responded by telling the class that he did not believe that I could tell the time and that we were going to try this activity in English for me and in French for everyone else. My teacher gave me times in English to put up on the clock face, which I could not do, and he had the whole class laughing at me. He ridiculed me for around twenty minutes. He kept giving me times, and got others in the class to give me times in English, to put up on the clock face. The whole class was laughing, and the teacher was loving it like he was getting the opportunity to become a comedian. The teacher became really impatient telling me that I was an idiot for him having to show me that this was the minute hand and that this was the hour hand. I was feeling so reduced and shown up; feeling and hearing myself speaking with a trembling voice. After he had had enough showing me up in front of my peers, all he could do was tell me to get back to my seat, telling me that I was in secondary school next year, reminding me that I could not tell the time and telling me that I was pathetic. I couldn't get over this. I felt so humiliated and just wanted the ground to open up and swallow me. I went to my next class with my mind totally pre-occupied with what had happened in the previous class, and came home thinking about what had happened, too embarrassed to share my experience with anyone. I had the experience on my mind while trying to get to sleep. As a boy who was having a seizure every 36hrs on average, I am quite confident to say that the experience in the classroom that day would have either given rise to an upon awakening in night or first thing in the morning seizure the next day.

CHAPTER 10

During my first year of secondary school I was swimming in a house race. At my school we had what was called "houses", and every pupil belonged to one of four houses that competed against one another at sports. I was made to swim, which I could do, but I only felt comfortable and confident with swimming breast stroke. During this race, everyone did front crawl, but I did breast stroke, and because of this I came last. When I was swimming, the whole swimming pool was surrounded by spectators and those waiting to take part in their race, and everyone started making retarded noises at me as I swam my two lengths. Some people ran up to the edge of the pool and started shouting abuse at me, calling me all sorts of names. If you were one of the couple hundred people around the pool, you were either making retarded noises, shouting abuse, or laughing. It was loud, and I felt so shown up in front of a huge number of people. I have a clear memory of people coming up to the edge of the pull, pushing their lower lip out with the surface of their tongue; making retarded noises while slapping one wrist with the other hand. I returned to the school after the swimming race and joined my modern studies class. I just sat there feeling despair, and feared the prospect of having to walk into the lunch hall as well as the tuck shop later on that day, and face the same people who had given me abuse only forty five minutes ago. I did not sleep that night as a result of overwhelming feelings of humiliation and despair. I just tossed and turned all night, until finally falling asleep at around 6am; to be woken up by my father at 7am, telling me it was school and I was to get up. Get up I did, but in a very sleep deprived state. Fortunately for me, there was no seizure the next day, despite the strong odds of having one in my first two hours of being awake as well as the possibility of a daytime seizure.

I have only mentioned four events in my life, that happened during my formative years, that have left me with scars; that have had detrimental effects on me academically, vocationally and socially. These incidents which I have described four of, were so traumatic that they left me with a condition called 'Social Anxiety Disorder'. This is a condition that can cripple your ability to integrate in all social settings. It can also be a condition that cripples you in only certain social settings. In my case it crippled me only in social settings that involve an element of performance which is why in my case its other name is 'Performance Anxiety'. This condition is very similar to 'Post Traumatic Stress Disorder' in that it has been caused by trauma, you re-experience symptoms in settings similar to the settings you experienced the trauma in, you demonstrate avoidance, you have dreams about the traumatic experiences, persistent remembering of the traumatic events etc. The difference between social anxiety disorder and post- traumatic stress disorder (PTSD), is that one of the diagnostic criteria for PTSD, under the DSM 5 (Version 5 Diagnostic Statistical Manual of Mental Health Disorders), is that you have been exposed to a major stressor that could have caused or involved: death, threatened death, actual or threatened serious injury, or actual or threatened sexual violence. I think that what I have, could be described as post -traumatic stress disorder, if the suicidal ideation, due to the social isolation brought on by performance anxiety caused by childhood scarring in performance settings, could be described as "threatened death". The question is, does the 'threatened death' have to happen on the day of the trauma itself or can it happen many years later?. As a scientist I would say that all the boxes of PTSD are ticked in my case, and that there is no difference between a trauma that causes near death at the time of it happening; and trauma that causes near death a number of years later. They are both traumatic experiences that can go on to cause "near death". I do believe that the interests of industry and authority have shaped a lot of psychiatric theory, and call me cynical, but I do sometimes believe that social anxiety disorder was created to reduce the number of claims made against third parties, who were responsible for events and circumstances that led to one developing an anxiety disorder; disabling enough to meet a diagnosis of post- traumatic stress disorder. A school experience that causes enough phobic behaviour in a person, where that person can find themselves never working and being dependent on the benefits system to make a living for their entire working lives; has been crippled by trauma more so than someone who will never be able to drive a car again due to a previous road traffic incident they were involved in.

As the events at school had resulted in me developing social anxiety disorder, I blame what happened to me at school for the social isolation I have had to endure, which has had its impact on seizure control. I have always avoided activities that involve performing with and in front of others, especially where intrusive thoughts can get in the way; such as activities that involve eye ball coordination, manual dexterity and judgement, thus, ruling out so many sporting opportunities. I also because of classroom experiences have avoided activities that involve being shown instructions or explained rules through fear that I will not understand the rules and then humiliate myself. It's the avoiding of such settings that has made it impossible for me to meet new friends as there is a reliance on being able to attend performance related activities if you are going to meet friends in later life. It is, as a consequence of the distress caused by the social isolation i.e. burnout resulting in problems with concentration and memory, that I have been bad with medication management and have unfortunately had seizures brought on by missed doses. Social anxiety disorder has also had me waken up in the middle of the night with night time symptoms of panic, full of worry over how I am going to cope living in a world with no relationships, where I can go up to three weeks without a conversation, thus, bringing on night time epileptic seizures and morning awakenings with unexplained large areas of bruising. I also waken up with strong feelings of agitation that bring on a feeling of mental nausea, where I feel myself experiencing the same feelings that someone feels when they have been going round and round pointlessly on a roundabout, where I feel myself wanting to get off this roundabout but can't, making me feel as though my mind is wanting to be "sick", combined with feelings of hopelessness and helplessness as a consequence of being in the knowledge that you are on this mental roundabout where you will continue to feel sickly for an indefinite period of time, making that corner in your life even tighter; bringing on feelings of panic which can bring on a night time seizure. The only difference between this mental nausea and its physical version is, with the mental nausea there is no remedy such as going to the toilet to be sick. You instead find yourself having to get up, sit on a couch and focus on calming down. This mental nausea is accompanied with a strong overwhelming feeling of burnout, which is made up of feelings of nervousness and mental exhaustion, which makes you feel that you are not going to have enough energy to do something as simple as put on a pair of trousers. I have also woken up with symptoms of panic, as you see no end to the suffocation; as you have no friends, no family, no acquaintances and therefore know of no one who can remove you from your isolation. It is also made impossible for you to remove yourself from isolation as a result of everyone being so hopeless at making new friends outside their existing clique of friends, which too often is made up of who they went to school/university/college/work with; and who the parents of their child's friends are. Anyone you do meet has no time, as they are always at work or at home with the family. This feeling of panic makes you feel dizzy and gives birth to more agitation. It is on these mornings that I get out of my bed and come through to the lounge and start meditating. A forty minute meditation session brings an end to these symptoms, and I am calm. No need for medications or psychiatrists. I do ask myself though, how I would have coped without the meditation practice, and the answer is I wouldn't have coped. I would have been incapacitated and spent my life in mental health residential care, prison or I would have committed suicide. I would never have taken medication for these symptoms, as not only do I not want the pharmaceutical industry to profit from my trauma, but I on principle also refuse to take and become dependent on medications since these fits of agitation have been entirely preventable, and have been allowed to develop as a result of family neglect and abandonment. My so called, "family", didn't just refuse to prevent such mental health symptoms from occurring, but have also just sat back and watched them develop, as my cries for help have just continued to fall on deaf ears. These mental health symptoms could also have been prevented but for us living in a one size fits all society, as well as virtually everyone in our society living a "formulated life", that can be described as: birth and kindergarten, followed by school/higher education into job, followed by marriage with children, followed by lifetime commitment to job and family, followed by retirement for the remaining years ahead and then death. It is the case that people meet their friends through living this formulated life i.e. through school/higher education, work and family; and if your needs make it impossible for you to live this formulated life then it should be no surprise to you that you will be without friends and family. You will effectively become a social outcast, causing you to live the life of a "one man band", where there will be a reliance on you developing very good coping skills if you are to face the demands placed upon you through living life in such a way. You have no one to hold your hand when facing any life stressor, you have to remain in good health as you live in a world where people would walk over your dead body in the street; and that includes health and social care services. I had worked in homes where there were clients who did not have relatives, and these were the ones who were neglected and allowed to just be forgotten about. A resident in a home I worked in had a vagal nerve stimulator where you used a magnet and swiped the area just below his collar bone to bring him out of a seizure. This man had no relatives or friends who visited and was just allowed to sit there and have seizures with staffs' backs turned to him with no one swiping his surgically inserted coil that lay just beneath his collar bone. This is why I eat my apples and walk my miles and get to the gym as well as meditate as I wish to keep such neglectful people out of my life when I am old. "Smokers", put that fag out now if you don't want to spend your later years wanting to get even with a social worker!!!

I have often asked why we are so cold and cruel to one another when I reflect on the incidents that happened to me in childhood and adolescence, as well as when I reflect on the experiences that I observed others have to endure. Since starting meditation I have managed to find answers to these questions through my own reflection. What I have learned is that the human race likes to ridicule and humiliate others over their weaknesses as it makes them feel much better about their own insecurities. I have learned that if you ever come across someone being nasty to someone, as they see that someone being vulnerable due to a weakness, then they are being nasty because they are trying to remedy an insecurity within themselves. Laughing at people and slagging off people is not a pursuit that those with high morale and self-esteem engage in. Confident people don't need to belittle and demean others. The belittling and demeaning of others is a pursuit for those who feel small and wish to make others look smaller so that they will look and feel bigger. A healthy attitude is one where, someone who feels small and does not like this, will go out of his/her way to become big; as opposed to making people in their eyes appear smaller than them, through the use of belittlement, giving them a feeling of being big. Unfortunately, there are very few confident people to act as good role models to those with little confidence, but plenty of people lacking in confidence to act as bad role models, which is why this behaviour we see coming from other people is so prevalent. I do believe that the belittling of others to make oneself feel big, by making others look small, is evidence of lacking an essential life skill that one must possess if they are to live a truly fulfilling life, bringing to fruition their full potential. 'Self- Directed Personal Development' that grows you is a life skill, and in my experience few people have this life skill and cope with the lacking of this life skill, by turning to jealousy and bullying of others who have made an achievement that evidences the possessing of this life skill. Look at weight loss for example, too often people cannot be happy for their friend who has lost a lot of weight through successful dieting and exercise, and respond to their own desire to lose weight by bitching about their friend. From my own observations, I have come to the conclusion that most people choose to live in the comfort zone, which is evidence of little self-directed personal development being used throughout the course of a lifetime, evidencing this life skill to not be very abundant in the mainstream population. I have noticed both as an advocate as well as a symptom management trainer that there is so much evidence of learned helplessness in our society, which is why there is so much bullying of others, belittlement, jealousy, two faced behaviour and a secret desire to see other people fail; including friends and family.

CHAPTER 11

When I left school at the age of eighteen, I had decided that I was going to pursue a degree in biology because I wanted to be a forensic scientist. I went to St Andrews University in Fife, Scotland, where I spent the first two years of my four year biology degree. I left school having proven so many of my teachers wrong, as I had been told I was "thick" by my teachers. I will never forget how my former Latin teacher came into my maths class when I was in my final year at school and had said to everyone, "Where is Mr Evans". We replied, "Back soon". My ex-Latin teacher just informed us that he would wait for my teacher to return. During this teacher's short stay, he said to everyone, "Guess what everyone! Bone got a B in higher physics" and then said, "And we all thought he was thick!". The class laughed, and I thought to myself, "You're just angry that your claims about my intellect can be evidenced as wrong and probably a touch embarrassed as well". I was laughed at and dismissed by teachers who discovered me with the 'UCAS form', that students fill in to select the universities that they wish to apply to. I am glad to say that this was not the case with all my teachers. There was Mr Turner; my headmaster and standard grade maths teacher, Mr Menzies; my biology teacher and Mr MacInness; my physics tutor, who had every faith in me. The other science teachers remained impartial. Science teachers seemed to have a more mature attitude towards D-stream boys, had a greater appreciation for how things can improve with time under the right conditions, and how confidence and performance can erode with time under the wrong conditions. People with science backgrounds do appreciate the "Artifact effect" where uncontrollable circumstances e.g. pollutants can affect experimental conclusions. There is no better example of this than education, where the conclusion to be drawn is the IQ of a person as well as academic ability; the education process is the experiment and the uncontrollable circumstances are for example an overbearing parent or an unhappy home that can impact on what one's ability and IQ can appear to be; therefore, science teachers are not so quick to form judgements of ability and IQ from a student's performance.

I look back at my school years and I think of the abuse I received from the age of five up to the age of eighteen, and the crippling effects that it has had on me academically, vocationally and socially; and   I think to myself that this was mental abuse that had the prospect of developing into permanent scarring that could have seen it impossible for me to hold down a job, support a wife and family, be condemned to a life on benefits, commit suicide, end up in prison or dead through mixing with the wrong company. This mental abuse was as bad as being sexually abused. I look back at my teachers and I firmly believe that the abuse they gave me was as bad as being raped, in terms of both the magnitude and severity of the immediate damage and collateral damage it was capable of causing, and was therefore worthy of imprisonment. I asked my doctor for a referral to psychiatry so that I could sue my former school for the development of my social anxiety disorder. I wished for such a referral to psychiatry, as I have never been given a formal diagnosis of social anxiety disorder, which I believe considering the extent it has affected me to should be diagnosed as 'Post Traumatic Stress Disorder'. I was given the referral to mental health, but cancelled it as I had done a lot of advocacy work that had educated me on how judgemental these mental health professionals can be, and as I said previously, if I was a betting man I would say that the community mental health team would use me as a scape goat, as it would never blame society's failings for my mental health problems. My inability to adjust would always be put down to 'Personality Disorder' due to my history of epilepsy, and that I could not be helped and had to accept that I was one of those people who unfortunately fell through the cracks. I had seen my clients, who had depression, be spoken to like this when I was a disability advocate. These clients were on Employment Support Allowance and did not wish to be; and instead had a preference to overcome their depression so that they could get back to work. My clients' community mental health teams had told them they could not be helped, and my clients' General Practitioners supported this verdict, telling my clients to come to terms with it. Fortunately for my clients, by approaching my advocacy charity, they ended up being referred to services such as cognitive behaviour therapy (CBT), after being told they could not be helped. I as a consequence of witnessing such behaviour, had no faith in my local CMHT being willing to help me, with myself being a very complex case, and also felt that I would not be able to handle the stress of following through with the necessary legal proceedings in my search for justice.

As a consequence of this abuse received at school, I went to university feeling inferior to all the other students and felt that someone like me shouldn't be at university. I had an attitude that a scraped pass was something for a person of my calibre to be over the moon about. I thought that a guy like me getting into second year with the bare minimum was like moving mountains. As I

approached my work with such an attitude, I didn't think big and only thought small, and as a consequence of this I only achieved small. I was not aware between the ages of eighteen and twenty- two about the relationship between your thoughts and your fortunes. I learned about this
when I taught the 'Expert Patient Programme' for 'Arthritis Care Scotland', but before then my worst enemy was the critical thinker in me, that was like a software package that had been put on my "mental hard drive" by my teachers and peers at school. I had many thoughts about failure i.e. the outcomes, failing i.e. the experience, and getting thrown out of university; and needed convincing by parents into staying at university and completing my studies. It is for this reason that university was a happy period in my life in terms of the friends I met and kept throughout my studies, but it was also a very distressing period in my life due to the lack of self- belief and the number of problems that I had invited into my life with this negative thinking.

My seizure frequency continued to be one every thirty six hours; with the notorious side effects of double vision, blurred vision, running vision, unsteadiness etc. I had to share a room with another student from Glasgow when I stayed in my hall of residence at St Andrews, and had many seizures in front of him that woke him up. Every second night, and sometimes every night; if my epilepsy was going through a really bad phase, I was wakening my roommate up and embarrassing myself in front of him. I would waken up in the morning feeling embarrassed getting out of my bed, not daring to ask what I had done during the seizure. It was for this reason that I had to move hall of residence to a single room as I could not continue with this live audience every time I had a seizure.

Seizures in front of friends was a very common occurrence when I was a student, and I will always remember a seizure that I came around from when I was sitting with two friends in a coffee shop. This seizure, like all other seizures, started off with a warning that terrified me; but had me not want to say I was going to have a seizure. You never want to tell someone that you think you might have a seizure as that is conceding to the seizure, which guarantees the developing of a full blown seizure; and because of the frightening nature of the seizure, you do not want to admit to yourself that you are going to have a seizure, especially when you know that your inner dialogue telling you that you are not going to have a seizure as well as concentration are capable of defusing them. The fear has you in a combined state of denying you're going to have a seizure as well as preparing for a seizure; and the prospect of defusing the seizure puts you off conceding to the seizure, thus, stopping you from asking for help. These two situations have the part of you that asks for help in a mental head lock. This mental head lock had me respond by standing up and walking towards the toilet, where suddenly I felt the world I was in with my friends drinking coffee; that the town of St Andrews is in, getting fainter, and fainter, and fainter; while at the same time the foreign world I feel myself to be in during a seizure becoming bolder, and bolder, and bolder; until there was no "Everyday world", and only "Foreign World", giving you a really strong "Ying Yang"; "out of body" like feeling, where I felt the blood rushing out of my face as well as an overwhelming feeling of vulnerability. The next thing I remember is being at a table in a café on my own. I was sitting there with this other table of people staring at me, and from what I remember I think they were asking me if I was okay. They were speaking to me from across the other side of the café, as my amnesia was lifting, and it eventually came to me after several minutes of sitting there that I was in a coffee shop, and the people sitting at the other table on the other side of the café were my friends. I recognised them, and went back over to the other side of the café, where I sat down and was nursed by them, until all the information about my whereabouts, myself and the others I was with came back to me. I was told that when I came out of the toilet during the blackout phase, I had walked out of the café and was gone for around five minutes and then came back in which is when I sat at the other table all confused. I had met my friends that morning at 9.00am for a 10.00am lecture, where I had not yet been awake for the minimum two hour period.

I was fortunate enough for daytime seizures to be very rare but I was always anxious about being in a lecture theatre because of the possibility of having a seizure and making a celebrity of myself for the wrong reasons. I do remember a lecture in my second year at university where I was sitting in the middle of the lecture theatre that had a seating capacity of around three hundred students. During this lecture I felt my seizure potential sitting just below my seizure threshold. This had me feeling the onset of fear rising to my head, subsiding; but not completely subsiding, before going on the increase again, back to subsiding; but not completely subsiding, before increasing again etc. I was also imagining the symptoms of a seizure; which makes a seizure more likely, which you start to do in the form of intrusive thinking. This went on for a whole hour, and this hour felt like ten hours as it was filled with the constant panic of having a seizure and showing myself up in front of a huge audience, that had me looking at my watch to determine how long it would be until I was out of this frightening situation. I fought this near seizure with constant effort for an hour and just wished for the hour to come to an end so I could get out of this very intimidating situation. I wanted "airlifted" to safety. I had never felt more relieved, when the lecture came to an end; and the lecturer said, "Okay, I think that is probably about as best a place to stop today, and reconvene on another day". As everyone stood up and put their books away, I felt I had quite literally been saved by the bell. I felt so fortunate that my reputation had remained intact, and I need not fear making it public that I had epilepsy. I came out the building feeling so traumatised by the whole experience, at the same time as feeling so relieved, and my confidence in lecture theatres did not return. I required someone to take notes for me and give me their notes to write up, as I had developed a phobia of going into lecture theatres. I coped this way for a number of weeks, and just forced my way back into lectures. Living with a condition like epilepsy has you living a life where every day you are outside of the comfort zone.

As one of the major characteristics of my seizures is 'Jamais Vu', where I lose familiarity with my surroundings i.e. the foreign world, one way I fought seizures was to picture in my mind scenes of places that I was very familiar with. If I thought to myself, in a Glasgow Academy classroom or a St Andrews/Glasgow University lecture theatre, of a scene such as a room in the house of a friend or the inside of a local supermarket that I frequented once a week; and pictured what was going on in these places in real time, it was as though I increased the potential for this world to hold on to me and weakened the potential the foreign world had of engulfing me. This is why you felt incredibly helpless at fighting seizures in places you were not familiar with, such as hotel rooms, as you were not familiar with the environment you were having your warning in, in the first place. You were trying to stay in an unfamiliar setting to prevent yourself from going into an unfamiliar world. It gave you that same feeling of going really deep under water, where you want to suddenly come shooting back up when the water starts to chill you and you get that intrusive thought of a ship funnel blowing. Going into an unfamiliar world from an unfamiliar setting, especially a few thousand miles away from home, made you feel even more vulnerable and scared between the climb from "1 to 6" i.e. before the point of no return. This putting my mind into thoughts of familiarity combined with positive self- talk; is how I fought warnings to seizures throughout childhood, right through to discovering mental arithmetic at the age of twenty. These thoughts of familiarity had a 30% success rate of defusing the seizure but they were hard work and you had to keep your wits about you.

 It was at the age of twenty- three, when I was daytime free of seizures, that I became a nursing student. During my nurse training days, I became extra anxious about seizures during the day and in staff handovers at 7am in the morning on the wards, even though I had been seizure free during the day since the age of twenty two; when I was put on two drugs that prevented seizures, and a drug that acts when you are about to have a seizure. Even though I was on a drug that acted when the seizure was about to happen, I never developed confidence in the drug, and believed that every morning warning would be my first daytime attack, where the drug had not done its job. I always felt that I knew that anxiety was the problem, and that this anxiety had caused my seizure potential to rise to just beneath my threshold. There were times in shift handovers on early morning shifts, while sitting in a small room or nursing station tightly filled with colleagues and mentors, that I could feel the seizure potential rising in the form of a wave of fear travelling from my stomach upwards; and the fear rubbing shoulders with just before "1", on the journey from "1 to 10" that a warning for a seizure takes. The fear rubbed shoulders with "1", and then after a few seconds the fear suddenly subsided as you felt the potential for a seizure drop, making you feel so relieved. Every rubbing of the shoulders of your seizure potential with "1", was a time when you felt your career and future employment were "walking on a tight rope". I used to think during the periods of relief, "Thank God, I am not under the care of that clinical pharmacologist anymore, as like the rest of his patients, he would have had me on everything and anything to make a name for himself amongst the drug companies". Even though I had many countless events, where the potential and threshold for onset of warning were near meeting, with the medication defusing the onset of seizures; and despite my medication having a 100% success rate in defusing daytime warnings, I never relaxed and I was always incredibly anxious when I felt the potential and threshold just about meet, as there is a first time for everything. A bit like being on a roller coaster and you are convinced you are going to fall out your seat, but at the same time you know you won't because you are "strapped in" by your medication. As I used mental arithmetic between the ages of twenty and twenty three to defuse the warnings to seizures, when I could never be

100% confident in the drug alone preventing me from having a seizure, I continued to use mental arithmetic, which helped me cope by being in the knowledge that I was on a drug that prevents warnings developing into seizures; as well as at the same time using a mental strategy that had an 80% success rate at defusing seizures. It is through this drug cocktail and mental arithmetic that I never had a seizure at work in my years in employment where it is an essential requirement for someone to be daytime free of epileptic seizures. There have, however, been a few daytime attacks since being put on this drug combination when I have either missed doses or have done high intensity workouts in the gym, where I have not slept the night before.

During my time at university as an undergraduate I did a lot of laboratory work. Unfortunately, my drug treatment side effects, my low confidence and mental health problems caused me to be very clumsy in the laboratory. I did not enjoy lab work and decided that I was not going to be a scientist, and just wanted to complete my degree, which I did with a third class Honours Degree in Molecular Biology. I graduated with this degree from Glasgow University as I had transferred from St Andrews University in 1995 due to the failing of a histology assessment which involved looking at slides under a microscope and being able to identify different tissue types and the different structures within the tissue. I found this a very difficult area to master as I had problems with my visual memory which is a symptom of having temporal lobe epilepsy. To get into Honours you needed to pass this assessment which I had not passed, therefore I was not getting into Honours. I had a meeting with university staff over my assessment and their refusal to let me into Honours. During this meeting the staff would not recognise my disability, would not budge on their decision even with a doctor's letter and just hounded me throughout the meeting. I was told that a "lad like you shouldn't be at university". I left this meeting with no joy, but Glasgow University let me into their Honours course in Molecular Biology. I unfortunately had to say good-bye to all my friends at St Andrews.

I was twenty years of age, and all my life I had only received criticism and rejection, and society complains that I am an angry guy and get defensive, and psychiatrists would say that because of these two traits I have a personality disorder. What a cheek, and what an insult. It should be obvious from these experiences why I would have never wanted an official diagnosis of depression and social anxiety disorder on top of the epilepsy. As you continue to read on you will increasingly notice the amount of grief that I have had to live with only having one of these three conditions diagnosed. To have the other two diagnosed would have been jumping from the frying pan into something hotter than a fire.

CHAPTER 12

When you are diagnosed with epilepsy at the age of ten, you are not informed about the repercussions that this will have on your prospects in higher education, nor are you told about the consequences it could have on you when looking for employment, and nor are you given any advice on how to survive in these settings. It is believed that as these two domains in life are years ahead, any kind of concern in these areas can be put off as though they will never arise. It is unfortunately the case that when you enter these two worlds, you are entering a jungle where there are previous victims of discrimination and prejudice that came before you, and that there will be many generations who become victims to these injustices after you. This is a jungle where you will have some friends and allies; however, from my experience those working in positions of authority are either the bad guys, and people you thought were allies will help the bad guys eliminate you if they are "asked" to do so. There are very few people on this planet who are bold enough to go to their trade union representative and say that their boss is asking them to fabricate evidence to constructively dismiss someone. They instead will just say, "Yes sir, No sir, Three bags full sir". You do not know how much I love non-conformists. There are few and far between. This is why I love comedians who offend. It is why I love going to watch Jerry Sadowitz, as he gives a middle finger to the world and its people. Jerry Sadowitz is Jewish, he had a loner childhood, never attended school and spent his childhood hanging around Tam Shepherd's magic and joke store, learning card tricks. I dare say that he received a lot of abuse at school as a result of his Jewish roots, and grew up angry with rage issues, which is why his comedy style is angry humour; and the people who like him are probably angry just like he is. I can certainly empathise with him, as I had my rage and anger before I discovered meditation. He's banned from the television because of his "inappropriate" humour which is a type of social exclusion.

 I have developed into a very anti-authority person, and I can understand why one in fifty people in prison have epilepsy. The treatment that I have received had resulted in me developing major depression, where the symptoms of the depression had surfaced as anger and rage, which became part of a vicious symptom cycle. This symptom cycle started with authority treating me prejudicially, and denying me things; as well as violating my human rights, causing me to experience rage and anger due to living without closure. This then allowed those in positions of authority to say, "You see, you're angry and aggressive and have a personality disorder", thus allowing future violating of my human rights because it's my word against theirs, causing me to experience further anger and rage. You would be surprised to know the roles that those in these positions of authority had held. Many of these people were those who were nurses, social workers, teachers, charity workers, disability advocates, university lecturers, parents and sisters. It was for this reason that when I went to my doctor with symptoms of anxiety, he referred me to the community mental health team for an assessment. I did not attend the appointment as I thought well its people in these roles who have caused this anger, anxiety and depression. These people will only defend their colleagues and put my problems down to personality disorder, as a consequence of having epilepsy. Psychiatry has it down in all their literature that personality disorder is very prevalent in epilepsy, and that in itself fills me with rage. Of course we have personality traits that are incompatible with living in society, when society raises you in this discriminative and prejudicial way. If a child is brought up being abused by its parents, will it grow into an adult that gets on with their parents? Of course not! So why should the relationship between us people with epilepsy and society be any different. It is these kinds of thoughts I find myself having when I see a police car, social worker, council tax officer, Department of Work & Pensions etc, or anyone in any role that involves judging people on their behaviours; and can persecute and compromise people, who they as judge, do not give a good evaluation of because of their behaviours. Psychiatry would fit that bill!! The term personality disorder is offensive and confrontational. It has the same effect on you as someone picking a fight with you; for the person calling you personality disordered to then say, "You see, you're angry, full off rage and can't be helped". This increased anger then exacerbates your depressive symptoms where one of the symptoms is; you guessed correctly, anger! It becomes impossible for you to hold down a job because you carry this anger around with you and can't take criticism of any sort of description, as society has provided you with nothing more than an overly critical life course, that stretches from childhood to the present day. My mother scarred me by fiercely criticising my teachers back in primary 3 onwards, which by doing so was criticising my work and performance, which is a major contributor towards the development of social anxiety disorder! Also known as 'performance anxiety', according to "Psychology Today" and other psychology articles/journals.

I am not medical but I have worked in health and social care. I am also a science graduate and have a wealth of life experience, and I do have my theory on how personality disorder came to be. We have two types of people in the world. One is the **follower** and the other is the **leader**. Fat cat capitalists are very intimidated by outspoken people. Outspoken people are often the advocates of the layperson, with them very often being lay people themselves e.g. William Wallace of Scotland, Tommy Sherridan (Former Leader of The Scottish Socialist Party), Scottish Nationalists (Winnie Ewing) in the era when there was next to no support for Scottish independence etc. These outspoken lay people do not tolerate second rate treatment of anyone, and nor do they allow anyone to walk over their human rights as well as the human rights of others. These types of people are a threat to the boss in the workplace. They are the kind of people who will use their leadership skills to start an uprising in the workplace when the pay is cut, when the work conditions become substandard or when one lot of workers are treated less favourably than another lot of workers. They are the ultimate "thorn in the side" of the "Fat Cats". The "Fat Cats" have a vested interest in shutting up the leader by discrediting him in front of the workforce so that the followers will not listen to him. This has been achieved and been made possible by the invention of the term "Personality Disorder". I believe that personality disorder was originally an invention of Occupational Health (maybe?), to say to the workers, "Don't listen to this guy, he is mad". It was a way in saying to the workers, "He's anti-social, self-destructive, lacking in insight, impulsive, paranoid, narcissistic, controlling etc". By labelling the leader all these things, he would become stigmatised in the workplace and no one would listen to him as a consequence of everyone believing him to be disordered, thus, silencing his voice; making the workforce much more easily exploited. This is how I believe personality disorder came to be, and worked its way into psychiatry; and there are many people out there with leadership skills as well as a great amount of potential, being sin-binned by being labelled with personality disorder, which disempowers and discredits the person in their own eyes, thus, destroying confidence, morale and self-esteem; causing all sorts of anxiety and depressive disorders. It is manipulating the soul, against the soul. It allows people in power to silence the outspoken, so that those under their power can continue to be abused, exploited and manipulated without any fear of an uprising, or any other type of social unrest stemming from the interests of others' human rights. A good example of this is 'Anti-Social Personality

Disorder', that many non-conformists are diagnosed as having. Non-conformists are independent minded people who can't be swayed into buying the latest gadget or spending their money on what everyone else wants to spend their money on, and refuse to obey some laws probably because so many laws are unfair and lacking in logic, making them very rational people that can't be manipulated or scared by others into behaving in a particular way, which is exactly the type of person the fat cat capitalists don't want you being friends with; so it is arranged for the non-conformist to be stigmatised, so that no-one will hang out with them or listen to them and therefore won't pick up healthy behaviours from them, that the fat cat capitalist would lose out from others adopting. These people are therefore stigmatised by labelling them with personality disorder.

I believe that 'Paranoid Personality Disorder' was invented to label those leaders who were telling others not to trust those who were exploiting and abusing them. The kind of modern day thinking you would hear coming from a leader, that in a previous era would have resulted in him being stigmatised by being labelled with paranoid personality disorder so that others would not listen to them, is something such as: "Don't trust these people. They say by being out of Europe you will earn more money because of more flexibility doing trade deals, when in reality it's about not needing to comply to European legislation, thus, affecting your worker rights that will mean pay cuts and redundancies". This of course is only my theory and you may have yours. The theory behind the other personality disorders is just the same. In other words, personality disorders were created disorders that are used to name "square pegs" who let logic guide their behaviour in a world that is run illogically, and therefore call a "spade a spade", and make a lot of enemies with those who use this illogic to manipulate others into buying the next gadget, or just accepting the next rule or regulation which are designed purely for the benefit of those who create them. According to a philosopher called Olivia Goldhill, President Nixon of the USA, who was the 37th US President between the years 1969-1974, had wished a disorder called "Personality Disorder" to be invented to make it look like all the protestors of his time in power, who protested as a result of their discontent with government policy over housing, education, transport and other areas of social policy; had a mental health condition. This finding of mine about President Nixon was made on the 7th October 2019 at the time of editing this book whereas my theory on personality disorder was something I had put together using my own logic combined with the world becoming a more transparent place through my meditation practice back in March 2018. These two theories are very similar.

If you ask me, Psychiatry is a science of many vicious symptom cycles. I have all the time in the world for Psychology as that is the science of mind, and how the mind works, where the skills they teach people to get out of these vicious symptom cycles are of sound legitimacy which I have used myself; but as for psychiatry it certainly hasn't proven itself fit for purpose in my experiences. It would appear it encourages these symptom cycles to the point of drug dependency benefitting the pharmaceutical industry. It leads to a life of dependency. Psychology leads you back to independency. As will be further elaborated upon in a later chapter, I am a meditator and this has opened my eyes as to how we function mentally and how things came to be. The world is becoming increasingly transparent to me in the form of "spiritual awakenings".

There are reputable mental health professionals who do not have the time of day for psychiatry. There is reference material on the internet saying that psychiatry is damaging and does more harm than good. Dr Allan J. Frances has posted an article in 'Psychology Today' back in 28th October 2013 titled *"Does it make sense to scrap psychiatric diagnosis"*. A doctor called Dr Lucy Johnstone comments in this article that, "Now, with some of America's most senior psychiatrists admitting that psychiatric diagnoses are not valid, that we haven't actually found the faulty genes or brain dysfunctions, and that medication can actually worsen outcomes, it may be on the brink of collapse" Dr Lucy Johnstone says in this article that psychiatry takes a biomedical model towards understanding mental health. It is looking for a "scientific" reason for people being depressed, anxious, etc and that that model of approach to understanding mental health problems is very limiting, and that psychiatrists have to look towards better understanding that not all depression and anxiety disorders are caused by something scientific, but instead caused by the resulting effects of loss, trauma, abuse, poverty, discrimination, domestic violence, the failings of our politicians, capitalism and so on. People are put on anti-depressants and tranquilisers as they are said to be suffering from "poor mental health", when in fact they are suffering from "Living in an intolerable society". Poor mental health is a "Rug", psychiatrists are a "broom", and the drugs they prescribe a "sweep"; for the purpose of our politicians getting re-elected, and our fat-cat capitalists continuing to earn huge profits in a world with an ethos of inequality; covering the cracks (which psychiatry is a tool used for this purpose) and getting more than your fair share. They say Islam is the world's largest religion. I would disagree. I would say it is "Demonism!" That worships three gods: Pride, Greed and Status. I do believe that good people are saints living in hell.

CHAPTER 13

I had decided to become a nurse back in September 1998 as I wanted to help those who had been and were medically disadvantaged like I was. I had an empathy with these people and also had a passion for helping such people. My intention was to one day be a specialist nurse helping those with epilepsy, or at least helping those with a chronic health condition that required long term medical evaluation. As has already been mentioned, during my years at Glasgow Academy I had experienced a lot of ridicule and humiliation both during and after school hours. This crippled my confidence which unfortunately had a transferable effect, thus, affecting my vocational life. I grew up to become someone who had developed what is called 'Social Anxiety Disorder' of the 'Performance Anxiety' type. In a similar fashion to epilepsy there are two types of social anxiety disorder. There is 'Generalised' social anxiety disorder where you fear all social settings, and there is 'Partial' social anxiety disorder where you only fear a specific social setting. This second type of social anxiety disorder was the type that I had developed, and as is the case with generalised social anxiety disorder, it is a condition that one develops as a consequence of an overly critical childhood. Throughout childhood I received too much criticism in the classroom as well as from my peers. All the incidents mentioned in the childhood and school section contributed towards the development of this condition and it caused me so much distress during my time in nurse training. During this time I had great difficulties performing on the wards and was often ridiculed, called names, put down on the wards by people making comments such as, "I wouldn't want you on my ward if you were one of my nurses" and mentors as well as university staff laying into me because of the quality of my work for someone at my stage in his training. The further anxiety as well as depression, that this treatment on the wards had resulted in, caused me to drop things, knock things, catch myself on things, forget to do things; resulting in further condemnation as well as put down, and resulted in me experiencing bullying and harassment. I would lose my temper, and I would then be reported to the university, where I would receive abuse from the staff saying that this happens over and over again. I had some good mentors on other placements, but so many mentors were bullies and could not cope with having a student with learning difficulties. I must stress that these are "learning difficulties", and not "learning disability". It's important that these two terms do not get confused. Despite not sharing with the university the fact that I had social anxiety disorder, as at that time I did not know that this was a condition, I never told the staff of the university that this was what was wrong when they used to take me into tutorial rooms in private and give me dogs abuse for the difficulties that I was having. Even though I did not share this with them, it should have been obvious that something was very wrong, especially in front of nurses who are supposed to have had an adequate amount of training in mental health to know that this disorder exists; and therefore, they should have at least queried the possibility that social anxiety disorder could have been a reason behind my difficulties on the wards. Instead of querying social anxiety disorder, they just labelled me a difficult student with an attitude problem due to my defensiveness; eventually resulting in me having to leave the course. This was the first dose of vocational rejection that I was to receive.

I decided to move south to the midlands after my nurse training and started teacher training. Of all the professions/vocations that have been oppressed by political correctness, teaching must be the worst. Political correctness had also contributed towards my rage levels. When I entered teacher training, I could not get over how liberal the schools had become with discipline; and nor could my friend Richard from Northern Ireland. On the first day of being introduced to the form class by the class's form teacher, the first thing the boys down at the front said was, "Oh no! We don't want a jock and a paddy, please".

When Richard and myself took a GCSE chemistry class, where Richard did the theory and I did the practical, the pupils were all talking over Richard; not listening to a word he was saying. The boys were having their conversations and the girls were having theirs. My mentor just stood there and watched the class deafen Richard. I was amazed that he was prepared to allow this class to continue talking over Richard. My mentor just laughed and said, "Poor Richard. The boys are talking about football, the girls are talking about shampoo and Richard is talking about chemistry". I thought to myself that when I was at school if we spoke over a teacher training student in the presence of our teacher he would have gone through the roof with rage and had all of us stay behind that afternoon after school for a double period. My teacher would also have targeted a few of us and made examples of us by having us on Saturday detention where we helped the janitor clean the school and any other given task. It was therefore the case that Richard and myself struggled to adapt to this change in classroom culture that we did not approve of. It therefore came as no surprise, during our fifth week on placement, when Richard picked me up in his car and made me aware that I would have to make my own way to school the next day as today he was only coming in for one purpose; and that was to hand his notice in. While driving his car that morning, Richard was waving a letter in an envelope and said to me that he had had enough of the cheek that kids get away with these days and that he did not have the patience nor the tolerance for such attitude. Richard and I did not share the same ethos that the education system in England had in the year 2001. The human being does not understand the word "Moderation". I was certainly not an advocate of the education system I had come from but the education system I was training to be a teacher in was one that had gone too much the other way. There is never a middle ground that we can stay in. The human being does not understand the concept of "Balance". He swings to the left breaking everything in sight and then swings to the right breaking everything in sight as opposed to remaining centre and still. Political correctness and political incorrectness are very good examples of this.

 On arrival at the school Richard handed in his notice saying that he did not wish to teach and was gone. I survived the upper secondary school placement teaching GCSE students as well as A-Level students, and I passed the placement.

 It was the case that during this placement I had a seizure in a staff room packed with teaching staff one morning, when the headmaster was briefing the teaching staff on some matter. The next thing I remember is coming round from the amnesia in a seat, in a near empty staff room, with just a couple of staff supervising me during my recovery. The school phoned my Dad who found himself speaking to the person in charge of training teaching students on the school site. This member of the teacher training team said that as I was training to be a biology teacher, there was obviously health & safety implications with me being left alone with students who would be doing lab work. The member of teacher training staff said that I would obviously need a classroom assistant. It was made possible for me to continue the placement with supervision, and I passed my assessed lesson where a member of the university teaching staff comes round to assess your ability to take a class. At the end of the placement I thanked my mentor for his time and commitment, but since the seizure, his attitude towards me had changed in terms of the tone of voice that he spoke with as well as his body language. When I left, having thanked him for his time and commitment, he wished me luck with the next placement as well as my teaching career as though someone had just died. I believed at the time that I must have said something that upset him, or maybe he didn't think I should have passed the placement.

I was then to start another teacher training placement, where I was now teaching the pre-GCSE years, and for the first two weeks of the placement I was getting along fine with my mentors. My mentors were what I would have described as being very pleasant and friendly, and my only complaint would be that the students I was teaching were much more disinhibited and unruly, but manageable. It was during the third week of the placement that my university mentor came round and said that he would speak about my progress, as well as the progress of another student on my teacher training course, just to see how we were settling in. After my university tutor had spoken to the two mentors that we had, I was invited in to just speak with my university tutor. My tutor, Invited me to sit down. He had a facial expression that gave nothing away about what he was thinking or the nature of what had been discussed with my mentors. When I sat down he looked at me, and quietly as well as curiously asked me how I felt I was settling in. My tutor asked me if I was finding the staff good to work with. I replied to this by saying that the mentors were very helpful and that they gave me good feedback and advice. My tutor then said, "Interesting". My tutor went on to say that he had been speaking to my two mentors and that they told him differently. He told me that my two mentors had actually communicated to him that they had great concerns about me. This was said to me by someone who came across as a really bad actor. This bad acting in itself was like a confession to me that this was not genuine and that someone was doing the dirty on me which gave me that feeling that I was right in the middle of a confrontation. I was shocked by this. It felt like a bucket of cold water had just been thrown over me. It was that kind of shock. It was unexpected and totally out of the blue. It felt like a really good friend had spoken about you behind your back. I felt betrayed and made a mug of. It was the same kind of feeling where you get talking to a stranger for a couple of hours, they give you a beer, you think they are a really decent guy who you are really enjoying the company of and then suddenly during a quiet moment in a quiet place he suddenly takes a baton out of his jacket and pushes you up against a wall putting the baton to your face telling you to give him your wallet. I know this feeling well since this described scenario is one I have had experience of in a park called Maxwell Park on the southside of Glasgow, when I was sixteen, after drinking a can of lager with a stranger on my way home from school on a bench by the pond. I can say that the feeling of betrayed trust is similar in both scenarios.

 In response to this hostile surprise I said to my university tutor that this was a total surprise to me. I asked what it was that was worrying them. My tutor replied by telling me that they thought that my teaching was too old fashioned. I said that I was not told this at my previous placement, and I said to him that I was firm with the kids but not aggressive. I said that this was required as the kids could be quite unruly because of the over top political correctness that has been allowed to plague the profession. The tutor said to me that it was necessary for me to speak with him back at the university. I agreed to this and attended the university teaching department a few days later to have words with my tutor. I told him that he was the first to learn about this complaint by my mentors and usually it would be the student. I told him that my mentors had never complained to me about my teaching style and that this unexpected sudden change in attitude towards me had most likely been because of the seizure that I had back at the school where I did the GCSE and A-Level placement. I told him that as someone with a history of being discriminated against, he as my tutor had a job to do to convince me that this sudden change in attitude towards me was not because of the epilepsy. I told him that it would be wrong of me to not recognise this as being a potential factor. The tutor did not want to discuss this with me and told me to get out his room if I were going to get emotional about the issue. I went back to the school and continued teaching but upon my first class after the criticism being made about me by my mentors, the unruliness from the kids escalated to a level that was too great for me to handle. Classes became demoralising experiences and my mentor used to stand there and say things like, "Well Mr Bone, they find your lessons boring, what are you going to do about it?" and in disbelief I asked my mentor if he was just going to stand there and let these kids speak like that to me. What kind of preparation is that for the world that these kids are expected to leave this school and enter into. I told the mentor that it was an abuse for him to just stand there and let me become demoralised and soul destroyed in front of everyone, and in some ways it was an abuse of the kids to let them behave in a way which if they behaved like in the workplace they would be sacked, if they behaved in the street they would get their head kicked in and if allowed to believe that they can get away with behaving like towards an authoritative figure could possibly cause them to behave in ways in front of other authorities that could result in them becoming majorly compromised or even prosecuted. My mentor shouted at me and said out loud, "Abuse is a very powerful word Mr Bone, you watch what you say in here!". I replied and said, "Whose the one doing the shouting now!". I gave up that placement and demanded that I got another, at another school; but it was just like the school that I had just come from but worse. I was very depressed but I stayed on and the obnoxious behaviour of the kids and my depressive symptoms did not get along and I was accused of being too strict. I was told that I was angry and aggressive but I disagreed. I would say that, yes, I felt these things but I channelled it as firmness which is not aggressiveness. Either the schools deliberately tried to spin my firmness as aggressive, or firmness is a shade of grey that most people don't see. The school system continued to say that I was aggressive, and because the pupils were getting the backing of the teachers when the pupils told me they were not listening, as what I was teaching was boring, a boy felt at ease with squaring up to me in the playground on my way home from the school with his friends. The kid put his finger in my face and threatened to beat me up with his friends if I ever told him off in the class again. I couldn't believe this. In my day, sure kids waited outside the school for one another when one was responsible for the other getting into trouble, but never did a student wait outside the school for a teacher. There was a hill behind the student at the time of squaring up to me, and I felt myself about to shove him down it and beat an apology out of him, and then tear his trousers down in front of everyone; and leather him with my belt in front of all his friends so he didn't look "the big man" that he believed he was being, and that was when I just quickly marched home away from the temptation, thinking to myself how much I hated this country and its culture, and that over the top political correctness; and others' conformity, had created this reality, and therefore, handed my notice in the next day. This political correctness has filled me with a rage being a very principled person, and the irony is this political correctness was supposed to protect people like me, but it was actually allowing mainstream people to beat me over the head with emotional batons; and for me to pick up the blame. Political correctness does not protect the person with the hidden disability where you don't look vulnerable, nor do you appear to have any limitations to the naked eye; therefore people believe that no tolerance need be shown towards any hidden disability related difficulties

;however, there is a consensus in our society that all children are vulnerable and therefore we live in an age where it is the fit looking adult's word against the fit looking child. This has just added to the anger over the years. When I was a disability advocate between the years 2014-2017 I met with a gentleman with autism and we were standing in Glasgow Central Station where a charity worker approached both of us wanting to collect money for children. We both looked at this man and both told him to shove off as there was not enough help for adults.

One thing that really gets me mad is the fact that society, and so many of its people, cannot tell the difference between 'firmness' and 'aggressiveness' in all walks of life, and not just in teaching. Firmness is assertiveness, and not aggressiveness. Assertiveness has boundaries, whereas, aggressiveness has no boundaries. I teach a course for 'Epilepsy Connections' in Glasgow, where I teach a session on assertiveness. As the slide says in my powerpoint presentation, assertiveness is based on balance which is what my teaching style was like, it was maintaining a classroom atmosphere where there is a mutual respect between teacher and student, as well as student and student. Aggressiveness on the other hand is about winning. Making the score 2:1. It's about "You damage me, so I will damage you more". This was not my teaching style. Hearing fully grown up adults say, "You're aggressive", when you are being assertive, reminds me so much of the kid that accuses his or her parents of not loving them because they are raising their voices when telling them off.

I have to stress that what was to come in future years ahead of me leaving teacher training right up to the present date does back the theory that I was discriminated against on the grounds of my epilepsy; as I left teacher training in September 2002, and upon my return to Glasgow, I became an Expert Patient Programme teacher for 'Arthritis Care Scotland', a teacher for 'Disability Information Greater Glasgow'; where I designed as well as taught a self- management course for those with disability, became an 'Expert Patient Programme' trainer for a charity in Slough, have been a rescue medication trainer for 'Epilepsy Scotland' as well as the 'Epilepsy Society', and I am currently a life skills trainer as part of the 'Epilepsy Futures Course', run by 'Epilepsy Connections'. All of these achievements certainly have the claims made by those in teacher training go against the majority's claims about me as a teacher, and it is interesting that the communities that have given me their approval in terms of my suitability to be teaching, are communities that are tolerant of someone having epilepsy, whereas, the jury is out on whether teaching is tolerant towards epilepsy, and it will always be out, as there will never be a time or an opportunity for teaching to demonstrate any tolerance that it may have, and therefore whether the teaching profession has a tolerance towards epilepsy will very much be down to the interpretations of different peoples' experiences with the teaching profession when disclosing their epilepsy; however, from my experience of having a seizure in a teaching staff room, followed by sudden changes in reception from university staff, teaching mentors and students combined with the achievements made since 2004 that conflict with conclusions made about my suitability to be a teacher, I would have to conclude that I was discriminated against as the evidence is more supporting of that theory. The change in attitude and reception of others, that I was on the receiving end of, during my time in teacher training was so digital after the visiting of my university tutor and the meeting he had with my placement mentor that it is safe to say that something was shared about me. As it was the mentors whose attitude suddenly changed towards me, if anything was shared, it was the university sharing it with them, and one thing i.e. the only thing that the university would have known that my mentors would not have known would have been that seizure I had in the staff room during the previous placement.

CHAPTER 14

After teacher training I moved from Loughborough to Nottingham where I worked for a learning disability home. I was looking after residents who had moderate to severe learning disability. The residents were great. I had good relationships with them. I did question the logic as to how they chose to run the home. There was a resident called Leroy who always went missing on his skate board where we would get a phone call from the British Transport Police from time to time telling us that Leroy had been found skate boarding in London. Leroy had a habit of doing this and the home eventually decided to give Leroy a bike instead of a skateboard. This is a good example of the political correctness crisis that this country has been going through and continues to be going through. It is also another example of something where I am at odds with the world around me and its people. It is very difficult being a logical person living in an illogical world!

I was given the responsibility, with another member of staff called Amy, to take Leroy and a resident we called "Little John" to Cleethorpes for a weekend holiday. Unfortunately, during this weekend holiday, I had a night time seizure in my bedroom, and during the confusion I was found by Amy to be wandering around. Word of this seizure got back to the managerial staff of the residential home. On the day of my first shift back from Cleethorpes I was given Leroy as my client for the day to work with. While all staff and residents were out for the day, I was left on my own with Leroy to supervise him in the back garden with him on his bike. Leroy was cycling around the back garden doing wheelies and jumping off raised parts of the lawn onto the lower lawn on his bike. The large back garden of the home had been converted into a mini-bicycle obstacle course.

When you work in these residential homes you do drink a lot of coffee, therefore being on an anti-convulsant drug that is also used for treating people with kidney disorders, one of the side effects that I have to live with is frequenting the toilet, especially when drinking compounds such as   caffeine that like the 'Diamox' has a diuretic effect. Hangovers after nights out on the town were horrendous as you passed larger volumes when you were drinking alcohol combined with Diamox. This extra dehydration then acted as an ally of the alcohol withdrawal, making you much more prone to a seizure than you would be experiencing alcohol withdrawal alone. Alcohol could effectively turn your anti-convulsant medication into a convulsant.

As a consequence of the diuretic effect of the diamox I had to go to the toilet, as the only one looking after Leroy, with no one in the home to watch Leroy while I was away visiting the toilet. It was for reasons like this that many in the home believed that Leroy should have been 'two to one care', and not 'one to one' care. However managerial staff see you as telling them how to do their job when you bring up such a suggestion at team meetings. Maybe we should have told the managerial staff to never make Leroy 'two to one care' to increase the odds of it happening.

After being away at the toilet I walked back to the back garden and on my entry into the back garden I discovered that Leroy had gone missing. I thought to myself "Why do these idiots give Leroy a bike", "He escapes to London on a skateboard, the British transport police have us come to collect him after discovering him skating up and down a platform on the underground and then on his return the manager gives him a bike", "If he can get to London from Nottingham on a skateboard, then he could get from here to Cairo on a bike!", "Guess what, the result of this risk assessment that management never carried out, and not listening to staff who look after and work with Leroy; is not going to fall on the head of those responsible, and instead will fall on the head of a foot soldier scapegoat, who will be me". After having these thoughts in response to Leroy's disappearance, I went to the manager's office as she had just returned to the unit, and told her that Leroy had gone missing. As I have already mentioned, I always felt that Leroy should have been two to one care, and not one to one. The manager said that it was my fault and that I shouldn't have gone to the toilet. I told the manager that every member of staff had been away from the home at this time with their resident so there was no one I could have got to ask to keep an eye on Leroy when I was visiting the toilet. The manager did not see this as a valid reason. I then asked the manager if she felt it was a good idea giving Leroy a bike when he had a history of absconding to London from Nottingham on a skate board. The manager responded by saying, "Do you not think Leroy should have a bike?" and I said, "No, I think it's illogical to give Leroy a bike considering he escapes on his skateboard the whole time to London"; and she replied, "You're fired". I could not believe it. Her body language, tone, disproportionate response to my disagreeing with her and the fact that Leroy had gone missing under the supervision of other staff momentarily contending to other things when the home wasn't empty of other staff, convinces me that this firing wasn't because of Leroy but was either a hot-headed impulsive decision made by the manager that was ego-driven or because of the seizure that I had had in Cleethorpes. I believe that this was a case of opportunistic dismissal and that I agree in that I did not disclose that I still had that 1 in 10 night's seizure on my application (as I had just put down that I was controlled epileptic) so I was not covered by the Disability Discrimination Act 1995 if a disability related issue were to arise that affected job performance. In theory, the occurrence of the seizure in Cleethorpes affected my ability to do my job as it meant I could not do sleepovers when taking clients on holiday, but in practice it did not affect my ability to do my job as other members of staff could be allocated the role of taking clients on holiday and my job did not require me to do sleep overs in the residential home as they had agency staff to do that as opposed to permanent staff, therefore, this was a case of discrimination not covered by the Act, as they should have responded to the seizure that I had had in Cleethorpes by writing to my doctor for confirmation that I was being truthful with them over having no seizures while awake, which they had decided not to do, as well as refused to do the honourable thing, and that was enable a man to keep his job by being prepared to make a compromise that would only show its head once or twice a year where they would be one member of staff down in the number of staff they could choose two staff members from to take clients on holiday. Maybe if society were to be more tolerant towards epilepsy, I would feel able to put down on my application that 1 in 10 night time seizure. The   Equality Act 2010 still gives the employer that liberty to fire someone if there is no disclosure of a disability before appointment to post, if a disability related issue that gets in the way of job performance arises, but how can you expect people to disclose if they know that disclosing will stop them getting a job, where other reasons will be manufactured for not giving you the job.

After losing my job in Nottingham I returned to Glasgow to try and re-enter nurse training, but again the confidence issues caused by the social anxiety disorder rose their head again and I ended up giving up and pulling out of the 'Diploma in Adult Nursing' with nothing after a disastrous placement in the community, where my mentor and her colleague were telling me to get back on the wards to complete my training as they both stood there and ridiculed me over my bandaging, as well as knowledge on surgical procedures. Nurse training in today's world is no longer clinical in nature. In my time in nurse training, which was close to three years, we had never had a lecture on any medical condition. At no time in these close to three years was the word "Epilepsy" ever discussed as the theme of a lecture or a tutorial. The same could be said for all other medical conditions. All we got in three years was a module on human physiology, which taught you Standard Grade/GCSE level human biology, and hospital placement time was spent doing auxillary nursing; and being let home early. Any other coursework was just essay writing on daft subjects such as "The nurse's role in health promotion", and attending tutorials where the boredom made you feel you had done nothing productive with your day whatsoever. If I had asked any final year nursing student to provide me with the information on epilepsy that is at the beginning of this book they would just have stared blankly. I do not know what the nurse training in the year 2018 is like but this was what the nurse training of 2004 was like. I remember my peers in nurse training saying, "My placement is great!. They let you home really early". Some placements had twelve hour shifts and they were letting nursing students go home as early as three hours into the shift. I therefore ask you, to ask that question: "What is epilepsy?" to the next nursing student you come across, and then have a good time quizzing them over all the other medical conditions to get your own back on them on behalf of me!

I was introduced to a man called Sam Whitmore, who was from Epilepsy Connections, just after I left nurse training in 2004 as I was starting to get suicidal ideation for the first time in my life, where I saw death not as something to be scared of and instead saw it as a place away from greed, self-interest, bullying & harassment etc. I remember standing in the Royal Exchange square Starbucks, in Glasgow, looking out the window, standing there with my Dad awaiting my coffee and thinking to myself: It must be great to be away from here. When Grand dad died did he say, "Thank goodness for that". I thought to myself how great it must be to be away from money, war, persecution, stigma etc and to never have to read about it, hear about it or rub shoulders with it ever again. It was because of this thinking that I was meeting with Sam Whitmore to see what opportunities he might have for me. Sam made me aware of an 'Expert Patient programme' that I could do on a voluntary basis, where you teach those with disability symptom management strategies, such as pain control and mental health symptom management. I became a volunteer trainer, and for the next three years I taught these eight week long courses that gave me purpose, greatly enhanced my quality of life and boosted my confidence, because it opened my eyes up to the strengths I had, which was teaching, presenting/public speaking, leadership, life experience etc. During my training to do this voluntary work I was told that I had great presentation skills, articulated myself well and was a good motivator. I was offered a job as a training development officer by a charity called 'Disability Information Greater Glasgow' (DIGG) and was given the opportunity to design my own course which was a self-management programme for young people with disability.

During the first couple of months of working at DIGG, I designed a course that had four sessions on: Working with your healthcare professional, Education, Employment, Dealing with negative emotions. After designing the course, my supervisor wished to meet with me so that the course content could be approved and finalised. Upon meeting my supervisor, with the course content completed, I was told that the course was too negative and needed revamping. When I asked what was negative about it, my supervisor told me it was full of information on anxiety and depression; and that because I teach the Disability Discrimination Act, it would give everyone attending the course the belief that they will experience discrimination. My supervisor said that the course had to be more positive as we did not want a course that would depress people. I responded to this reaction to the course content by saying, "Dianne, are you telling me that I am to design a course that says living with a disability is a great experience"; I said to her, "I will tell those attending what it is like and what they need to know so that they have the life skills and knowledge to be able to take the precautions they need to take to protect their interests". I also said, "I will teach them the mental health strategies for combatting symptoms of anxiety and depression". Dianne said to me, in a really objectionable way, "Do you have this problem in other jobs, Tim?", "I bet you do", "Something tells me this is not the first time this has happened". I just denied any previous problems in the workplace as I did not see them relevant. This brought an end to the confrontation. The next day I got a phone call from the boss who had inherited money to start this charity. He told me that I was to not worry about the attack made by Dianne, and that I was to just go ahead with teaching the course that I had designed. For the remainder of the two years, I did my own networking and taught the course to a number of charities and some local authority area disability/further education services. My boss never enquired about my work, but showed a lot of interest in the others' work, and throughout these two years, my work was never discussed at any of the team meetings; and then towards the end of the two years, I was told that I was not going to have my post funded as well as be out of a job come May 2007, despite the good course evaluations provided by those attending my courses; as well as the charities, local authorities and other organisations who allowed me to teach the course to their clients. To "rub salt into the wound", I opened an e-mail on the same day as learning that my contract was not going to be renewed, and learned that it was from Diane who had correspond copied me into an e-mail to a Disability Employment Advisor down at the jobcentre, saying that DIGG had this employee with epilepsy and a personality disorder who will find it difficult because of these two conditions to find and possibly keep employment. The e-mail said that Diane would be referring this soon to be former employee to the Disability Employment Advisor and it would be appreciated if they could advise on appropriate jobs, working for appropriate understanding employers.

Diane was from a psychology background where she was trained in the era where she would have been educated about the "Epileptic Personality Disorder", where it was believed that our personality traits such as defensiveness, argumentative, angry, rebellious etc, were down to something biological within our brains; when in fact many of today's health professionals are increasingly recognising that this theory of epileptic personality disorder is absolute nonsense, and in fact these personality traits are down to the person with epilepsy living in a society where they have received very right wing treatment from many people, experiencing many traumatic events as a consequence of the world being so right wing. In other words, they have the personality traits that anyone would develop living in such a world.

 I was outraged by this e-mail, but especially outraged by the fact that my boss was not going to reapply for funding when I was the only person working for the charity who actually saw clients and worked with people with disability. The course had been given very good ratings by those attending, especially in both the "Dealing with negative emotions" session, and the "Working with your health professional" session. Many clients attending became aware of how they had been discriminated against without realising it, when I was teaching them about the Disability Discrimination Act. Many clients also shared with me how they had been forced into taking medications against their will by doctors, when teaching the "Working with your healthcare professional" session that covered the 'Patient Rights Act'.

The other two workers, who I shared an office with at DIGG; with all respect, just answered phone calls providing information to people with disability over the phone, which was information those phoning could have got from their citizen advice bureau, and most of the time the information that was being asked for was information neither of the two workers knew as they received no personal development. I felt, and so did others who knew this boss of mine for the reputation that he had, that this charity was being used as a front to access his father's left behind money; that his father had left behind for charitable purposes, and he was putting in minimal investing into the growing and developing of the charity's services. His son loathed him and told me to watch out as his father was a "total bastard". His son had developed problems with alcohol addiction due to the trauma of being raised by this man, who labelled his son learning disabled despite never being diagnosed with such a condition, and it doesn't surprise me at all that the charity is now all boarded up after him bleeding it dry of money. This man just used people with disability who would struggle to get jobs to fill these vacancies to complete the front that he had chosen to set up. This man was a former consultant in public health who had just retired and this I was told was how he was planning on spending his retirement years i.e. living off his father's left behind money. As I was the only employee whose role required the spending of money on resources other than salary his decision to get rid of me, but not the others, was consistent with the widely held belief amongst others that this man wanted the money left behind for charitable purposes for himself, spending as minimal as possible on the front that he had created to access the money. It shows you what kind of bosses you can gravitate into the hands off when you live with a disability and will struggle to get a job. I feel that this was being half way towards being involved in organised crime. It does not surprise you that 1 in 50 people in prison have epilepsy, if people with disability can find themselves being employed by fronts due to poor employment prospects. It doesn't surprise you either that those with my type of epilepsy are thirty two times more likely to commit suicide than the general population due to poor future life prospects and opportunities. One of my bosses was judgemental towards me, and the boss of bosses only prevented this judgementalism from causing me to lose my job, as he at the time needed me to fulfil all requirements to access his father's money, where one of the criteria for accessing his father's money was probably to employ a certain number of people with a disability, as when I left the charity I was replaced by another disabled young man who was filling a new post that was office bound where he was seeing no clients.

CHAPTER 15

I had no job, when I left the job that I had as training officer for Disability Information Greater Glasgow, and ended up going into social work training at Glasgow Caledonian University in 2008. This course was a post graduate course. It was one year in duration, and it was part university and placement based. I started a placement in 'Adult and Elderly Services' at Glasgow City Council, where for the first couple of weeks I got on very well with my mentor, whose name was Douglas Gray. We had great conversation, we got on like a house on fire, we had a great number of shared jokes and I informed him of my reasons as to why I wished to be a social worker. He told me that I had made a wise decision and that I would not regret it. I thought to myself, "what a great guy". I thought to myself, "Why couldn't the nursing mentors have been as good as the social work team". I didn't just get on with my mentor but I got on with other staff in the office as well. There was a carry- on kind of guy that had you in stitches, that I also thought highly off.

 It was on the Thursday of the second week of being on placement that I was out with Douglas Gray, driving from one client's home to another; and he asked me what made me wish to become a social worker after doing a degree in molecular biology as he was driving. I told my mentor that I had grown up living with disadvantage all my life and that I had used statutory services all my life, as I had lived with epilepsy since childhood and that making it to where I was had been a nightmare for me despite being seizure free during awake hours since 1998. I told my mentor that society had disabled me more than epilepsy had. I went on to say that there are many societal ills that people with disability find themselves up against and that I wished to pursue a career helping people overcome these societal ills. I continued by saying that I could not think of any better career than social work for someone wishing to help those with disability overcome many of the societal ills. I said that social work was both community as well as meeting unmet needs of others and therefore it was a great career for anyone with a self-empowerment ethos.

On the Friday of the second week of this great placement my mentor asked me if I wanted to do a day down at one of the other social work offices in the local area. I said, "yes" to this and he gave me the phone number of the office to arrange to go down there for a day. It was a Friday afternoon and I phoned the other office, which was an elderly social work office. A lady answered the phone and said they would be pleased to have me for the day, and that I was more than welcome. I was given instructions to pass on to my mentor when I was on the phone to the other office arranging this   visit. These instructions were for me to be there for a certain time on a certain day. I informed my mentor of these arrangements, and my mentor on the day of the arranged visit said after my arrival at work, "Come on, let's take you down to the other Shettleston Office" as he picked up his coat and briefcase and said, "My colleague will be coming down with us as well". This other person, whose name I can't remember, was really comical in the car while I was being driven down to the other office. When we got to the other office my mentor did a kerb side park. My mentor said, "There you go" and I got out the car. My mentor then said to me, while I was standing on the kerbside with the door open and he sitting in his driving seat, "We will see you later on back at the office, after you have spent the day at this office and you can tell us how you got on". I replied by saying, "Thanks for the lift and will see you back at the office" shutting the car door. I walked up the path to the office and looked over my shoulder and saw a side-on view of my mentor pull away, where he looked tense and anxious as he put his car into first gear and drove off like a criminal trying to get out of the area as fast as he possibly could. I will never forget his body language, and the way the car just drove off like a car wanting to get out of the vincinity as soon as possible, and without delay. I thought, "Strange" and walked up the path to the office door and rang the bell. The person who answered   the door said, "Hello, can I help you?". I said that I was Tim Bone the social work student who had been invited to come down today to work at this office. I was told that they had no record of this. They said, "Sorry what's your name?". I answered, and they said, "Come in". I entered the office and made the lady aware of the phone call that I had given on the Friday of the previous week when it had been arranged for me to work from this office on this day. The lady said that she had no record of this phone call that was made. The lady who had let me in was now on the phone to my mentor enquiring as to why a student social worker had arrived on their door step claiming that it had been arranged with himself over the phone for him to come down today and spend the day in their office. The lady who had let me in was now on the phone enquiring as to why a student social worker had arrived on their door step claiming that it had been arranged with himself over the phone for him to come down today and spend the day in their office. My mentor had said over the phone that he was no wiser than her and that he had only been acting under the instructions that I had given him. The office I was standing in denied ever receiving a phone call from me and passing instructions onto me, for me to pass on to my mentor. I was collected and brought back to the office. Upon our return to the office I sat at my desk which was in another room to my mentor's desk. After about ten minutes my mentor said, "Tim, could you just come into my office for now". I went into his room where he sat down behind his desk and I was encouraged to pull up a seat and sit down at the opposite side of the desk in this grey walled dark office with the dark grey sky outside. When we were both seated, he sat there leaning on his left forearm with his hands clasped together with his left shoulder slightly higher than his right and he asked me in a very nervous unconvincing manner if I had a fear of the telephone. He went on to further say that I need not worry if I did have such a fear as he knew many people who had a terrible fear of the telephone. My mentor then said that he very often heard me say 'Excuse Me' when I was on the phone and someone answered. I replied by saying that I did not have any phobia about using the telephone. I informed him that I used the telephone when doing voluntary work at Epilepsy Scotland back in 1993, had been using the phone as part of my job as a support worker at Thelmer Turner Homes in Nottingham in 2003 as well as Fair Deal in Glasgow in 2004, and had spent two years in a job as both a disability information provider and symptom management trainer; where I was answering and making calls every day, and that my use of the words "Excuse Me" were just being used as a figure of speech whenever someone picked up the phone at the other end. He then responded to this by saying that there may be difficulties in allowing me to see clients. I told him that he didn't express any concerns about my suitability to be a social worker the first week I started my placement right up to asking me on the Friday of week two to phone the other office as he felt it important for me to see the other client groups I might find myself working with when I qualified. I told him that right up to this morning there had been no instances where he had expressed doubt in my suitability nor had anything happened that would give one reason to think I was not suitable. I asked him if this set up over the appointment, the accusation of being paranoid with using the phone and then expressing that there will be difficulties allowing me to work with clients had anything to do with the fact that I had disclosed to him that I had epilepsy when giving him my reasons for going into social work the previous week. My mentor responded to me asking him these questions by saying, "Wait Here!". My mentor stood up, walked out the office, was gone for about five minutes, came back into the office with his boss; and his boss stared at me and told my mentor to give me my jacket and get me out of the office. My mentor picked up my jacket, gave it to me, and then ushered me out of the office; walking up behind me with his arm outstretched, forcing me to keep walking or get trampled over, just like a doorman in a nightclub throwing out a drunk customer before things get physical; as I walked ahead of him towards the office door, down the staircase, through the reception office, out into the foyer and door slammed shut behind me. It was done in the most dismissive way with no explanation given. I will never forget how he just did a u-turn at the door of the reception office while closing it, walking away back towards his office, displaying a body language that told you he no longer had any reason to feel any concern, and that he could now get on with the rest of his life as though it was business as usual for him from this moment onwards, and that I had become a memory in his mind that had less presence than a memory of twenty years ago. I was left standing outside of the social work office having learned one thing from my time on that placement and that was that I was no longer a social work student. To this day I was never given a formal explanation as to why I was put off the social work course. It did turn out that when I researched the mentor's background he was in fact not a qualified social worker, and was instead a mental health nurse who I have no doubt held a judgemental view towards those with epilepsy. It is also interesting that there was a lady who worked in the office that also had epilepsy and did not see clients, that I had been introduced to the week before this incident. I had not yet disclosed at this time my epilepsy to my mentor or other social work team member, however, the university knew about it, and I wonder if there had been a prior arrangement between university staff and mentoring staff to play this stunt before I had started placement; and that this lady being in the office was their way in trying to look both anti-discriminative as well as convince me that people with epilepsy not being allowed to see clients was a legitimate city council policy so I would be put off taking any legal action as well as convincing me that it would be my word against theirs since there was already someone else in the office with epilepsy denied the right to see clients. It was an attempt to say they had been here before with someone else and won, so they will most likely win again. It did come out when my father went to the university to speak to the course organiser, Tim Kelly, that my mentor had mentioned that I had paranoid delusions and that there was nothing the university could do to help. My father came back from the meeting he had with Tim Kelly with a copy of the letter sent to the university from the Shettleston office, with it saying that they were cancelling my placement as they believed me to suffer from paranoid delusions. This event that occurred on this social work placement, happened in March of 2008, and I have had to live without closure to this date; which before me taking up consistent meditation practice, contributed towards me having to live with anger and rage; contributing towards the development of my major depressive disorder. The anger and rage made me feel I could not cope, which brought on night time anxiety and suicidal ideation. One thing that eventually allowed me to cope, and I mean helped me cope a lot, up until moving away to Chalfont St Peter in October 2009, was telling myself that I would wait a few years until I was forgotten about and that I would in ten years' time, turn up on Douglas Gray's door step and say, "Do you remember me?". I would say, "Did you think you would treat me like that and get away with it?" and murder him on his doorstep, attaching a label to his body that would have something like "Child Abuser" written on it, that would be a label that would go with him to his grave; and have others talk about him in their gossip long after he was gone. I told myself that I would have him remembered as a child abuser and that two people could play this game of false accusations that he had just irreversibly begun. I was so grateful that there was such a thing as "the other side of the law!". I was also grateful that there were manufacturers of firearms. Revenge is a "dish best served cold!!!!!"

I moved to Chalfont St Peter to work at the Epilepsy Society in 2009, and between October 2009-March 2012 my mental health symptoms improved dramatically, as I was in another part of the country which acted as a distraction in itself from all the grief in recent years I had been through back home in Glasgow. The polish, Lithuanians, other eastern Europeans and Africans are far friendlier tolerant people to work with. During my time working with non-British staff, which was a little under two years, my life was discrimination free and I got on with everyone until my job moved into a different residential unit in June 2011 which was full of British staff. British culture is very unfriendly.

After my return to Glasgow in July 2012, having lived in Slough between the years 2009-2012, I had a relapse in depressive symptoms including symptoms of rage, hatred, feelings of misanthropy flowing through me as well as suicidal ideation as a consequence of memories of how bad the experiences in Glasgow had been with nurse training and Social Work, and I was back to wanting to murder that "Social Worker" on his doorstep, thinking to myself, "Only six more years to go"; but I started meditating in Sept 2014, and since September 2017 I am now a consistent morning and night meditator which has resolved the anger and rage, defusing within me any need to murder anyone on their doorstep, but I believe without my meditation practice I would have murdered this man and I don't think I would have waited the remaining six years. I doubt, I would have been a suspect, due to the amount of time that would have elapsed, but I, none the less, could have still ended up in prison doing a life sentence, where I would have done the full 25 years for killing a social worker, if there were to have been any witnesses or glimpses of me on CCTV. I would say that authority makes criminals of people by behaving criminally themselves; and the way people in positions of authority have treated myself is evidence that there are people in caring roles who do not have criminal records nor any tainting on their character in any way, when you screen them through criminal disclosure Scotland; who should not be trusted to be working with vulnerable adults, and are probably more dangerous to be working with vulnerable adults than people who are serving prison sentences at this present moment in time. Who is the worst person?: The social worker who sets his student up to make him look like he is too cognitively disadvantaged to be a social worker as a consequence of having a neurological disability, therefore has him put off the course by making false accusations of suffering from paranoid delusions; or a son who ends up in prison as a consequence of being witnessed punching a man, who had earlier on assaulted his elderly mother unwitnessed? Criminal Disclosure is a farce, and is as good at weeding out the untrustworthy from trusting roles as sitting down and having a bowl of cornflakes does!. They should just empty the prisons and allow us to live in an 'every man for himself' society, but keep the cells for the sex offenders. Having been a student with epilepsy and social anxiety disorder on health and social care courses as well as an employee in health and social care roles, I have seen so much law breaking by supposedly "honest", "law abiding", "honourable" people who are forever breaching the human rights act.

It is now October 2019 at time of editing this chapter and I can say that two years of consistent morning and night meditation has allowed me to focus on the present with the aim of giving myself the best future I deserve, thus allowing me to let go of the lack of closure caused by what happened in 2008 at the Glasgow City Council Shettleston social work office. It is the case though that between 2008 and a few months ago I have been told so many times by people in positions of authority that I am an angry, aggressive person and using it against me to their advantage. I look at social workers, police officers, council tax people, housing officers, DWP, DVLA etc and think "One half of you make me angry and fill me with rage, and then the other half of you persecute and penalise me for being angry and full of rage!". I see a police car, child protection social worker, a discriminatory boss etc and I think, "You criminalise us, then you slam us up for being criminal". The judicial service is a "clueless dog chasing its own tail".

CHAPTER 16

As already mentioned, in 2009 I moved to the Epilepsy Society in Chalfont St Peter to become a residential support worker. As my epilepsy was controlled when awake, and my job did not require me to do sleep overs as they brought in agency staff to do that, there were no Occupational Health issues, and I started work that October. During the three years that I was at the Epilepsy Society, I worked in a challenging behaviour unit where those living within had a number of different seizure types as well as profound learning disability. I worked in this unit for two years. This was good. There were no issues, I met a partner and we moved in together in Slough. During these three years I did live with depression but I could control the symptoms with two fifteen hundred calorie workouts in the gym per week, enabling me to fully function. As I was approaching two years of working in the residential unit, I started to suffer from burnout, and was beginning to have an increased seizure frequency of one every three nights. The reasons for this burnout was because the care I was providing was so institutional, and all the days were "carbon copies" of the previous days. The residents in the home just sat on the couch watching television programmes such as 'BBC News 24' which was of no relevance to them. The residents couldn't have told you who the prime minister was for Christ's sake. Not that they weren't capable of knowing who the prime minister was, but more because they couldn't care less, as to people like them who live in a society that has been allowed to forget about them by caging them up in residential units and throwing the key away, it is of no relevance to people like themselves whether a right wing government or left wing government is in power. I can say as someone with the same disability as they, that judging by the reception I and they have had from society, in response to our disability; all western societies, whether its May or Coburn voters, or Obama or Trump voters, are right wing when it comes to other peoples' human rights. The only argument the left are interested in, is the argument concerning financial inequality; however, you never hear the left concern themselves with the inequality in human rights in the context of disability, and when you do hear them concern themselves over other inequality it is almost always in the context of gender inequality. There is some attention given to racial and sexuality discrimination; which are areas of discrimination where people get beaten up, set on fire and murdered, but this attention is given to a much lesser extent than gender discrimination. I have to be honest with the reader and say that you get all these feminists on the news who say women are discriminated against as they are on £25,000 pa, but men are on £30,000 pa; or women are discriminated against as there are not as many women in science, engineering and technology as men, but I cannot take that seriously as being discrimination, having had the experiences that I have had, and others like me have had, as a consequence of having a disability. There are people with first degree burns out there because of racial or sexuality discrimination for heaven's sake. In the context of gender discrimination, you have an example such as women being on £25,000 pa and men on £30,000 pa, but in the context of disability you have someone being wrongfully accused of challenging behaviour by social work, so that they have an argument for putting that person in residential care, so that the house that person lives in can be given to a family of three; as the person with the disability is not seen as being a good investment due to their inability to work and inability to make an economical contribution towards society, but the family of three could have two people in the same house who do work and are both making an economical contribution towards society. People such as social work will effectively imprison someone for the rest of their lives in residential care because they have a disability and are seen as being a drain on the shortage in housing due to their disability requiring a house with more than one bedroom to store equipment such as hoists and wheelchairs. This example of disability discrimination is on a completely different level to the example of gender discrimination mentioned, and those in such positions like social work who would do such a thing to a person in a housing association home with a disability, would describe their politics as being left wing.

Another example of disability discrimination would be someone with a disability working in a company where they hold high position, but have to be off work every Wednesday afternoon to attend a hospital clinic. As a consequence of this, something at work is reported as "stolen" and this "stolen item" is then found in this person's desk and they get fired. As a consequence of their age they cannot get another job and are living on Job Seekers Allowance for the long term where their job has become filling in job application forms, but not getting interviews. This scenario has started off as disability discrimination and has now evolved into age discrimination. This does put the complaints of women only being on £25,000 when men are on £30,000, as being a case of discrimination into perspective. To me it sounds like spoilt jealous school children bitching about one another over their toys. It is "discrimination very light weight" and it gets a disproportionately greater amount of attention than the "discrimination heavy weight", where people are set on fire because of the colour of their skin. All I can say is "COULD WE PLEASE WAKEN UP AS A SOCIETY AND ADDRESS THE BIG ISSUES AND STOP GIVING DISPROPORTIONATE AMOUNTS OF COMMITMENT TO THE SMALL ISSUES". This giving disproportionate amounts of time to the smaller discrimination issues is done purely for the sake of winning votes as well as acting as a distraction from the obligation to address the big discrimination issues. I am sure that there have been many feminist women who have developed disabilities and experienced discrimination such as losing a job, being prosecuted, losing a house, being expelled from a university course, neglected by family and friends etc because of their disability and have thought to themselves "and I thought I was getting a really bad deal being a non-disabled women!!" I do agree though that there are women who get bullied and harassed in jobs due to their gender, therefore it would be wrong to say that gender discrimination is without its big issues, but the ratio of big issues: small issues; is much smaller in gender discrimination than it is in disability discrimination, evidenced by what I watch on the television, read in the newspapers, come across on websites as well as evidenced by my years of running an advocacy charity for people with neurological disability.

During my time of being a support worker in the residential unit that I worked in for just under two years, our manager used to say to us all on a regular basis at team meetings, if we could just try and look busy for the benefit of the institution looking like it did things with its clients, so if there were a visit from the care inspectorate or relatives came round they would believe the residents to be in receipt of good quality care. The residents became very frustrated and there were temper tantrums on the unit. I on a frequent basis got punched by the client I was the keyworker of and had plates of food thrown at me by a resident who was my key client's rival on the unit who saw me as some kind of ally of my key client. For two years I put up with this and I never once lay a finger on a client in retaliation. The only thing I ever practiced was restraint which discredited the claims made by previous people that I had some kind of problem with rage and anger that made me dangerous. I am a person who if you treat me well, I will treat you well. My motto is: "Speak to, and treat others; the way you wish to be treated and spoken to yourself".

I could make an exception for the client's disrespectful behaviour, as it was part of their learning disability; as well as the frustration of living with no quality of life. Clients were just pumped up to the eyeballs on anti-convulsants and sedatives. It was no surprise their seizures were poorly controlled considering my night time seizures started to increase to two per week, from one every ten days. I used to waken up in the morning before my 7am shift with a mental nausea, where you don't feel you are going to be sick; but instead feel you are going to collapse with low motivation, no interest in anything at present, with nothing to look forward to in the future. It feels like you are just going round in purposeless circles, where you are in exactly the same place today, as you were this time yesterday, and that you will be in exactly the same place, at the same time tomorrow. The only difference you feel is that the circle of repeated routine has a narrower diameter each time you circulate it, thus restricting your breathing space and making you feel that your mental corner is getting tighter and tighter as you become closer and closer to mental breakdown. Life becomes a chore. It feels like you are waiting for a bus, and you have been waiting and waiting and waiting, but the problem is there is no bus coming because you are not waiting for a bus. That "Come on when is the train arriving!" feeling, but there is no train. There is no clock to look at and say, "five more minutes" as there is no train coming, because you are not waiting for a train, you are just feeling like you are indefinitely waiting for nothing; bringing on feelings of panic as there is nothing to bring your wait to an end. I had to be signed off sick. I am so surprised my day time seizures never came back, and the irony is I have to thank so much my neurologist, whose name was Professor John Duncan, for putting me on that drug combination back in 1998 that rid my life of day time attacks; who had worked at the very centre that was giving me my burnout. If I had been having daytime attacks on top of all the chaos created for me by others, since leaving Glasgow University back in 1997, that would have just been dynamite, but then if I had been having daytime attacks as well as performance anxiety; I would have just been kicked out into the street after university and given no opportunities whatsoever, and either be dead or in prison.

As a consequence of the burnout, I asked if I could be moved to another unit on the campus and work with another client group where there might have been more variety. I was put in a unit which was just like the unit I had come from, but the only difference; which is quite a big difference, is that it was not challenging behaviour. Despite this however it was still repetitive and I just continued to experience burnout. As there was no challenging behaviour the job was less challenging and just accelerated the rate of burnout. I had jumped from the frying pan and into the fire. I managed to last a year in this unit before instead of burnout ousting me out of the job it was instead discrimination, but not of the disability kind, but now the gender kind. To administer medication, you had to be drug trained, which required to be shown how to do the drug round and then required you to have a supervised drug round. The manageress of the home, had all the drug trained staffs' names in the staff rotas highlighted; and they were all women. The manageress never drug trained any of the men, and the reason for this was because to get promotion at the centre you had to be drug trained; and it was her way in keeping all male staff at the bottom of the staff hierarchy.

Residents with very poorly controlled epilepsy had two types of medication. They had their usual routine anti-convulsant medication, and what was called 'Protocol Medication', which they were put on when their routine medication had been ineffective and they had had a really bad spell of seizures. There is something called 'Status Epilepticus', which is where a person goes from one seizure into another without regaining consciousness. This is a very dangerous state for a person to be in and it can cause death. During status epilepticus, emergency medication is administered; and after recovery, they are put on protocol medication. When a client is on protocol, they have a sticker on their locker saying "On Protocol" for the next shift doing the drug round. A client can also be on protocol without there having been status epilepticus, when they have had a bad spell of seizures.

When I was doing my drug training, my trainer said, "Let's go into John's room and do his medication". In we went and I got the drug Kardex out, read out the drugs he should be given, put the anti-convulsants into a pot and gave them to John. The lady from training said, "Well done" and signed the little box where I had put my initials. Later on, that afternoon; a member of female staff came in to the lounge where myself and clients were sitting and said, "Tim, did you do this morning's medication round?" I told her that this was the case, emphasising that it was a supervised drug round. This member of staff just dismissed that it was a supervised round and said, "So, you would have given John his medication". This woman was standing there with her hands in her denim jean pockets with a big grin on her face looking so smug. I said, "Yes, that would be the case". This was followed by the female member of staff asking, "Did you give John his protocol today?" and I said, "No, he's on usual routine medication"; and she said, "Well he's not. You did not notice the protocol sticker on his locker". I said, "That protocol sticker was not there when I administered the drugs". I said that the drug trainer had been in the room with me supervising me. There was no recognition of this fact. I was accused of endangering life and that I was not fit to be administering anti-convulsants. I was full of pent up rage when I got home. They had deliberately put a sticker on John's drug locker after I left his room to stitch me up. This injustice on top of all the other injustices I had to put up with over the years had nearly pushed me over the edge. My partner was away that weekend and I had no one to share this experience with. I woke up that night in a fit of rage. I started to have a panic attack as I did not feel I could go back into work, and work with either one of these women. These women being the sexist manageress as well as the member of staff who chose to be a part of the setup. I thought that I would murder that member of staff who came in with that snearing grin, enjoying telling me that I had endangered life. I was teaching the Expert Patient Programme in Slough at the time, just like I had done in Glasgow, and I remembered giving a lesson on 'Meditation'. I thought it was now time to practice what I preached. I looked up meditation on the internet that night in the dark on my mobile phone and learned about its therapeutic effects for anger and rage. I went into the toilet and sat there for 20 minutes just relaxing my body, getting rid of all muscle tension, I slowly breathed through my nose focussing on the speed, sensation and depth of my inhalation and focussed on the same things during the exhalation, clearing my mind and just letting the thoughts about what happened flow through my mind as opposed to engaging with them. I did this for twenty minutes morning and night so that I had had six meditation sessions by the time I got back to work on Monday, where I came across this manageress and felt no rage nor anger, and was instead calm and enjoyed smiling and saying good morning to her. The meditation had saved me. It stopped me from losing my job and possibly ending up in trouble with the law, as I was experiencing virtual breakdown when I came back home on the Friday evening. Meditation is certainly a practice that I would recommend to anyone who has experienced a serious injustice that causes an acute amount of rage that is too overwhelming to cope with. Meditation could be used to save a marriage, or like in my case; a job, and treat a huge number of other emotional ailments that get in the way of someone being able to function in any setting such as work, family, social, educational etc. I once read a Lee Child fictional novel, where a man who had worked for an oil company all of his life had just suddenly been made redundant. This man felt so betrayed by his company, considering he had put a lifetime's work into the company, and went on a massive arson attack. I thought to myself "This man should have meditated to defuse that rage". Meditation would defuse a rage of that magnitude.

A few shifts after returning to work, after that weekend of defusing my rage, the manageress of the house did take me aside after the night shift had handed over to the early shift that I was on. I was told that she would like to see me at lunch in private in her office with no explanation given. I was so anxious about this and had to put in a full morning's work thinking to myself what on earth was this woman was up to now. I knew from her body language and her facial expressions that this was not good news and that this was possibly round two of chasing me off site for good. This was to be another social work training experience. It was to possibly be another major injustice to have to live without closure on. When I visited the manager in private in her office at lunch time, I was told by her that she felt that I had issues with concentration as well as memory, and that I was to go on medical leave while occupational health questioned my fitness to continue working as a support worker. I could not believe it. It was social work 2008 all over again, in the year 2012. I went home and sat around my flat for a few days continuing to meditate morning and night to cope with the anxiety, rage and depression that I was experiencing because of my experience with the world and with people. I remember my old university friend Alan saying to me back in 2009 in a pub when he was up in Glasgow visiting his mother, "What do you want friends for? People are complete Shits". He was right as far as my experience of the world was evidencing people to be like. This attempted injustice happened at a time when British history only has to look back two years to remember a taxi driver in Cumbria who shot dead twelve civilians when he went on a rampage in his taxi shooting people dead while hanging out the driver seat of his car. He even loaded a gun, got out of his taxi and put a bullet in the back of an old lady's head. The newspaper had reported that before the rampage he had had an argument with his brother over a will that his ill mother was leaving behind. It turns out that he shot dead his brother as well. My experiences with people and family were certainly giving me an insight into how someone could develop a loathing for people, and become judgemental towards people, believing that they are all the same, and feel a strong appetite to randomly taking peoples' lives. I don't know what happened here but from my own life experience I could certainly paint a scenario that should leave people open minded when these things happen. It is too easy to say, "Head case, should have been locked up. What a low life for going around killing innocent people. Well if there's a god he will have gone to hell". I am afraid to say that from my experiences that is the opinion and conclusion that the vast majority of people would make without being able to evidence it. My attitude is, yes, that conclusion drawn by the majority could be the case, but it could also be the case that this man suffered from depression as a consequence of low morale and self- esteem caused by being overworked, low paid and having to deal with abusive, aggressive drunk people who he had probably had to take years of insults from, sitting in the back of his car; possibly had even been threatened and attacked on a good number of occasions as well as become very disillusioned with the world and its people. This is especially the case if he was a principled man and felt a loathing towards humanity, as he felt he lived in a world surrounded by double standards and cowardly as well as selfish behaviour. This depression probably got in the way of his relationship with his family members. They probably misinterpreted his depressive symptoms as being aggressive, anti-social as well as awkward; which led to him having ill feelings towards family as a consequence of them being unsupportive and unempathetic, leading to a good number of years of being excluded by the family, resulting in him being excluded in the will or the will leaving him something which when compared with what the others were being left, certainly had his mother spell out "I only leave you something on principle". This was probably as much as he could take from the bad experience with the human race that he had had to endure for a number of years, resulting in his hatred for people becoming too great to handle, resulting in a mass killing spree. All I can say is that if it had not been for my meditation, I could have very possibly gone that way. This potential injustice, on top of years of abuse as well as previous injustices, would have been too much for me to take, and my hatred towards humanity would have become too great, possibly resulting in such a behavioural response from myself. I was thinking, if it were not for my meditation practice I would be probably getting sectioned under the Mental Health Act, where a psychiatrist would be saying that my aggression, anti-social misanthropic attitude and views were down to me having a personality disorder, and that this made me a risk to the health and safety of myself as well as others. Under section 22 of the Mental Health Act, I could have been given a 'Compulsory Treatment Order', which could have involved me being sectioned as I certainly would have been an uncooperative patient looking for the opportunity to carry out mass destruction.

When I eventually got a phone call occupational health appointment, that the manageress at the residential unit at the epilepsy society had arranged, the doctor asked me questions testing my memory and concentration and concluded the assessment by saying to me, "I think it's time to get you back to work". When I got back to work I decided to hand in my notice as I was never going to rise within the organisation due to the medication training and with the previous injustices that I had experienced I knew this was an attempt to constructively dismiss me as they could not legitimise failing me on my administering routine medication training and at the same time the training department keep using me as a rescue medication trainer of other support staff i.e. buccal midazolam and rectal diazepam, due to my previous experience of being employed by Epilepsy Scotland to train support staff to administer rescue medication on the West Coast of Scotland. I feared that they would probably find something else to use against me to fulfil their goal of constructive dismissal and then be accused of having paranoid personality disorder co-existing with temporal lobe epilepsy when legally challenging the decision to dismiss me. I worried what the next thing would be. Would they next accuse me of doing something of a sexual nature. The problem with learning disability is that those with it are very easily exploited by others into saying things and doing things, and I did not put it past the feminist staff from manipulating a client into saying that I touched them inappropriately while washing them. It could also be the case that the manageress had decided to make me paranoid by referring me to occupational health with the intention of putting these fears into me on my return to the workplace that would cause me to hand in my notice. Well if that was her intention then it would be fair to say that it had worked.

CHAPTER 17

On my return to Glasgow in July 2012, I worked for a support work agency, where I got a role working in the Mirren Centre in Paisley, which was a day centre for those with moderate to severe learning disability. The female staff did not like how much a female client saw me as her favourite support worker, and that I had been told previous to this dislike that there had been a number of male staff in that work place who had had others make sexual allegations against them and were currently under investigation. I was told that I was filling in for a male support worker who had been suspended from practice whilst he was at the centre of an investigation concerning sexual allegations. It's a real danger being a man in the United Kingdom today. It was through fear of such an allegation being made against me at the Epilepsy Society that I decided to leave and move back to Glasgow with my partner, as I had no idea what stunt these women would play next as a result of not being successful in their accusations of me being too cognitively impaired to be a support worker.

After four months of being at the Mirren Centre, somebody high up in Renfrewshire Learning Disability Services came to the centre; and after taking me aside into another room, said that there had been concerns over how close a down's syndrome girl called Jennifer was becoming to me. This woman took me aside after witnessing Jennifer pull me up out of a seat and start dancing with me at a Friday dance session by asking me to come into a room. Upon entering the office of the community centre the door was shut and I sat with this member of staff who said she had great concerns about this down's syndrome girl always wanting to dance with me and that I was to watch it as it could raise suspicions of sexual interest. I couldn't believe this. I felt very vulnerable and decided to have no contact with this client which disappointed her. A few nights later I had a seizure in my bedroom in the middle of the night which I have no memory of at all. This is the seizure where I walked into the bathroom in the morning and found blood all over my face when I looked in the mirror and then found my wall mirror behind the door of my bedroom shattered into many medium to large pieces.

When I went to work at another community centre, managed by the same council as the previous community centre, the manager noticed the wound to my head above my right temple sustained during the seizure that involved the smashed mirror in my bedroom which has left a scar. This seizure happened a couple of days after being assaulted by a client at the Mirren centre who gave me a blow to the head with a billiard ball in response to me telling him to put away the billiard table. This was the reason for being moved to another community centre to cover shifts. This was a client who once dropped his change when buying a CD in a music shop. When told by me that he had dropped his change which involved me tapping his arm to get his attention, he turned round and pointed at me leaning his face into my face and said, "Don't you ever tap me again!!". There are some people with learning disability who you think, "Maybe they got it wrong with this guy and that he should be in residential care and not living in the community". The country is in denial. Everyone is going to get a degree and have a graduate job! Every person is fit enough to be living in the community! What a load of politically correct garbage and it has the potential to cost lives.

The manager of the community centre that I was now working in asked me how I got the injury to my head, and I told him that I woke up one morning to the sight of my face that I saw in the mirror, the discovery of my mirror smashed all over the floor and I therefore must have had a seizure . You hope they ask as you worry they think you've been in a fight. After telling this manager how I sustained the injury, I never had another shift allocated to me by the agency ever again, to work at this community centre or work anywhere else in residential as well as community care services. As well as that, I also at the time was doing a zero- hour contract for an organisation that rehabilitated ex-young offenders living in the community. When I informed the boss there about how I got the injury I was again never given a shift. This is where the Equality Act 2010 section on employment is completely inadequate. Any agency or zero- hour contract employer can get around it. Any other employer can set you up to do something or appear to have done something that "legitimises" sacking you. In other words, all the Equality Act has done is given employers an incentive for going down the road of constructive dismissal. Making discrimination illegal has only made the experience of discrimination harder to live with, as you see those who get away with it as getting away with a crime, making the injustice even greater. If society is going to have a law then society has to use it.

The care agency that I had worked for knew that I had seizures upon awakening and that they were complex partial seizures. The problem with those who have a knowledge of epilepsy is that their knowledge is very textbook in nature, and if you were to define complex partial seizures in words as they would understand it as being, the definition would be something along the lines of " complex partial seizures do not involve injury as person does not fall over and bang their head off hard objects. Subject will stray, remain standing, go from standing to sitting or will crouch their way to the floor". This is the case when you are only taking into account the biological nature of the condition, but it is not the case when you take into account the nature of the environment in which the seizure takes place. You may not bash your head during a complex partial seizure due to collapsing but you could bash your head through tripping over an environmental hazard such as shoes, missing a step in the dark, being up a ladder, driving a car, falling from a height due to losing your balance for the same reasons anyone else may lose their balance e.g. alcohol intoxication, simple human error etc as could have been the case with myself with the balcony incident in the holiday resort of Rhodes.   Head injury could also occur in the form of being assaulted by someone during the seizure or depending on what country you live in; head injury could result from rough treatment by the police. Not only could you sustain a head injury during a complex partial seizure, but the incidents that can give rise to head injury can also give rise to a multiple number of temporary as well as permanent injuries such as fractures, dislocations, back injuries, paralysis, other spinal injury, scarring/scalding from burns and other trauma etc. When I took a client with complex partial seizures to a café in slough, he picked up his mug in mid conversation and poured the coffee over his head. This is how susceptible you are to burns if for example you were sieving pasta at your kitchen sink or you had a hot kettle in your hand.

As most people in health and social care only have a text book knowledge of epilepsy; when the care agency were informed about the incident in my bedroom by the community centre manager, as well as the incident that had happened in the previous community centre involving the client with the billiard ball; it was immediately assumed that the assault had caused an injury in me that had caused me to develop a different seizure type, and that I now had either developed tonic-clonic epilepsy or I now had an epilepsy that started off as complex partial seizures that evolved into what are called secondary generalised tonic-clonic seizures, that are tonic clonic seizures that begin as complex partial seizures. The secondary generalised tonic-clonic seizures start off affecting only the temporal lobes and then the electrical disturbance in brain activity spreads from the temporal lobes throughout the whole brain. Since my very earliest memories of having a seizure forty years ago I have never had a secondary generalised tonic-clonic seizure, but I did once waken up with a bad friction burn on my forehead one morning that I cannot explain, and have wondered if the friction burn had been sustained from another seizure type that caused my head to rub against the head board of my bed which is made of vertical bars. I have also woken up in the morning on maybe three or four occasions where my bed room lamp, alarm clock, bedside table and all other things that I put on my bedside table have been found to be lying all over my bedroom floor to the right of my bed, where I have no memory of the bed side table going over in the middle of the night, nor do I have any memory of any noise being made by the items spilling off its surface. I don't think these were secondary generalised seizures as there was no next day post-ictal symptoms such as exhaustion and headache which would usually be present after a night time generalised seizure, but I do believe that they may have been epilepsy related. How can you have no memory of getting a friction burn as well as no memory of your bedside table with all its contents going over in the middle of the night?

As it was most likely believed that my seizures had worsened in nature, as a result of me coming round a few mornings after the assault with heavy bleeding from the right temple after a seizure; there were probably fears that I would now be having seizures during the day, and it was for this reason that neither the council that ran the community centres, nor the agency, wished to have me on their books resulting in them making a point of never giving me another shift. As well as never getting another shift with the agency, I also heard nothing more about the post that the council had previously wanted me to apply for. I don't believe that the assault was a reason for not hearing back from the council about the job, nor being given another shift again, as I had worked at the community centre for six months with no history of not getting on with clients, and if they wanted rid of me over the assault then they wouldn't have moved me to another community centre since they were at liberty to just tell the agency they no longer wished me to work for them if faith in me had been destroyed by the assault. If the workers who work in both healthcare and social care roles got an epilepsy in the real world training, then they would know that it is possible to have a complex partial seizure and come round from it with sustained injury, thus preventing them from jumping to their medically inaccurate conclusions on my epilepsy worsening to another seizure type.

I shared with a friend called Frazer all the recent experiences that had happened at the community centre; as well as at the rehabilitation of young offenders establishment. I had met Fraser at an 'Epilepsy Scotland' support group back in 2009 just after the discriminative experience I had had on the social work course. Fraser responded to what I had shared with him by saying to me, "Tim, Get out of that kind of work. These people are the biggest discriminators of all the discriminators". If I were to write a character reference on social workers, support work organisations, social care/health care educators, disability charity workers etc I would have to say they are discriminators or they sit back and allow the discrimination to take place. If these people, in these roles, do not like my analysis of them, then all I can say is that I am allowed my analysis as that is my experience, and I welcome them to find someone with my issues to counter my reference of them. Everything I say about those who play these roles, both in the statutory as well as voluntary sector, can be evidenced by experiences that I have been on the receiving end of. As has already been commented upon, you may as well get rid of the criminal disclosure Scotland system as far as I am concerned, because the system is just full of criminals anyway. These people have constantly demonstrated themselves not to be fit to be an employer, colleague or an educator of a vulnerable person, therefore they are certainly not fit to be the carers of, or play a caring role in the lives of vulnerable people, and I say this as someone who ran an advocacy charity, where one of my clients was forced on a regular basis to lie on the ground in her lounge experiencing incontinence as a result of her husband not being in to carry her up the stairs to the toilet, after the local council refused to install a chairlift into her home. This lying on the floor incontinent of both urine and faeces as a result of not being able to get to the toilet from the lounge when her husband was not at home, had been going on for months before my advocacy charity intervened. Such treatment of someone is criminal and is worthy of prosecution.

CHAPTER 18

I decided after the seizure that resulted in injury to face, that I was going to start an advocacy charity that protected the human rights of people with neurological disability. For those who do not know what advocacy is, it is helping those with disability voice their concerns, beliefs, values to those in positions of authority such as housing officers, doctors, social workers etc as well as ensuring that those with disability get access to their entitlements and are not denied anything they are entitled to. I started this charity and ran it successfully for three and a half years. I resolved 120 cases being a one man band who could only get three years of funding for 15 hrs/week, and my plan was to demonstrate effectiveness as well as there being a need for the service, so that I could apply for more funding. I had resolved cases such as getting clients new boilers put into their homes that housing associations had been denying them, getting occupational therapy to install chair lifts into peoples' homes who had mobility issues and were relying on relatives carrying them to the toilet upstairs where the client was not a stranger to lying on the floor suffering from urinary incontinence when there was no one at home. I had also resolved cases such as getting a man's bathroom converted into a shower room as he had balance issues; getting fines dropped that people with disability had been charged for parking in disability bays despite showing their blue badge; preventing patients being forced by their doctors to take medications that they did not want to be on; ensuring doctors carried out all the tests before arriving at a diagnosis and not cutting corners in the diagnostic process; getting the sheriff court to recognise that a person with autism could not do the practical part of their community payback order due to oversensitivity to sound; preventing social work from cutting care budgets; dealing with antisocial neighbour complaints etc. It was a charity that could have grown and myself and the directors were in the process of speaking to a fundraiser who was going to help us find more funding. Unfortunately, my style of advocacy was disapproved of by the Scottish Independent Advocacy Alliance. They said that I had had too many complaints from social work for the size of the charity that we were. I disagreed with this as the number of complaints over 3.5 years had amounted to a total of 4 complaints after being told on a previous occasion by a team leader of another advocacy charity that if you are receiving complaints from social work then you are doing your job well, as your role is certainly not to be their friend. The problem is too many advocacy charities that are members of the SIAA receive government funding as part of the Mental Health (Care & Treatment) Act, where they in return for government funding make mental health advocacy a priority, as this act gives every person with a diagnosed mental health condition a legal right to an advocate if they need one. This means that the advocacy charities are receiving funding from the very people who employ social work and occupational therapy and all the other authorities that make up the statutory sector. I believe this affects the independence of your advocacy charity and makes it too easy for the council and the Health & Social Care Partnerships to have your charity on their lead. This is why we would have never accepted government funding. It is too convenient for government to be providing the advocates of people with mental health problems with money to provide advocacy in an area of health and social care where demand for resources is at its greatest ever and is only going to keep growing in the future and government are expected to fund it. This looks more like to me, money that will silence advocacy as opposed to providing advocacy. The SIAA were wanting to mentor me so that I towed the line with the other advocacy charities and danced to the tune of the SIAA. This I would not do and I decided to close the charity as these people were too powerful and could have created so many potential situations for us to have our charity vanished. It was also the case that many funders were wanting to divert their funding from new charities to much larger as well as longer established charities. What is painful is that the funders couldn't afford to provide funding to charities like mine, that was making a real difference to peoples' lives, simply so charities like epilepsy connections can afford their expensive office space in the centre of Glasgow. Many clients were upset by our closure and I have remained in touch with a couple since the closure.

At the time of closure of my advocacy charity I had had a number of cases that were going to have to now come to an end. One case was a woman suffering from a depressive disorder which was making it impossible for her to keep her flat clean. When I went round to her home you could literally not see the carpet. The place was full of old newspapers, magazines, clothes, dirty crockery and much more. You had to literally kick things out your way to make a path for yourself. This was a lady who lived on her own, was around 35 years of age and had no supportive family or friends. This lady had been to her doctor who refused to diagnose her with depression, she had also been refused services from the 'Community Mental Health Team' as a result of the refusal to recognise her as being depressed, thus, giving social work reason to refuse to appoint a cleaner to come round and help her clean her home, as living in untidy dwellings is a classic symptom of depression. As a consequence of her untreated, as well as undiagnosed depression, she had found it impossible to clean her flat, causing the housing officer of her housing association to tell her to have it cleaned by certain dates where a home inspection would be carried out. This lady has found it difficult to keep it clean and could risk facing eviction. When this lady went to her General Practitioner to make them aware of the consequences of her depression not being diagnosed and how it could end up in things happening to her such as eviction, all the G.P. could say in response was, "Elaine, let's face it, you are one of the ones that just go through the cracks" holding her fingers up and doing a kind of scraping of a blackboard motion. I thought that if this is how she speaks to Elaine with me there, then how does she speak to her when I am not there. Elaine was obviously very distressed when we informed her that Fairway Advocacy was going to close and that every other advocacy charity had a very long waiting list, and that they were all receiving statutory funding and therefore had a vested interest in siding with the housing association, the G.P. and the Community Mental Health Team etc. I am still phoned today by Elaine to resolve cases for her even though I am no longer a practicing advocate, and Fairway Advocacy no longer exists.

Another case I had was a case where a client with autism was doing a 'Community Payback Order'. The client was put in a workshop to fulfil the community service component of his community payback order, where there was a lot of noise, which people with autism are very sensitive to. He could not work in this workshop as it was causing him a lot of distress. The social work department were going to refer the case back to the sheriff court and my client could have ended up in prison as an alternative to the community payback order, which was a likely outcome as a result of social work claiming that they could not find an appropriate workshop for him. My client had already had a spell in prison due to his condition causing him to cross social boundaries that are not obvious to those with autism. The crime cannot be made reference to as it would breach the Data Protection Act and make my client easily identifiable. All I will say is he distracted a police man on duty causing alarm. It would have been the easy option to have replaced his community payback order with a prison sentence after the social work department referred his case back to the sheriff court as a consequence of not being able to find a suitable work environment for my client elsewhere. I fortunately wrote to the sheriff court and explained the effect his autism had on him, and the end result was for him to just have to complete the supervision part of the community payback order   and never mind the work placement. My client said when we came out the sheriff court that never would the outcome of the re-referral to the sheriff court have been what it turned out to be if it had not been for the contribution made by Fairway Advocacy and that he would just be going back to prison. When we closed, the last I had heard of this client was that he had been evicted from his homeless shelter, which social work would have been made aware of, and I have no doubt that this could have been used to put my client back in prison, which Fairway Advocacy was no longer around to try and prevent. Eviction would have allowed for the social work to say that he had not satisfied the supervision part of the order, by being an anti-social resident, and re-referred to the sheriff court causing my client to go back to prison. Fairway closing made this client very vulnerable especially when social work had been pulling him up, during his supervision meetings that were fortnightly, for being seen by others going to gay nightclubs; which according to social work, someone doing a community payback order should not be doing. This told you three things. One of these things being that the judicial social work department were judgemental, my client was being followed and that they would have used anything against him they could find to discredit his character that could have had him back in prison.

Another case is a gentleman with high blood pressure living above an antisocial neighbour who had been keeping him awake at night as well as antagonising him during the day by knocking on his ceiling with an object causing vibrations to go through my client's floor. I had arranged to see the housing officer of his housing association concerning the bullying, who had been refusing to do anything about it when my client had been trying to complain himself. My client has to go to have his blood pressure reviewed on a regular basis at the Glasgow Royal Infirmary as he suffers from high blood pressure and has experienced blackouts. My client was getting nose bleeds with the stress caused by his neighbour, which was hiking his blood pressure up to values that could cause a stroke resulting in death, paralysis, loss of speech, epilepsy etc or events such as silent strokes, which over time can lead to conditions like dementia. Unfortunately, I had to bring his case to a close when Fairway Advocacy closed. This issue like the other two mentioned ended up unresolved. One major life skill that seems to be absent in our society is the ability to budget and spend money wisely. How the funders could not keep funding our charity and instead choose to invest in charities that provided jobs as opposed to meaningful services is beyond belief. It is the case that you have a charity like mine preventing disabled people from having accidents in the home by accessing what they are entitled to from Occupational Therapy, and you have the other charities that just bring in people with disabilities to have free thinking sessions about pink elephants, and it is the latter that the funders give the funding to. A senseless and very illogical world.

These are just three example cases that demonstrate that the issues that people with physical disability e.g. hypertension, mental health issues e.g. depression, and learning disability e.g. autism, are very similar and cross many paths. I get fed up with all these charities in the voluntary sector that say they exist to meet the needs of those with disabilities and yet they sit back and let authorities treat people with disability in this way; and I especially hold a serious disliking, which would be a resentment if it were not for the meditation, towards the Scottish Independent Advocacy Alliance who could see that we were resolving many cases, meeting the needs and wishes of those with disability, successfully addressing the injustices that those with disability were coming to us with and making it possible for clients to access their entitlements; and yet accuse us of providing a service that was giving advocacy a bad name and that they now wanted to mentor me at the same time as social work putting in a fourth complaint about me. It is my opinion that the Scottish Independent Advocacy Alliance bend over for the social work departments and other statutory organisations, for the statutory funding that they get in return from government. It is this type of silencing of the small guy by the big guy, through the misuse of power to abuse and punish others who are just innocent people born with or acquire during the life course a disadvantage, that has had me grow up into an adult aged forty two, going on forty three, who hates authority. I hate the police, the council, the bank, the Driving Vehicle & Licensing Authority (DVLA), occupational health, the armed forces, the dragons on Dragons Den, the institutes of higher education and many more. I felt, and continue to feel that I owed society no good civilian as a consequence of how I have been treated by society's authorities, and how I would be treated by the ones I have yet to, and probably will never come into contact with. I felt that society should not expect people to be good civilians unconditionally. I believe that if society demands you to be a good civilian by meeting certain demands, then it is only right that society meets certain demands, such as the right to be treated with respect, that also protects your right to self-dignity, as well as right to all your promised entitlements. I believe that there is a partnership between you and society, therefore if society treats you badly, then as part of your adapting to living in a society that has chosen to be more your enemy than your friend, it is right that you treat society more as your enemy than your friend. I remain very open minded when I read about people who are involved in organised crime and have decided to make careers out of conning, hurting others and murdering. I can understand why some people would become angry enough and feel that they had been treated badly enough throughout their formative years to be of a "religion" that has an ethos of "zero-morality" where they can con, hurt and kill with a free conscience. Society criminalises, then punishes people for becoming criminal. Society is a dog chasing its tail with crime, just like it is the same dog chasing its tail with automation, global warming and health i.e. we complain that everyone is coming down with type 2 diabetes yet at the same time we sell huge 850g bars of chocolate for £1. Our society is a complete "Numpty" (Scottish word for stupid person), therefore is it any wonder that it's health, social care and education system has judgemental views towards a person with epilepsy and social anxiety disorder; as well as show an ignorance towards raising a child during its formative years, as a result of a lack of knowledge in subject areas that these sectors would claim to be their expertise.

In the days before I started meditating, if I got a late council tax payment letter, I would feel the need to go ballistic with a person who held an authoritative position. I would be straight on the phone cursing at the person on the other end of the council tax payment line even though I knew I had not paid my council tax bill and that there was nothing unfair about the sending of this notice. I basically saw the letter from the council tax department as being an opportunity to pick a fight with an authority to try and remedy the lack of closure I have lived with over previous experiences with authority.

The injustices that I had experienced up until March 2015 had made me so hot headed that I had such a low tolerance threshold that had transferable effects in other areas of my life such as neighbour relationships. I found myself feeling intolerable feelings of rage towards neighbours playing their music. When I complained to the factors about the music I was told in a very dismissive letter that this was not a problem for the factors to resolve and that it was my problem. I thought "Damn Authority!!". I felt a rage and a resentment that had me respond to this by printing off copies of stories from newspapers off the internet that had headlines such as "NEIGHBOUR STABS NEIGHBOUR OVER NOISE POLLUTION", "NEIGHBOUR SHOOTS ANTISOCIAL NEIGHBOUR", "MAN KILLED BY ANTISOCIAL NEIGHBOUR IN STREET FIGHT". I wrote a letter as well to my factors saying to them that the noise affects communal areas such as the close which could affect someone's ability to sell their home, and therefore they should play a role in defusing this noise. I also said that they had a role to play in defusing the noise due to the building's sound insulation being poor quality which was a structural issue shared by all living in the close. I had already had an antisocial neighbour the year before living below me and had to get the environmental protection services to deal with him after being threatened by this neighbour outside a newsagent I was coming out of because of a letter of complaint I had put through his door. This guy was evicted.

 I told the factors in the letter that I could not just keep reporting neighbours to Environmental Protection Services and that due to a lack of sound insulation throughout the whole building the closes were at risk of becoming dangerous places with neighbours standing on other neighbour doorsteps where the break out of fights was becoming a possibility. I finished the letter saying that if someone were killed then they could not say that they had not been warned and could not have played a preventative role. I travelled to the factor's office in Glasgow and placed the letter and headlines on the receptionist's desk and said, "Get your bosses to read that!". When I got home the phone rang which I answered. A voice on the other end of the phone said that it was the police and that I was guilty of causing alarm after handing in my letter and headlines into the factor's office. I was told that this was a breach of the peace and that I could be charged. I thought to myself "Oh Fuck, this is the next nightmare of my life" and I let out a huge sigh of relief when the policeman said, "Fortunately for you, your factors do not wish to press charges". The police said that this better be the last of the complaints received from me regarding the noise from neighbours' homes. The phone went dead and I sat down and thought to myself what caused this to happen. I then realised that my letter and headlines were a knee-jerk reaction to my rage with the letter from the factors and that this rage was a symptom of my depression. It was now my depressive symptoms that could have had me put in prison or more likely in today's world a six month 'Community Payback Order' which sitting beside the epilepsy would not enhance my employment prospects. I had been meditating at the time and thought to myself without the meditation I would have most likely blown a fuse with the police officer over the phone. I have already said that the meditation defused my anger towards what happened to me over the drug training at the Epilepsy Society over a period of a few days, however, the anger and rage I was feeling when I read the letter from the factors was an anger and rage symptomatic of a depression that had been engrained in me for many years, probably most of my life. This wasn't an anger and a rage that would take days of meditation to remedy but an anger and rage that would most likely take months of consistent meditation practice to conquer. This was March 2015 and I started meditating in September 2014 but inconsistently i.e. sometimes twice daily but mostly once daily. It's now March 2018 and I have been meditating since September 2014 but have only been meditating consistently morning and night since August 2017. I must say that six months of meditation morning and night has really improved my rage to near zero. The meditation is now at the stage where you feel the scars being removed. I do unfortunately have a tendency to relapse when I am with my parents as our relationship is not good but the relapse only lasts for as long as I am in their company. The effects of relapse don't linger for hours afterwards like they used to. You will find out more about this in later chapters.

After Fairway Advocacy's closure I was left without a job until November 2017 when Epilepsy Connections offered me a job as a Self -management trainer as part of their 'Epilepsy Futures Course'. I am currently a teaching this course at the time of writing this chapter. Time will tell where this moves onto. I am a fighter and I remain positive. One thing I can say is that I have never given up and I see each past bad experience as a blind summit towards the top of the mountain that success resides at the top of. There has been a lot of life skill acquisition, life knowledge, character building etc over the years. No pain, No gain.

CHAPTER 19

I have briefly made reference to the acquisition of life skills and life knowledge over the years. This chapter will inform you of all these gains that I see myself as having gained and all the negatives that I see as having turned into positives.

As has not been mentioned, back in nurse training I did suffer from an anxiety disorder, on top of my social anxiety disorder, where the symptoms were very 'Obsessive Compulsive Disorder' like in nature. As my epilepsy comes from the left temporal lobe of the brain, I am very susceptible to developing anxiety disorders. The anxiety disorder that I had was an anxiety disorder where I was having unwanted thoughts as a result of intrusive thinking where I would tell myself to give up things I did not want to give up as well as tell myself I hated things I did not hate. I couldn't stop these thoughts. This anxiety is typical of someone who has temporal lobe epilepsy since the temporal lobe is responsible for thoughts and emotions. For eighteen months my life felt intolerable. This anxiety was literally on 24 hours per day, seven days per week; and I felt in July 1999 that the corner that I had been getting squeezed into since January 1998; which was when this anxiety disorder began, could not get any tighter. The pre-cursor to developing an anxiety of this theme i.e. giving things up I didn't want to, was my mother forcing me to do an MSc in Rehabilitation Science which trained you to be a physiotherapist. The internal cynic in me couldn't stop saying, "You are only doing this course because your mother forced you to". This anxiety was true, I had been forced through manipulation by my mother to become a physiotherapist, because she liked me massaging her back as a kid. The problem was this message discredited every future decision that I made about what I wanted to do with my life, so that when I did make a decision on my career, where I lived or who I dated; I would always find myself uncontrollably saying the words, "You don't want this, You really want that"; making me feel false, and giving me that feeling that I was about to uncontrollably give something or someone up that I did not wish to give up. It was very distressing, and it was like living twenty four hours per day, seven days per week with that feeling you get standing at the edge of a cliff or up something very high; like scaffolding, looking over the edge and getting uncontrollable thoughts of jumping, giving you that feeling that you are about to lose control which freaks you out, making you want to stand back, but you can't stand back because there is nothing physical to stand back from, causing you to live every awoken moment with nervousness and feelings of panic. I had lived with this feeling for eighteen months, twenty four hours per day, seven days per week, and in July 1999 I felt I had met my breakdown threshold and that I could not fight this anxiety alone and therefore it was time to concede by going to the doctor for a referral to psychiatry, or at least be put on tranquiliser medication. The next words I thought to myself were, "I am mentally unfit" which then had me question my physical fitness. It was this questioning of physical fitness that then had me remember a teacher of mine at school saying, "Boys, if you are physically fit you are mentally fit" in a physical education lesson, as we were having a debate with him over the significance of physical education. At this lesson we were all saying that there was no qualification in physical education and therefore what was the point in doing it. We were saying that it did not boost our employment prospects. Our teacher responded by saying that exercise makes you more productive and then finished off by saying, "Boys take a look around the room and notice every person sitting here. One in three of you will have a mental health problem at some time in your life, and that it is so true that if you are physically fit, you are mentally fit". I responded to this memory by buying a tracksuit the same day that I admitted to myself that I was mentally unwell and took out graduate membership of the Glasgow University gym after Googling "exercise and anxiety" on my mobile phone for a good number of hours, reading lots of scientific papers of studies done, where exercise had been used as a replacement to tranquiliser medication and anti-depressants. What my physical education teacher had said was true. I exercised on a treadmill for three hours per week and within five weeks my anxiety symptoms had disappeared. I felt like I had got out of prison. I felt like I could breathe again. I was free of these uncontrollable thoughts. I did these workouts on the treadmill three days per week, and then my attendance fluctuated from three times per week to twice per week with the occasional two consecutive weeks of only getting there once a week. It was during these consecutive weeks of once per week that my anxiety symptoms returned, but once I had a week of two visits, I was anxiety free again. When I was getting there three days per week, I got wonderful feelings of euphoria and confidence that was like a 24/7 high. It was great. Just a shame the discipline just wasn't strong enough to get their three times per week, however, twice a week was enough to rid me off anxiety and panic as well as reduce my depressive symptoms between 2003 and 2014 from severe to moderate.

Without the exercise anxiety would have given me a breakdown and I think depression would have killed me. That lesson at school was the most valuable lesson I had ever attended in my life. I have been keeping physically fit since July 1999. There has been one ten week period away from the gym, due to a slipped disc on the squash court, in these nearly twenty one years, at the time of writing. Up until 2013 you could quite literally count on one hand the number of weeks that had elapsed without me exercising. Even on holidays I would be using the hotel gym. I had managed to sweat anxiety out of my system. I had managed to sweat half of my depression out with two visits per week. I have had many mornings ("many" is an understatement) where I waken up with a very strong euphoric feeling, where I feel a very strong motivation and feel that I am wakening up in a world full of opportunity, and I have a strong desire to get out of bed and make the most of it all. This is a regular when I am exercising two days per week and walking everywhere I go. I burn off two half marathons worth of calories in the gym per week, plus walk twenty miles per week. Each half marathon workout is made up of four and a quarter miles on the cross trainer, and fifteen and a quarter miles on the bike (three and a quarter miles as part of a warm up and the twelve miles after the cross trainer), remembering that a gym bike unlike a road bike has no free cycle, therefore your feet are pedalling for the full distance covered. This total distance comes to just over three thousand miles per year. This is a mileage greater than the distance from Los Angeles to New York which totals 2,797 miles. I see these three thousand miles as being a coast to coast route across an America which is "My America". From "My Los Angeles to New York". I see my life as covering a distance per year that is a virtual reality of being out in the wild with hot days and cold nights, away from everyone and everything, that hardens me as a person and has a huge confidence building effect, and gives me a huge sense of self. I have also wondered how much the seizure frequency reduction has been down to the exercise. Exercise encourages the production of two chemicals in the brain called 'Neurotransmitters' that are responsible for electrical conductivity. Dopamine is produced by exercise which brings on feelings of reward, motivation and confidence. Serotonin is the other neurotransmitter that brings on feelings of euphoria, tranquillity, good mood and feelings of re-assurance. These two neurotransmitters have got me through all this grief and kept me strong and resilient enough to face the challenges that people have thrown at me. I have never taken anti-depressants nor tranquilisers, as they are just an industry, and debatably the biggest industry in the world, and not the information technology industry. Any activity that results in the production of these neurotransmitters such as exercise, meditation, reading, eating apples/red bell peppers/tomatoes/green tea also help to prevent dementia and Alzheimer's disease. The exercise protects me from stroke and circulatory disorders and therefore in a perverse kind of way the grief thrown at me has created habits within me that will minimise chances of stroke, heart disease, cancer, alzheimer's disease and dementia. Talk about turning things on their head.

As already mentioned there has also been social anxiety disorder that I have suffered from, where I have avoided sports and performance settings. This is anxiety related to trauma, and unfortunately, I have not been able to lift this with exercise and it has unfortunately caused for me social isolation. It is not an anxiety that you constantly feel i.e. chronic, but an anxiety that you get, in the anxiety provoking situation i.e. acute.

 I have no friends as they all left after my university years to other parts of Britain or the globe to never be seen or heard of again. I have had great unmet social needs and I have been living a loner life pretty much for the last twenty years but for the three years at the 'Epilepsy Society'. I have not had supportive family. As already mentioned, my sisters have been unempathetic and think I am attention seeking and have been too much of a burden for my parents. I never see my brother in laws and do not know my nephews. It terrifies me and has had me waken up with panic in the middle of the night thinking who will be here for me, to fend for me when my parents are not here and I have no one. They say there is a social isolation epidemic in the United Kingdom at present amongst the mainstream population therefore it is not unique to social anxiety disorder. At the time of writing this chapter I am meeting a local authority councillor on the 21st October 2017 to discuss the problem with social isolation and how there needs to be a community centre for isolated people to go to where they can meet. It is not just a problem that the elderly suffer from. It is impossible to meet new friends in adulthood. The formulated life of getting an education, a job then getting married and having children is such a prescribed way in living that leaves no room for getting to know new people if you are a person who lives a non-formulated life as a consequence of having needs that society does not cater for. You cannot rely on getting to know your neighbours or people who live around you as everyone is into social media and talking has just disappeared. I have lived in

Nottingham, Loughborough, Slough, Glasgow, Helensburgh and I have not been able to make a single friend, quite literally a single friend, in twenty years. It can't be said it is me as there are seven billion people on this planet. Even if I were the most objectionable character you came across, there are certainly enough objectionable people to become friends with. I will make verbal mincemeat of the next person I ever hear say, "Oh, they are so clique" when making reference to someone else. My experience is that everyone is clique. To become someone's friend in adult years requires you to convince them into wanting to add a new member to their existing clique of friends. To achieve this is like trying to break an 8 digit security code in one attempt. The furiously rigid and non-flexibile attitudes of people to get to know new people and form relationships with new people has left me thinking "will I ever have a future relationship of any description ever again?".

When I moved up to Glasgow in 2012 after living away in Slough for the previous three years, where I had been working at the Epilepsy society, my attendance at the gym became poor. My attendance at the gym had dropped to once per week and I started to get strong depressive symptoms as a consequence of being socially isolated. I was overcome by feelings of rejection and not knowing why I was rejected was causing great frustration. This frustration exacerbated existing depression and I lost the desire to share the world with the human race. I did not want to live, I suffered from intense suicidal ideation and I didn't want to go to the gym because I saw it as being good for my health which was only going to be prolonging an agony called life. It was no longer unusual to go more than a week without going to the gym. The depression was snookering me from getting to the gym to burn it off. This is when I decided that I was going to go back to my meditation practice that I used when I was set up over my medication training.

From Dec 2014 up to present, I have been meditating every day where I have built my meditation practice up to two lots of forty five minutes per day since September of 2017. It was the case that for the first three years of the practice I had gone through phases where I had done it twice daily, where I experienced the therapeutic effects of the meditation and there had been no depression nor night time anxiety. Unfortunately, my practice had also slipped and I had gone days only getting the night time meditation in, resulting in continued depression and night time anxiety. I have not just been overcome by depressive and anxiety symptoms when not meditating twice daily but I have also had cognitive problems where I have suffered from problems with concentration, processing and memory due to the depression. As a consequence of depression, I lost my literacy skills. When meditating twice per day consistently, my literacy skills come back, I can read an article and tell you what I've read; but meditating once a day, I am just reading words, and that is it. If I'm not meditating at all, I am not even reading words. My mind is too anxious about not remembering what I have just read to be able to give what I am currently reading any focus. It is the case that the depression causes literacy issues brought on by cognitive impairment but then you become highly anxious about this cognitive impairment, which further jeopardises your cognitive faculties. It starts off as a symptom of depression and then becomes as much a symptom of anxiety, so you are now at war with two conditions that have hijacked your literacy skills. The depression affects the processing, and then the recruiting of anxiety affects the concentration, with nothing about what you've just read registering in memory. It's like the armed robbers robbing the security men of the money before the money is put in the safe. The "money" being read information.

In August 2017 I had lost so much faith in memory and processing that I now could not even have confidence in being shown how to work a coffee machine in a friend's home and remember what I had just been shown. I thought "God, I am dementing". It was at this moment that I got a real fright and started meditating twice per day without fail. I therefore decided that enough was enough and started meditating twice per day without fail, and found both my literacy skills and processing return, and my anxiety disappear, meaning that I now have unaffected concentration. If it were not for the meditation and the exercise, I would not be here writing this book. Suicide is an ending that 1 in 7 of those with my type of epilepsy will make an attempt at trying to achieve, and over the last three years, during times of slipped meditation practice and slipped attendance at the gym I have felt myself so close to bringing it all to an end.

Social Isolation, lack of any relationships, the baggage from past, lack of future prospects, lack of family interest, lack of evidence of care or compassion in the world, lack of hope in things ever improving; has caused me on many an occasion to be so close to ending my life. The thing about suicide is that you don't want to die, but you find yourself in a position where the continuation of life becomes impractical. What you do want is for life to change so that living becomes a practical option for you. You long for the life where the living conditions make the continuing of life a practical choice. Therefore, you can "Want to die" at the same time as "Want to live", but the life you want to live is not the one you are living. Therefore, don't be fooled into believing that someone is lying about their desire to commit suicide because you see healthy behaviours. It could be the case that on the days you see "Healthy Behaviours" they have hope that they can have the life that they want to live, but on the days they talk of suicide they are having a day where they are convinced they will never live that life, and they will always live the life they are living. When someone is having such a bad day, they are 100% convinced by the arguments that life will never improve, and that any future feelings to the contrary will be nothing but false hope, and therefore they will not be swayed into not taking their life because they might feel differently tomorrow. It is therefore possible to find someone talking about suicide today, being found eating a healthy baguette as part of a calorie controlled diet tomorrow, and being found to have taken their own life the next day. The relationship between suicide risk and lifestyle choices is not as black and white as most people believe. This is one of the reasons as to why people find themselves saying: **"He was appearing all happy the other day, had just proposed to his girlfriend, talking about all his future plans that he and his wife to be were looking forward to, and was later found dead".**

Depression and Anxiety have been two conditions that I have never received a formal diagnosis for as I have always turned down appointments with mental health professionals. I have already expressed my own personal thoughts on psychiatry and I do believe that whether they are aware of being so or not, I do see the mental health professionals as being the advocates of a society that has made me depressed and been the cause of my crippling performance anxiety. It is because of both the abuse I had been on the receiving end of as a child, and as an adult, that I live with the trauma that causes me my symptoms of social anxiety disorder and depression. Psychiatry from my understanding always looks for the root of the problem to come from within the person. Psychiatry would never even accommodate the theory that the root of the problem comes from within society. To the world of psychiatry, the world is a place of "normality", and if you do not fit into this normality then you are "subnormal". From my experience the world is anything but normal, and you just have to switch on the news to see that the world is in fact a gross cocktail of abnormalities made up with man's obsession for power, greed and status with major insecurity being a precursor for all three. I see a bomb drop from a plane, land, kill innocent civilians; and I am to accept that that is normality, as no psychiatrist or other mental health professionals are coming forward and saying these people who are in power, who are choosing for all these countries to go to war and kill many innocents are clinically unwell. Surely, we should be allowed to believe if there were a mental health condition that caused you to declare wars and have innocent civilians killed, the mental health professions would be up in arms. The very fact that we do not hear a squeak of concern from mental health professionals when heads of state misbehave in narcissistic as well as both egocentric and megalomaniac ways, is confirmation of their belief that such behaviour is not evidence of being of unwell mind, thus, discrediting their definition of 'normality'. I think, "well if that's normal, I do not wish to be", and I also think "If that is what psychiatry would use as a model to help them navigate me towards normality then I would rather they did not try". My opinion on the matter is, anyone who is of a mentality that causes them to drop bombs from the sky causing the death of many innocent civilians for the purpose of increasing power or telling others who is the "boss", is of very unwell mind. According to the Mental Health Care & Treatment Act 2012, anyone who is deemed to be of a state of mind that makes them a risk to themselves or others, should be given a compulsory treatment order if they refuse to take treatment that could involve sectioning against one's will. Is it therefore not the case, according to the "Laws of Psychiatry", which includes the definition of 'normality', that the behaviour of dictators is excessive, stems from both insecurity and ego therefore making it the case that their behaviour is abnormal, which puts others at risk, and therefore the behaviour of these dictator should warrant compulsory treatment and that these dictators could be forced to take this treatment with or without sectioning under this Mental Health Care & Treatment Act 2012 or equivalent. I therefore ask where are the psychiatrists when we have "Saddam Husseins" running all over the place. Do the laws of psychiatry somehow not apply to the dictators i.e. the megalomaniacs? Normality exists one minute for one lot of people and then doesn't exist the next minute for another lot. Normality is an illusion, a bit like a seizure! Psychiatry does a lot of research into what they call "Abnormality" but they do no research into what they call "Normality". How can we draw conclusions on whether something is normal or abnormal when there is no scientific consensus on what "normality" is? Psychiatry is a spoof science. In the field of neurology, we know when electroconductivity in the nervous system is abnormal as we know what normal electroconductivity looks like. In the field of cardiology, we know what an abnormally developed heart looks like because we know what a normal healthy developed heart looks like. We can't know what an abnormal mind is like, as we have no idea what a normal mind is like. Would you share with a psychiatrist every thought that goes through your head? Are you open and honest about every opinion/view/belief you hold with other people? Let's not forget that homosexuality was once considered a mental health condition, but now that we live in a more liberal society, many more people are open and honest with one another about their sexuality and we now know that most people are attracted to members of the same sex, and homosexuality is no longer considered a mental health condition. Psychiatry is a specialty that is anti- individuality and forces anyone who does not conform to wear labels, as these people are seen to be a threat to a society that functions through the abuse and exploitation of those who feel the need to conform and fit in; hence, the fact that one of the diagnostic criteria to label someone as 'depressed' is a person who thinks the world is a terrible place as well as its people. The beginning of seeing the world's people as being a terrible lot is the beginning of one choosing to no longer conform.

I avoided psychiatry as I knew they would always say that my depression and anxiety come from within me; and they would give it another name such as "Personality Disorder", causing me to feel substandard, thus reducing my morale and self- esteem; destroying my confidence, which would only make me more depressed. It would have also made me more angry having to live with these labels, and resentful of others as I would have seen myself as being used as a scapegoat for all the symptoms that I was showing as a consequence of others treatment towards me throughout my life. The Psychiatric world is always looking for a biological reason for why a person with epilepsy is angry and depressed and has great difficulty settling when it has nothing to do with biology and instead has to do with others attitudes towards the person with epilepsy and the trauma others create for that person throughout their life. This results in the wearing of highly inappropriate as well as inaccurate labels which if were allowed to be found out about by the wrong people could be used against me to their advantage or to bully me with. For example; if I got married, had a kid, got divorced and it was to be determined what parent the child stayed with, my so called personality disorder would have been brought into the equation. Social Work can use the fact a single mother has a personality disorder to strengthen their case into taking away her child. Another example of how such a label such as the one of "personality disorder" could be used against me would be if I ever took an employer to court for unfair dismissal under the Equality Act 2010 as a consequence of sacking me on the grounds of my epilepsy. My employer's lawyers could say that I had a personality disorder that made it very difficult for others to work with myself and claim their reason for sacking me to be down to poor working relationships with colleagues. To seek help from mental health services would only have been putting myself at future risk of becoming trapped in a vicious symptom cycle as well as becoming trapped in a vicious persecution cycle. As has already been mentioned at the beginning of this book; conditions like epilepsy, anxiety and depression cause battles, where 85% of these battles are political/social-cultural and the remaining 15% are symptomatic battles.

My attitude has always been that the best mental health therapist is in your own mind. Psychiatry was a service that I saw as being something that would disempower me and cause me to develop a dependency on drugs and professionals for the rest of my days whereas the alternative therapies were what I saw as being the remedies that were long lasting and self-empowering, resulting in you becoming a more and more independent adult. This is why I have always resorted to meditation and exercise to conquer these two ills, that my own life experience has taught me other people are too often the cause of. In my view, it is our society that is dysfunctional; and not the individual by default, who might have become "damaged" because of him or her being shaped by a dysfunctional society. Why would any person turn to the dysfunctional society for help that was the cause of their damage? That is absurdity and that is what I would have called turning to psychiatry. If car mechanics were like psychiatrists, they would look at a car that had been vandalised by baseball bats and say, "You see, you shouldn't buy that make of car. You'll see that it comes with a smashed windscreen, huge dents and requires a major paint job. You should instead buy a make of car that leaves the factory in the perfect state." Totally sweeping the real issues, that are both political and cultural in nature, under the carpet; such as angry young people with poor employment prospects, on the receiving end of a prejudicial education system as well as on low incomes, turning to alcohol consumption to cheer themselves up, resulting in anti-social behaviour such as vandalising cars.

As I have already mentioned, the best mental health therapist is found within your own mind. You just need someone to teach you how to use it. You can learn this yourself by reading up on the subject over the internet, or you might just to get you started require a therapist; or probably even better, a person who has actually used these therapies themselves and managed to overcome these mental health problems i.e. Peer Support, to introduce to you some of the techniques that you can use to treat symptoms of depression and anxiety. I learned about meditation, positive thinking and visualisation through the teaching of the Expert Patient Programme. What is it they say, "If you have walked the walk, then you can talk the talk".

CHAPTER 20

I was first introduced to the world of practicing alternative therapy when I started working as a symptom management trainer for the charity called 'Disability Information Greater Glasgow', that provided disability information, back in 2005. During my two years of working at this charity I had to work with a boss who was very unpleasant and had a very short temper. If you needed showing how the fax machine worked, he would get very angry and aggressive. I was friends with his son and his son shared with me how his father had broken his nose at the family dinner table over a dispute where his father put the palm of his hand behind the head of my friend, and slammed his face towards the table thus breaking his nose. I was on a drug called 'Lamotrigine' at the time for my epilepsy and one of the side effects of Lamotrigine is anger and irritability. Everyone else at work was fearful of what this man might do; however, because of the medication I was on I was much more fearful of what I was going to do in response to him doing what he might do. At times you would ask a question and you would get spoken back to like you had asked a stupid question or you would get a very impatient answer. You stayed out of this man's way as much as possible. I was the only man working in our office and he was a terrible womaniser. I had heard from others that my boss had, had sexual relationships with a couple of people he held professional relationships with who had dealings with the charity and also attended the team meetings. During these meetings he would flirt with the ladies that he had previously had sexual encounters with and on a daily basis he would show favourable interest towards the female staff. Never did my boss ever show any interest in any work that I was working on. My boss never made any enquiries regarding my work, and despite me having so much to feedback on with regards to the progress made with the course I was designing and who I was teaching that course to, he never showed any interest and just wanted to talk about the other business my female colleagues were working on which I had no involvement with. I would sit there quietly throughout the meetings while the women had loads to say. I felt devalued, belittled, offended, shown up and I went home harbouring anger and rage on top of the side effects of my lamotrigine, combined with symptoms of depression. I panicked as I felt that I was never going to be able to hold down this job. I had images of shouting, "Fuck Off" in the boss's face and swinging a punch at him. I was so pent up with rage. I was wandering around my flat cursing to myself and dreaded going back to work the next day as I would have sub-zero levels of tolerance for him if he were his usual self. It was then that I told myself that I was new in the job and I could not just leave and that I would have to stay for a couple of years if I were to leave and it not look bad on my employment history. I then decided that if I were going to continue in this job then I would have to stop feeling this way. When I got home from work I asked myself, "What made me feel so angry and frustrated?", and my answer was "Because of what that boss did today". My next question was to ask myself, "How angry am I now in comparison to how angry I was back then?". It was after answering this question that I discovered that there had been an increase in anger since my boss sinning like he did and me sitting in my lounge that evening. I then asked myself, "What has happened between coming home and sitting here with greater feelings of rage and frustration?". This is when it came to me that it was not what happened that caused my anger levels, but my thinking of events afterwards that had caused my anger to rise. It was the thoughts triggered by the events that caused my anger, and not the actual event itself. It was thoughts such as, "This is what I should have said" and "This is what I should have done" as well as thoughts of seeing me do these things, such as having fly on wall images as well as through my own eyes images of me beating him up, that only filled me up further with pent up rage. This is when I first became aware of the relationship between your thoughts, emotions and behaviours. This is when I learned that to not get angry and remain relaxed, I was to not allow myself to think about the job, the people, or anything that happened that day other than stuff I might need to remember to prepare me for a future day at work. I also learned that how we think is habitual and the last habit I wanted to get myself into was coming home and thinking about what happened, what I should have said and done as well as what I would have liked to have done. This is an error I had been doing all my life and it was what had allowed the nurses on my nurse training course to bully me and pull my strings causing me to have arguments with them giving them the ammunition to accuse me of having an attitude problem and require me to get unions involved to stop me from being thrown of the nurse training course.

It was after this discovery of the relationships between thoughts, emotions and behaviours that I discovered the skill of using 'ESCAPISM' as a means of ridding myself off; and preventing further anger caused by my workplace. When I came home, I decided to start reading fiction books. After reading for two hours my mind had had two hours respite from thinking about anything to do with work. I had been in an angry thought free zone, and after putting the book down, my mind continued to remain in this zone. If I ever found thoughts to do with work entering my mind when not at work, I just blanked the thought by having my inner dialogue say it could not join in the discussion as it did not know what the thought was talking about. My inner dialogue would just say that it had never heard of any of these people and knew nothing of these past events. This caused me to drop all thinking to do with work outside of work. As a consequence of this I had not developed brewed anger at home, thus, preventing me from blowing a fuse at work; and if anything bad happened at work, my inner dialogue could like a sports coach tell me not to respond, as within a few hours from now I would be in the midst of a plot thousands of miles away from here in another city, in another country; and all the people around me at present would be totally irrelevant. This escapism from the reading fiction prevented the terrible side effects of lamotrigine from taking home baggage from work, amplifying the emotional effects of that baggage at home; and then emotionally exploding the next day at work. I managed to keep this job and endure two years in the post before my boss chose to neither apply for, or did not get the funding to renew a two year post. As has already been discussed in a previous chapter, it was believed by many that the charity that was set up by my boss after retiring from the health board was possibly a venture used to access money left behind by his father who had expressed a wish for his money to be left behind for charitable purposes, so my bosses priority might have been to open a charity that would give him access to the money. The priority of my boss was possibly to keep the charity running, spending as little money as he could get away with spending on any service that was provided by the charity. If this had been his plan, then my boss would have seen my role as a threat; as another man, who I cannot name, who was big in the world of fundraising, thought that my course on disability symptom management, as well as human rights, was a great course and that I should put a bit more on benefits into the course. This same man said that my boss should be looking to invest his funding, as well as apply for more funding, to finance my role of training officer and the teaching of my course. I believe that this other man had been appointed as a director of the charity, who might have been made a mug off thinking that he was a director of a charity with a legitimate cause.

Since this era in my life, I have read crime and espionage fiction; and have very recently greatly increased the amount of time I spend reading to cope with social isolation, as again the effects of social isolation are environmental, and reading can have you sitting in your home on your own one minute and being a fly on the wall watching Mexican drug dealers making attempts to eliminate CIA officers, as well as become Mexico's biggest drug lords, for the next three hours, seven thousand miles away. Reading has the same "Getting Away" effect that a holiday has, and the characters in the story can act as a substitute to real life companionship. These books are also therapeutic if you are anti-authority, as the characters in these books are all guys who have been let down by the education system, the welfare state, housing, private health service, family, the judiciary! I hope members of the judicial service reading this paragraph take note!!

CHAPTER 21

As a consequence of the social anxiety disorder preventing me from joining clubs and society's, I have remained socially isolated for many years. My isolation, when I am not at work, goes back twenty years. When I have not been under the employment of others it has not been unusual for me to have a three week period elapse in my life where I do not speak to a single person. The closest thing I got to a conversation was: "Do you want space for milk?", with a bit of three minute banter. In other words, the only conversation you get is with someone taking your order in a coffee shop or with someone dishing up a black pudding supper for you. You can go to the pub and spend all night talking to a stranger but then you are relying on alcohol which is not a good idea. Social isolation and alcohol could be the beginning of a slippery slope which is not good if you are on anti-convulsant medication and have seizures.

If you discount the phone conversations with my father. The amount of isolation in my life has been excessive and has caused me to develop symptoms of panic, and if not for the self-management tools I have learned, this isolation would have had me diagnosed with 'Panic Disorder' and on prescribed medication which would not have been without their strong side effects.

It was in September 2009 that I had my first ever panic attack. It came on suddenly within a matter of seconds when I was walking back from my local gym. It was terrifying. I suffered from symptoms of 'depersonalisation' where my mind and body no longer felt connected. I felt that the connection between body and mind was disappearing and that something tragic was going to happen once the connection between body and mind had totally disappeared, such as death or loss of all self- control. I was getting out of body sensations, thinking I was about to die from loss of self- control and start freaking out throwing everything around the place. I was terrified. My heart was racing and I was ultra- paranoid. I wanted to walk on the other side of the road to any passers-by just in case I jumped on them. I phoned my Dad who was a doctor and I was speaking to him over the phone with the same anxiety levels as someone being chased by a mugger with a knife. I told my Dad over the phone that I was getting out of body sensations and thought I was a dying man walking and that I was going to lose control and start attacking people.

My father told me that as distressing and as realistic the symptoms were I would not end up losing control, I was not going to die and that I was to just walk to the Western Infirmary; which I walked past on my way home, and tell them at the accident & emergency (A&E) that I was having a panic attack. I entered the A&E, and I was sat in a cubicle and given something to calm me down. I asked the doctor what had happened to me and the only reply was, "You have a personality disorder". This came as a real shock to me as I had never been diagnosed as having a personality disorder. It wouldn't surprise me if they had been looking at the wrong notes, as a few years later I was in the same accident & emergency department when I slipped my disc on the squash court and had been told that I had sprained a muscle and sent home in a taxi with no pain killer medication and slept the whole night in my bed with an untreated slipped disc. Proper diagnosis had to wait til the next day, when my Dad did a postural examination of me and said, "You've slipped a disc. It is not a sprained muscle". You can't trust a doctor nowadays!!

After being told that I had a personality disorder at the Western Infirmary, I replied to the doctor by saying, "No, I am a normal person who was psychologically scarred by his teachers and other children when he was a child and now has phobia of the opportunities that get you meeting people and forming relationships with people resulting in social isolation thus resulting in panic attacks at the age of 34". I don't have any more a personality disorder than the person that can't go into swimming pools because they at one time nearly drowned. If we lived in a society where everyone socialised in swimming pools, then people who have a fear of water would be socially isolated. If they don't understand you, then how can they help you? Their answer is always reactive i.e. here's a tablet to sweep the real issues under the carpet with, as opposed to therapeutic i.e. let's fix what's broken, because they don't recognise what's broken. I believe that psychiatry is just society's way in preventing schools, other statutory services, employers etc from being sued for the psychological damage they have created in others. Making a condition look like the cause comes from WITHIN you, protects those who are responsible for the creating off these psychological conditions from legal accountability, where the true cause comes from OUTWITH. Psychiatry makes states of mind caused by environmental trauma look like they are caused by something organic that went wrong in the womb. I could sue that French teacher, Geography teacher, PE teacher and many others!

Being a Biologist I left the A&E that night and went over with myself what was going on in my body and mind's mechanics during the panic attack. The answer I gravitated to, using all my taught knowledge, was the part of my Central Nervous System for the fight or flight reaction i.e. the 'Amyglada', also known as the brain's anxiety centre, had started firing off causing me to experience heightened anxiety; causing hyperventilation, thus, further increased firing of the fight or flight centre; thus, bringing on more heightened anxiety and hyperventilation, creating an even further increased firing of the amyglada; bringing on excruciatingly intolerable levels of sudden anxiety and hyperventilation, creating a vicious symptom cycle called a" Panic Attack". I deducted that this 'Fight or Flight' response could be defused by slow breathing, as this would fool my brain into believing that there was no risk, as it would detect that the breathing rate had gone down, thus, causing my brain's flight or fight system to gradually switch off, as the slow breathing became more established, thus, decreasing feelings of panic until all symptoms are gone. I learned that if this were to happen again, all I needed to do was breathe in and out slowly through my nose. You can't hyperventilate through the nose, so nasal breathing can defuse a panic attack. Since then all symptoms of panic have been controlled with slow nasal breathing. In theory, I had panic disorder; but in practice, I did not, as a result of the knowledge taught to me in human physiology at university. No need for "as required" medications which so many people are on, when all they need to do is shut their mouth and breathe slowly through their nose, releasing all muscle tension by dropping their shoulders and imagining themselves being all floppy.

Between July 2012-Dec 2014 slow breathing is how I coped with any onset of panic attacks brought on by isolation, and since Dec 2014; meditation has totally eliminated my life of ever having to defuse panic attacks when I have been consistent with my twice daily practice. I do however sometimes go up to three weeks without a conversation with anyone at the time of writing this paragraph i.e. May 2019, and find myself not suffering symptoms of panic during the day but can wake up in middle of night with symptoms of dizziness accompanied by feelings of agrophobia (because I feel a small isolated fish in a gigantic ocean where I know no-one) and claustrophobia at the same time as I feel the going without conversation without anyone for weeks pushing me into a tighter and tighter corner. I immediately respond to this by my inner life coach saying to me, "Shut your mouth, breathe slowly through your nose, now breathe slowly out, breathe in, now breathe out, ...Do you feel your symptoms subsiding?"; and what I feel is the dizziness disappearing, my mental tight corner getting larger and larger, my ocean shrinking into a pond and, thus, full recovery. Again, no need for highly paid psychiatrists, no need for referrals to community mental health teams, no need for judgemental General Practitioners like my doctor at the Helensburgh Medical Practice, no need for medications; and instead the learning of a life skill, the winning of a battle, and the building of confidence that is transferable to any challenge in life.

I have been plagued by feelings of anger and rage due to the injustices I have had to live with, where I have had to live without closure, and continue to do so to this day. I have coped with this lack of closure with meditation since Dec 2014. Up until Dec 2014 I had not learned about using meditation to address and remedy anger that had been engrained in me over many years. I had only used meditation to remedy an anger brought upon me by a one- off incident back in 2012 at the Epilepsy Society over the drug training incident. Up until turning to meditation to remedy this engrained anger I relied on another technique. It is to be remembered that the emotional turmoil created within me by others had to be endured on top of the side effects of the anti-convulsant medication that I was on. This high level of irritability combined with too much time alone, too much time to think, too much trauma to reflect on; placed on me many occupational/vocational, academic, social hazards. It was important for me to stop the rage and anger as the more you thought about it, the worst it got, where no appropriate outlet for this increasing rage/anger led to the further development of anxiety and depression. It was from the time where I learned about escapism that I became aware of your thoughts creating your emotions, thus, impacting on your behaviours. Your thoughts are your mental joy stick. I therefore, learned to not think the thoughts that brought on this rage and anger. As I have already said, thinking is habitual and you can condition a mind that has habitually negative thoughts into one that has habitually positive ones. I went about achieving this by paying more attention to my thinking, and whenever a negative thought entered my head that brought on feelings of rage and anger, I would immediately pause the thought and see the thought explode in my mind; and replaced it with a more appropriate thought. This required a lot of **pausing, exploding** and **replacing** at first, but the requirement for these three got less and less over a period of about three weeks until I was no longer having such angry thoughts, and I was no longer feeling such emotions. The only problem is though, when you are no longer experiencing angry thoughts, you become complacent with your thinking, as you start to take not feeling angry for granted, and this can allow you to start letting in the angry thoughts again; forgetting to pause, explode and replace, causing your anger to relapse. There is also a "reluctance not to feel angry" that you have to fend off, as you think that on principle you should be angry, and to not be angry is to let people get away with things that they have done even though you know the anger which has no outlet is suffocating you with anxiety. This reluctance can be resolved by asking yourself, "Is it right that what these people did to me be allowed to cause me angina, heart disease, stroke by allowing their treatment of me to make me angry?". I also ask myself, "Will I feel angrier or less angry if I find myself having carers come into my room in a nursing home; to wash me, dress me and feed me and sit me there all day; where I can't do the things that I loved, such as living a very active lifestyle, because I had had a number of strokes that left me paralysed down one side of my body, with loss of speech and visual impairment, because I allowed these bullies and bigots to cause me to live with chronic anger for so many years of my life?". This question is then usually followed by a "Pause and a Bang!!"

CHAPTER 22

Living with epilepsy will unfortunately throw hazards at you when you are having a seizure that you cannot take any precautionary measures to protect yourself against purely because of the nature of the seizure. As consciousness is not lost, but is instead impaired to a state which could be described as a blackout, you are prone to behaving in bizarre ways due to loss of awareness and orientation, and therefore cannot risk assess your behaviours before carrying them out, nor do your behaviours have motives or purposes. You neither have any knowledge of past, awareness of present, or concept of future; and your behaviour has become meaningless and purposeless, with you having no awareness of anything that you are saying or doing. As a consequence of this, you can be in a night club, where upon experiencing the blackout phase of a complex partial epileptic seizure you go up to a table and sit on it, pick up a bottle of beer, pour all the beer out of it and then throw the bottle like a bowling ball onto the dance floor. A doorman or those sitting at the table are more likely to think that you have taken an illegal substance as opposed to being drunk and certainly would never consider a seizure being the cause of the bizarre behaviour. This can inevitably result in the doorman being very rough with you or you ending up being assaulted by those sitting at the table. This assault could be anything from someone pushing you to the floor, to a serious head injury, or even worse; being murdered. Living in a society where there is a knife culture, this can be a very likely outcome. This could result in a person with epilepsy developing social anxiety disorder. It is not the cause of my social anxiety disorder, which was school, but it could be the cause of someone else's social anxiety disorder who lives with complex partial epilepsy, or any other type of epilepsy that can make you centre of attention, and result in personal injury/loss; or even death. One epilepsy charity in Glasgow does offer befriending services, and one of the reasons why this service exists is because so many people with epilepsy will have social anxiety disorder, or at least a fear of being out and about in public places, but do not want to rely on social work services for a support worker to take them out. The problem is this befriending service was only one day a fortnight for a couple of hours, just taking them for a pub meal in the afternoon and then home again. Completely inadequate. This was back in 2003, I don't know what the service is today, but I certainly know how this charity treat staff with epilepsy, which you will learn about later in the book.

Epilepsy cannot only get you seriously assaulted/murdered by a member of the public but if you are a woman with epilepsy, having a complex partial epileptic seizure, where you are suffering from serious confusion while being out and about on your own, then it is an invitation for a passer- by to sexually assault you. It is also an opportunity for a passer- by to rob you of your possessions. You could come round from the amnesia phase to find yourself without your wallet, jacket, watch, jewellery etc. As well as getting yourself sexually assaulted or robbed from during a seizure. A seizure can also make you look like the sexual assaulter or the robber, where you could find yourself in a public place during the loss of awareness and orientation stage of the seizure; and find yourself going up to, and putting your hand on a women's breast inside a pub/bar in front of her boyfriend or in front of her friends, and the doorman then detains you until the police come. I must emphasise that the touching of one's breast would have no sexual motive behind it. Remember what I said in the first paragraph of this chapter, and that is the bizarre behaviour has no motive or purpose behind it. As well as the prospect of being falsely alleged to have sexually harassed or assaulted someone, you can also be set up by a seizure to look like you have taken something that does not belong to you. During a seizure you could very easily pick someone's laptop up and walk off with it when the owner is at the toilet, or even worse take a child's hand and walk off with it, thus, resulting in any charge from theft to attempting to abduct a child. A shop is a very vulnerable place to have a complex partial seizure and shoplifting is very often a charge that one experiencing a seizure finds themselves being landed with. What can start off as a warning to a seizure in a café, ends with one finding themselves outside a clothes shop in handcuffs.

These previous two paragraphs have only mentioned a few examples of risk you are exposed to when having a seizure in public; but the list of things that a person with epilepsy could be seriously assaulted for doing, charged with by the police (remember 1 in 50 people in prison have epilepsy), left badly injured; or experience loss of life, is endless. What makes a person with complex partial seizures even more vulnerable is the fact that neurologists often advise those who have been arrested during a complex partial seizure for behaviours mistaken for being criminal in nature to plead guilty at the sheriff court and be let off with a caution, as they find it difficult finding a lawyer who will take on their case, since the lawyer does not think the pay cheque is large enough to make it worth their time defending such a client. I've been told that a lawyer gets paid £200 to provide medical legal representation in the case of someone being charged under the influence of a seizure; and they do not see this as being a large enough sum of money to make it worth their while. As a result of this, those with partial seizures who plead guilty and get a caution often find themselves back in the sheriff court on a later date over another incident they were arrested for, and this time they either go to prison, get a community payback order or a large fine. They also end up with a criminal record that further jeopardises their prospects of getting a job as well as causes them to lose a job, if they are in a job that requires them to have a clean criminal disclosure. If they are training to become a health or social care professional or some other vocational position that requires a clean criminal disclosure then they could find themselves being put off the course.

I have had my two experiences of having a potential run in with the civilian as well as my brush with the law. My first of the two experiences was back in 1990 on the island of Rhodes where me and my family were having our annual summer holiday. During this stay in Rhodes we stayed in a hotel where I had my own hotel room. My hotel room was six floors up and had a veranda. The room next door to mine had a veranda as well where there was quite a gap between both verandas. I was sleeping in the humid hotel room one evening and it must have been around 2am. I woke up in my bed and suddenly felt the feeling of strong fear coming on, rising from my gut to my head and the blood leaving my face giving me that draining/tingling feeling in the nose and cheeks as well as that constricting feeling in the gut. I felt "White". Suddenly the world I went to bed in started to become fainter and fainter, and the seizure world became more and more prominent, where I started to feel the room becoming crowded discrediting any theory of being in a previous world i.e. the Real World. The bedroom had become Vatican like in atmosphere "with other people there" that weren't there. Throughout this full blown psycho-hallucination I was in a state of panic as the world was so alien and there was no previous world that I had come from and there was no future world I was going back to and that this alienation was for ever and had been the only thing I had ever known with full blown anxiety and fear. Then it was the fogging out of alertness and orientation. During this stage of the attack I got out of my bed and went out onto the veranda and climbed from my veranda onto the other veranda. I could have fallen sixty feet as it was five floors up possibly resulting in spinal injury, serious head injury or probably not worse; death, as I would rather be dead than seriously head injured or spinal injured. I've seen it in homes where support staff have been trying to feed fully grown men with baby bibs, rocking their head violently from side to side, with the support worker with one hand, feeding the client with a plastic spoon, and with the other hand, they are wiping away food running down the side of the client's face.

Once I was over my veranda and onto the next veranda, I opened the sliding door of the hotel room next door to mine. I walked into the room, which was the bedroom of a young girl. During this visit I climbed into the same bed as this girl, and she woke up and became very distressed. The girl had got a fright and panicked and her father came running into the room. I have no memory of this event and therefore cannot tell you how I responded. All I remember is being in the corridor of the hotel recovering from amnesia and hearing the voice of my Dad, which I was not recognising, apologising to the father of the girl, with the father saying that it was okay and not to worry about it. I remember him saying, "don't worry about it; these things happen". At this time though, I had had no idea that I had had a seizure. I had no memory of climbing from one veranda to the other, nor any memory of getting into bed with the girl sleeping in her bedroom. I was lucky not to have fallen sixty plus feet, and I was lucky not to have been assaulted by the father of the girl as well as lucky not to have had the police called and arrest me. If I had not had my family with me, and instead had been on holiday with drunken friends, I think it would have been a very different story. I was also only fifteen at the time, where as if I had been the age I am today; 43, I also think it could have been a very different outcome on first finding me in bed with the man's daughter. This happened in a country where the prison sentences aren't as liberal as in the UK. In 1990 Greece someone falsely accused of attempted sexual assault and found guilty would probably have got around 7 years in prison with no such thing as time considered spent for "good behaviour". There would also have been trespassing laws that I would have been accused of breaking. All I can say is that I am a very lucky person, and unfortunately too many in my position are not so lucky, and end up in prison. The lawyers that do represent people with epilepsy often say to those with complex partial seizures, "plead guilty", which has the same outcomes that apply when neurologists tell their patients to plead guilty. Lawyers can also find it very difficult finding a neurologist who is prepared to come to court and give evidence on behalf of someone with epilepsy as they do not see it as providing them with a large enough cheque. Many neurologists are only interested in the cases that let them earn mega-bucks such as compensation claims after head injury. This often gives the lawyer no alternative but to suggest to their client that they plead guilty. Neurologists giving evidence today on behalf of those with epilepsy, tend to be retired neurologists; as today's generation of doctor is of a very different personality type to the previous generation of doctor. As mentioned in chapter 2, medical schools set high grades as entry criteria, meaning you need 6A's at A-level to do medicine due to its popularity. This popularity is because of the huge pay and socio-economic position that doctors get, so as a result of this, many of those that become doctors do so for their love of money and not the disciplines that make up medicine; meaning the commitment of the doctor towards the patient has become increasingly compromised over the last thirty years. Universities should think more about the personalities of those that get into medicine and not the grades. In my opinion the entry criteria should be how much evidence your curriculum vitae has on it that evidences you to be someone who is interested in the patient. Examples of such evidence would be voluntary work, campaign work, previous employment, personal experience, hobbies & interests etc. I've been told by a neurologist that you don't even have to be good at science to be a doctor! It's all knowledge, requiring no understanding; unlike science, that requires both knowledge and understanding. I was told by my father that doing medicine was no more difficult than learning a telephone directory. It's all flow diagrams i.e. if this doesn't present with the following, then it will be that; or, if X doesn't work, then try Y.

The next experience of a seizure in public coming close to having a long-lasting compromise on my life was when I did have my brush with the law. What had happened was back in the year 2001, myself and a couple of friends had gone out for an evening in Glasgow where we started out having a few pints of lager and decided to go over the road to a place called the Cathouse night club which is a popular hangout for students and young adults in Glasgow. It was a Tuesday night and was therefore very quiet and I had had quite a bit to drink. Aftershocks were only a pound; and me and my friends were doing the usual, "Cheers Boys", and throwing the whole glass back in one. I had to count to ten and distract myself by imagining the sound of a waterfall to stop the nauseating feeling from making me sick. This distraction technique I used to control my symptoms of Obsessive Compulsive Disorder between the years 1993-1997, before I discovered aerobic exercise in 1999.

A LITTLE ON DISTRACTION

It was between 1993-1997 that my symptoms of OCD had me believe that I had caught HIV off toilet seats and handles as well as caused me to imagine things had happened to me that hadn't happened to me, that had carried the risk of catching HIV. It's amazing how the mind can convince you into believing things happened, that didn't happen, due to overindulgence. I would worry for hours about things having happened that never happened, and overcame this anxiety by engaging in three to four hours of constant distraction that would give me up to three days anxiety relief, and then I would be using the distraction technique again, once the anxiety had returned, to defuse the next bout of anxiety.

After defusing the anxiety, you suddenly realised how irrational your anxiety had been. No one taught me this; I just discovered it myself when I went to university. I just decided that I was no longer going to have this anxiety and I rejected it, and it was through this rejecting of it that I discovered Distraction. I just heard waterfalls in my mind, and the ferocious splashing of the water hitting the pool that it was falling into when I was experiencing a strong bout of 24/7 anxiety. I just listened, and listened, and listened etc, etc, etc, for three to four hours, followed by the anxiety disappearing for around three days. As the theme of my anxiety had changed between January 1998- July 1999 from catching HIV to thoughts intrusively telling myself to give up things I didn't want to give up, I no longer recognised the distress this was causing as being a symptom of the same anxiety disorder I was affected by during 1993-1997, and therefore never thought to use distraction up until finally admitting to myself that I was suffering from an anxiety disorder in July 1999, and remembered my PE teacher telling us when I was seventeen that if you are physically fit you are mentally fit, resulting in me from then on using aerobic exercise to get rid of this continued anxiety disorder that had been putting on a different face for the previous eighteen months.

I misused this waterfall distraction technique by using it to stop me from being sick after downing the aftershocks, resulting in me being able to drink more aftershocks causing me to become very drunk and start truly enjoying myself, but my friends were whining saying, "It's too quiet, it's rubbish tonight, we're going home", and I said "Well I'm staying out, goodbye guys", and went to the dance floor, and started dancing. It was a buzz being in there on your own dancing. Upon 3am the doormen came up the stairs and said, "That's it guys, Could you please finish your drinks and leave by the exit to the staircase". I did what they asked and was walking down the stairs and started walking up Union Street seeing taxis pull away from kerbsides; drunks jumping into other taxis; people just acting like clowns on the pavement side with their pizza boxes and kebabs, where I suddenly felt fear starting in my stomach, rising to my face, and thought to myself "Oh my God! I have been seventeen hours without medication". It was as though I was a land animal suddenly discovering himself to be at the bottom of the ocean. There was a period of denial, but the transition happened and full blown seizure came to full fruition. The next thing I remember is being 200 metres up the road standing at the foot of the side entrance to Glasgow Central Station handcuffed. I had no memory of anything that happened before hand. I was just standing amongst this crowd of around four police officers waiting for a car to take me, the arresting officer and his colleague; as a witness of the arrest, to Cowcaddens Police station. I think that I must have had another seizure as by the time I arrived at the police station the amnesia was still lifting and the police station had the same atmosphere as the mental maze I am in when I am trying to find out day of the week, time of day, all information that defines me e.g. what I do for a living, where I am to be and when I am to be there etc. I remember from this evening being taken down to a room to pick up a mattress and a blanket and ushered into a cell which, if memory serves me correctly, had a red floor and white walls with a concrete bed along the far wall of the cell. I also remember a smell of disinfectant and throughout the arrest process I wasn't making sense of what I was being told I was being arrested for and what I had done. I was just being told to shut up as well as having my claims that I did not know why I had been arrested dismissed, and told to just participate in the usual protocol of an arrest. The police left me in a cell for a period of time I cannot remember being in the cell for, but the point is they left me in there without my medication, after possibly having two previous seizures, never mind just one. I had already had a seizure (possibly two) due to medication deprivation and here I was continuing to spend even more hours without my night time medication. I could have had what is called a 'secondary generalised seizure' if I had had another seizure, which is where a complex partial seizure develops into a full blown tonic- clonic seizure that affects the whole brain as a consequence of continued drug deprivation, as well as alcohol withdrawal. If that had happened, I could have died in police custody due to head injuries sustained from having a violent tonic-clonic seizure on a concrete floor with no one around to cushion my head. This does happen. If you search google you will find lots of stories of people with epilepsy who have died in police custody. Treatment of people with epilepsy in police custody is shocking. A story in the 'Independent newspaper' back in 2014 reports of a nineteen year old dying in police custody after the police failed to notice him have three epileptic seizures on their CTV system; in the same newspaper you only have to wait until the year 2016 to learn that a man with epilepsy died when he was restrained during an epileptic seizure and sprayed with pepper spray. In September 2014, a mother is reported as being furious over the death of her son from an epileptic seizure while being in police custody. I encourage you to search this subject as there is a huge amount to be found on it.

After my stay in the cell I was taken down to a room where I was photographed and fingerprinted. I was then taken out to the area of the police station you are discharged back into the community from to be informed that a report will be sent to the sheriff court and that I was being charged with breaking into a car and stealing the contents of that car e.g. CD's and other. The next thing I would hear would be contact from the sheriff court informing me of my date in court. After my arrest the charges were dropped which was probably because of the Prosecution's judgemental attitude which was most likely, "This guy is going into teacher training in a matter of a few weeks and therefore must be telling us the truth"; however, if I had not had an educated accent, nor was going into teacher training; the outcome I dare say would have been very different.

After learning that I was not going to be prosecuted, I wrote to the police telling them that their training on epilepsy was inadequate and that I wished to come along and give a presentation on epilepsy and my experience with the law. In their reply to my letter they said that their curriculum was full enough to make competent police officers and that they did not need me giving them lectures. Well they said this back in 2001 and these newspaper articles I informed you about where people with epilepsy had died in custody are 2014 and 2016. As has already been mentioned in previous reference to the police in this book "Ego costs Lives". Maybe, if I had been allowed to give these presentations in 2001, police forces all over the country would have been encouraged to invite me to give presentation by forces who had already attended my presentation, meaning that those police officers who oversaw the deaths of those with epilepsy in 2014 and 2016 would have been more aware of the dangers people with epilepsy face in custody and they would have kept a more watchful eye preventing these deaths.

My most recent two experiences of a seizure in public where I could have got myself either assaulted by a street civilian or been in trouble with the police were both back in 2009 where the first of the two incidents was an incident where I was walking home from a nightclub from the centre of Glasgow back to my house at 4am in the morning, which was a four mile walk; and I had not had my night time medication. When you're drunk you're "Mr Bravado", and you don't fear having a seizure because of missed medication. Your attitude is "I will worry about the seizure when it happens! Until then I don't have epilepsy".

 The only memory I have of that four mile walk is one of freaking out on two guys, where both guys were saying, "Calm down!!" repeatedly. If memory is correct the two men were very shocked themselves, as though they had been taken by total surprise. I have no memory of any event that led to this hysterical state. I was told by a doctor that I would have had a seizure where like all complex partial seizures I would have been walking around during the blackout phase with impaired consciousness where someone had obviously come up and asked me if I was okay and most likely put their hand on me to escort me away from a road. Like all seizures, you should not touch the person during such a seizure as this can cause the person to experience a state of shock bringing on challenging behaviour. This is also known as "disrupting the seizure" and is something that an observer must not do. Fortunately for me, the men that I had the seizure in front of had no criminal intentions when approaching me, as having a seizure in public does provide an opportunity for someone to rob me, and then feel the need to badly physically assault me when I "explode". I was also fortunate that they were understanding enough to tolerate my hostility, and not feel any wish to counter attack. If they had, with two of them and myself in a state of impaired consciousness, there is no having to guess who would have come out of such a confrontation the worst. I did have a client with autism, when I was an advocate, who because of his symptoms, became aggressive towards a group of teenage boys who had antagonised him, that resulted in the boys jumping up and down on his head and leaving him head injured. I remember going to the court with my client to give him moral support and the gang of boys all walked away from court with grins as it was deemed that my client had started the fight.

In 2009 I also had a seizure in the gym changing rooms. I had my seizure while I was undressing out of my gym gear on route to the shower. I remember staring into my locker to get my bag and towel and suddenly the onset of symptoms came on but very subtly. At first, I was thinking and feeling; "This isn't happening, and I am just imagining", and then it became "It is happening"; followed by "It is happening, but it's not coming"; to "Its coming, and it's now happening". There was no warning it was like for around one minute the real world was going from 100% to 98% to 96% to 94% and the seizure world going from 0% to 2%, to 4%, to 6%, unlike the usual transition that happens in increments of 10%. The seizure world was coming to fruition and the real world fading in very small increments of only 2% for the first minute. When the seizure world comes on in such small increments and the real world disappears in the same small increments you do at first think that what you are experiencing is maybe imagination and not genuine onset of seizure. After one minute the real world went from 90 to 80 to 70 etc and the seizure world 10 to 20 to 30 etc which is when you realise that it's not imagination and you are in fact experiencing onset of seizure. I then experienced full blown onset of seizure and the next thing I remember is the gym instructor shouting at me and following me while I was confused and walking away from him. I was being shouted at, at a time where I did not know I was in a gym, I had no knowledge of having recently done a workout and had no knowledge nor could make sense of what the gym employee was shouting at me for. All I knew was that I didn't know anything. At the time of fully recovering I was shouting at the gym instructor simply because he was shouting at me. The manager came into the changing room and demanded someone explain what had happened and what all the shouting was about. I said to the manager, "I have just had a complex partial epileptic seizure". The manager was very accommodating, and the fitness instructor's jaw dropped and suddenly started apologising to me saying he was really sorry and that he had never come across this before. I sat with the instructor in the changing room until I was recovered enough to get changed, and I went out to the seating area where they sell all the prospective members their new membership, and was told by the fitness instructor that I had gone into a number of men's showers while they were trying to wash. I said that maybe they should lock their shower doors, but dropped it as I was just glad I had not been assaulted or reported to the police. This experience would put anyone with complex partial seizures off ever using public swimming pools. If this is the reception one with epilepsy gets when walking into shower cubicles with fully grown men, then what would it be like if I were to walk into cubicles with children, or walked into the women's changing room, and got into their showers. It is my experience that people always like to expect the worst case scenario. People love to expect the best newspaper headline, and therefore even though you would appear confused, I have no confidence that this confusion would not be overlooked when determining a man's reason for going into a women's shower. The police didn't recognise my confusion during the arrest, nor the rate of recovery. The rate of recovery from the seizure should have told them that I was not under the influence of an illegal compound, nor did I do what I did as a result of ingesting something that impaired my cognition. They should have also known from my confusion that my decision to get into someone's car was not one I had made voluntarily, and that my meaningless, purposeless language was evidence of me not being under the influence of alcohol.

As a daytime seizure was unusual for me to have, and I had, had all my medications, and a good night's sleep the night before the seizure I had in the locker room of the gym in 2009, the only theory that would have explained the daytime event, would have been the food I had eaten in the last 24 hours having either the food additive 'aspartame' or 'monosodium glutamate' in it. I went home and took out of the bin an empty tin of chicken soup that I had had for dinner the night before, and looked at the ingredients label, and there it was "E621". This E-number, E621, is the E-number of 'Monosodium Glutamate'. As a consequence of this I now look at all ingredient labels of all new foods that I add to my diet. I must avoid this substance like a person with nut allergy must avoid nuts. It is dangerous, and its dangerous effects have been given great publicity in America but not in Britain, and many groups in America have tried to have it banned from all food manufacturing but with little luck as it gives people food cravings encouraging people to buy more. Monosodium glutamate is known as a "neurotoxin", and when MSG is put in foods in high doses, such as Chinese food; a full blown transition into seizure can just suddenly come on without warning within minutes of ingesting. When the MSG is used in low doses, such as in the soup I had eaten the night before, it brings on seizures hours after ingestion and the seizures come on without a typical warning in the same way the seizure in the gym changing rooms was described as coming on.

There have been a number of times since 2009 where I have had seizures in the gym. There have been around four daytime seizures, where on three occasions I have come round with paramedics and gym staff sitting around me; and on the fourth occasion I came round sitting on the floor with the gym manager giving me a bottle of fluids with salt, as he believed my reason for having a seizure was excess loss of salt during the workout. All these seizures were antagonised by missed doses or a missed night's sleep the night before.

I have had little momentary pinch transitions just lasting seconds without any warning on afternoons when I have been in the gym pushing myself, after having missed the night before meal as well as having had no morning breakfast. These pinch transitions happen because my sodium levels are low, as my salt intake has been nil, therefore the lost sodium in my sweat makes my sodium levels very low, and you will remember from chapter 1 that seizures are brought on by your cellular sodium levels going all over the place. This state where I have little transitions in the gym due to low sodium levels is called "Hyponatraemia", but it never brings on a seizure, just little momentary disturbing "suddenly in seizure world, immediately back in this world" transitions, where the transitions could be described as being "low volume". I can't describe in words what I mean by "low volume" but I believe it may be when the amplitude of the disturbed brainwaves is low just like is the case with noise i.e. a low volume sound, is sound waves with low amplitude. I will make an attempt at describing what I mean by "low volume", and that is I feel like I am a "spectator" of the transition, as opposed to be "being a part" of the transition, where I am both "watching and feeling" the real world turning into the seizure world, where I am removed from the seizure experience keeping me in the world I am in, cycling on my bike; but where I get a true appreciation for how convincing the seizure world is, to the point where the front of my mind is convinced and feels the seizure world to be undeniably real, but the back of mind knows that it is not, where I then experience the front of the mind becoming convinced of the seizure world being unreal as the seizure world I am "watching and feeling" goes back into real world. I get a "ying-yang" interpretation of the world that I am detached from, unlike when I have a seizure where I feel myself to be engulfed by this "ying-yang" interpretation of the world, however despite the ying-yang interpretation being something I am detached from it is still convincing. It's as though memory is the source of the experience I am   having and not present moment disturbance in electrical activity, which would explain why I don't feel myself being a part of the experience and instead feel more like a satellite looking down on the experience.

The problem with a complex partial seizure's symptoms is, to the observer they can be mistaken for a diabetic hypoglycaemic attack, which makes more sense for someone to be having in a gym, to a gym instructor who is not educated on epilepsy. As a consequence of everyone thinking "diabetes" everyone immediately jumps to the phone to dial "999" when all that is required, is for a gym instructor to follow me, making sure I do not stray into danger; explaining to people around me what I am having, and then reassure me until full recovery from the amnesia. It is the case that despite the aggressive nature of a seizure, regardless of seizure type, as well as the dangers to your health and safety that you are exposed to during a seizure, someone having an epileptic seizure does not constitute a medical emergency. An epileptic seizure only becomes a medical emergency if it is a person's first ever seizure, as it could be a sign that someone has just had a stroke, or when someone with epilepsy has a generalised tonic-clonic seizure that develops into another seizure without the person regaining consciousness in between seizures. This going from one seizure into another without gaining consciousness is called "Status Epilepticus", and requires the administration of emergency medication. A tonic-clonic epileptic seizure is also considered a medical emergency if the seizure lasts longer than five minutes and no one knows the usual length of time that a typical seizure in the affected person goes on for. All seizures become medical emergencies if there is any serious physical damage such as suspected head injury, spinal injury, burns, inhalation of foreign objects etc.

I am a non-pretentious person and I will speak my mind as living in an unaccommodating of epilepsy society has been character building, but can also be character destroying. It's character building for those who choose to not conform as by doing this you have to develop survival skills, knowledge, grow determination, perseverance and develop a high mental pain threshold and rid your fear of authority. All of these traits have made me a non-pretentious person who "calls a spade a spade". If someone is an idiot, I will say so, but my calling of them an idiot will be evidenced. If any person can evidence this person to not be an idiot then I will take back my claim of them being an idiot. It is for this reason that I will say the police are impulsive, ignorant, egocentric, narcissistic, bullies as well as intolerant. I have only seen evidence of them being of these traits in my experience. It's sounding like the police have a personality disorder. It sounds like I am angry. Yes, I am angry. Not nearly as angry as I would be if I didn't meditate. If I didn't meditate, I would be so angry that I would want to be authority's worst nightmare. The anger would have made me an anarchist. I would have been breaking the law "left, right and centre". It just shows you that the legal system and society as a whole criminalises people. It is assumed that only greedy bad people become criminals. This is not the case. Those who have been traumatised by bad people holding legitimate positions of responsibility and power in our society can end up in crime because the abuse received can have too scarring an effect on their character to be able to hold down a legitimate position in our society, and they end up gravitating into a role under the employment of someone who sees their temper and grudging of society as a vocational asset, and the affected person sees such a role as being an outlet for the anger and an opportunity for "get back at society time", for giving them such a bruising of an upbringing. Society throws bricks at these peoples' houses throughout childhood, adolescence and beyond, so what do you expect?. They are going to throw bricks back at society's house, which a career in crime gives them the opportunity to do. Psychiatrists have referred this throwing of bricks back at society by those with epilepsy as the "Epileptic personality". What an insult, doesn't it just make you angry and want to throw a brick!.

I as someone with epilepsy have to say that the charities don't address any of the issues that this book has discussed so far. Why am I the person writing to the police telling them they need a lecture on epilepsy. This is surely something the charities should have covered. Social workers don't even touch on the subject of epilepsy during their training, nor do nursing students; as unbelievable as this may sound. Support workers working in learning disability homes or working in the community get a one day training every year to renew their emergency medication certificate which is much better than any of the rest get, but still inadequate. When I was a nursing student I did three years at university, and if you had asked a final placement nursing student to tell you about epilepsy they would have stared at you blankly. You ask what were we learning during these three years. Certainly not value for money information for every tax payer with epilepsy. The same could be said for numerous other conditions as well. Instead we were taught things like "How to resolve an ethical dilemma", if you were studying social work; or "The nurse's role in health promotion", if you were a nursing student. It won't be long until they are training police officers at university where they will be asked to write 3,000 words on "The police man's role in the arrest process". The country has gone crazy and as a non-conformist I blame conformity. People just sit back and allow this madness to happen. Tony Blair was the worst thing that happened to higher education. He used human insecurity to make himself popular by promising everyone a university degree. A degree would have protected a person with epilepsy from discrimination and prejudice in the 1970's and 1980's. Tony Blair destroyed this lifeline causing those with epilepsy to find themselves swimming amongst the sharks. Socio-educational/economic status and wealth are the only left- wing issues people want to discuss. Why? Simply because they remedy human insecurity as well as vent a rage that is often justified but too often caused by an unsatisfied greed!!!

Much better education on epilepsy is needed amongst those who uphold the law, and that includes lawyers, police, social workers etc. These people also need an education on the psycho-social consequences of wrongful conviction as well as discrimination that can push a person with epilepsy and living with other disadvantage into crime. I appreciate that there are too many conditions to teach all these professions/vocations about, however, there is so much overlap in terms of the issues faced by those with these different disabilities, and it is the "overlap" relevant to their professions that they should be taught about. An absolutely useless education system!!! Those that uphold the law, design the infrastructure of our health and social care system, our education system as well as anyone who can call themselves an employer or educator, should all be taught about the **DAMAGE & COLLATERAL DAMAGE OF: BAD DECISION MAKING, IMPLEMENTATION OF ONE SIZE FITS ALL RULES & REGULATIONS, DISCRIMINATION/PREJUDICE, PUTTING CAREER PATHS BEFORE WELLBEING AND SO MUCH, MUCH, MUCH MORE!!!!!!!!!!!!**

CHAPTER 23

Relationships are important as the people you have relationships with are your allies in life. These are the people you are going to turn to during times of crisis. Your life is designed by the society that we live in to be a team sport, and that team is made up of yourself as the captain, your family and your friends. It must be stressed that this is not some sort of hierarchy. I am a sense of purpose person who is non-pretentious and regardless of rank, amount of power and number of responsibilities; if you have as much as one responsibility which if were not fulfilled by someone in your role, the shared aim and objective of the team would be unachievable, then you are as important as the captain. A good analogy to demonstrate this would be "What is more important? The engine or a couple of square feet of hull of a ship, in the fulfilling of the ship's purpose". Naive people would say, "The engine"; whereas logical people would say, "Neither, without one the boat does not propel forward, thus, making it stranded; and without the other you have sea flooding in, thus, sinking the boat.

I was born into a family which is made up of a mother, father, two sisters, two aunts, two uncles and four cousins. I come from a family where the aunts, uncles and cousins do not live locally. I very rarely see the uncles and aunts. I possibly see my uncle and aunt from my Dad's side of the family a few times per year when they come up to Helensburgh from Leeds where they stay for a weekend and I go round to my parents to meet them and spend around five hours with them having a catch up, a meal and then a walk or visit somewhere in the local area. I then say good bye until the next time. The uncle and aunt from my mother's side of the family lived in Aberdeen and in recent years moved to Ayrshire. I see them once every three to five years. The cousins on my Dad's side of the family I probably see once every seven years, as they live in Leeds and New Zealand, and the cousins on my mother's side of the family I probably cross paths with just as many times and couldn't tell you where they live. We are a family where certainly amongst the sisters, aunts, uncles and cousins, the priority area of concern for each has not been the mental and physical wellbeing of others. Family has not been seen as a team that help one another get through the challenges of life. Family has instead been seen as a group of people to celebrate novelty events with. We meet up, and it's the novelty of meeting one another for the first time in months to years that is celebrated, and is the only thing that family members are interested in. As a result of this, family get togethers are to be celebrations, and therefore anything that cannot be celebrated as it is an area of great concern is met with no interest, or if were to be shared, you would be accused of spoiling the event. This is evidenced by the fact that the only time we do meet with my mother's side of the family or cousins from my father's side is at Weddings, Christmas, New Year, birthdays celebrating landmark ages i.e. 50ths, 65ths etc. The only thing we meet for that is not celebratory is funerals. If someone said, "You meet with your cousins in a few weeks time" and I am told this at a time that is not in the run up to Christmas/new year, a birthday or a wedding; I would be thinking to myself "Shit, who died". At least my aunt and uncle from my father's side make the effort to visit every three months.

We are not a close family and one of the symptoms of depression is social withdrawal at group events. The depressed person will always sin bin themselves into another room because they just don't feel like partying or being part of the crowd. I at Christmas and New Year events, from the year 1997 to 2008, always withdrew and went to my room after a few hours of our family members arriving. I didn't speak much, and got irritable before withdrawing. I spent hours up in my room, and only came back down to say good bye; until the next new year day the aunt, uncle and cousins on my mother's side of the family would be back in Glasgow. I was like, "Yeah sure, see you next year". I felt betrayed by my uncle who was a psychiatrist who should have been able to recognise the symptoms of depression, as I didn't want to be a recluse at these parties but I couldn't help it. Cynics would say that I was an attention seeker. I would say to them, "You say that because that is all you know. You say that because you know no other reason as to why someone would need a member of the family's help to get them out their room and back downstairs". This might surprise you as it sounds like attention seeking but it is very different. Attention seeking is where you love attention, and you get enough, but you have a greed for more as it gives you are narcissistic trip. It is like the girl who knows she is very good looking and deliberately puts a picture of her body on facebook in the knowledge that she is going to get lots of positive comments about her looks and it is going to make her big head even bigger; and just like attention seekers get moody if they do not get their attention, the girl who knows she's good looking who puts her picture on facebook gets really moody and has a temper tantrum if no one has commented on how good looking she is. That is attention seeking's definition explained. You are looking for more than you need so your morale is not just high but very high. Attention seeking also involves an element of drama. A temper tantrum is usually thrown in front of everyone if attention is not received or a behaviour that shines the spot light on the person seeking the attention. Withdrawal is the opposite of shining a light on yourself. You withdraw because you feel drained by the company and find the company uninspiring and wish they would just all fuck off!.

Very often the attention, the attention seeker is craving, does not need to be of a healthy type. A mother shouting her head off at her attention seeking child is very often giving the child the attention they are seeking. Attention seekers will settle for any type of attention. In my case what I was needing was more attention than the others without compromising the amount of attention the others were currently getting because I had a low opinion of myself. I had very low morale and self-esteem and had sub- zero levels of confidence because of it. I needed to feel valued and recognised to the same extent as my sisters and cousins but because I felt much less valued and recognised than them because of living a very difficult life where people had been overly critical towards me throughout childhood and adolescence I needed more attention to get my feeling of being valued and recognised up to their feelings of being valued and recognised. My relationship with the world had been one of put down and constant criticism i.e. me-teacher, peers etc. This personal-critical had also come from cousins. As a consequence of this I was needing relationships that were   personal-praise in nature to compensate for the personal-critical, and family members were the only likely people of forming such a relationship with me. Attention; where quantity given is determined by need, is like a morale and self-esteem booster and some of us need higher doses than others, as well as different types, to remedy damage done by others, because we have had more attacks on our morale and self-esteem. Who does the medic spend more time with; the person who has passed the army medical assessment or the severe burns victim? Does a repair job on a home that has a crumbling wall, require the same amount of attention as a repair job on the reglazing of a cracked glass window pane? It is this kind of demonising the amount of time required to do the repair job that psychiatry is guilty of. The more damage done to you by others, the greater the amount of attention required by others to repair the damage, thus, resulting in the greater amount of demonising of you by psychiatrists through the diagnosing you with conditions that have the most offensive names. **Psychiatry is of the ethos that the most shameful thing in the world is the "self" and anything that affects the "self" regardless of who is responsible for it is a terrible condemnation of the "self" that the "self" should be seen as being the cause of. Psychiatry does not recognise the character shaping effects of both politics and sociology. It fails to recognise the flaws in our education system, family lives, one size fits all systems, benefits system, the failings of laws such as the Equality Act, the corruption of authorities such as councils/housing associations/charities etc that others become victims of and the issues they find themselves living without closure on, the sadistic streak that exists in humans (as it carries out no research into what is a normal person) and the perverse joy others get from traumatising others, the majority's susceptibility to low morale and self- esteem and how they resort to belittlement and confidence bashing of others to remedy this insecurity and many more. Psychiatry believes we live in the ideal world, that is a level playing field for everyone, where no one has any grounds for making complaints, nor feel negative emotions; and, therefore negative behaviours and complaints can be seen as symptoms of mental illness.**

Attention seeking is like an addiction where attention seekers want more attention to give themselves an ego trip, which is a very different mentality, where they become temperamental if they do not get that high they are after. They are narcissists with an aggressive streak in them. Attention needing is meeting a need, whereas attention seeking is feeding a greed. The two must not be confused. Attention can patch a wound. Unfortunately, attention can also be used for "cosmetic" purposes.

To demonstrate that I had this greater need than my cousins and sisters I will describe the difference in fortunes that we have had in life. I don't wish sympathy but what I would hope for is that those reading this will learn from it and have a greater insight into how as a society we can treat people better during their formative years, as well as the importance of not using a one size fits all model of family. I would then hope that this information would then be applied to practice in the everyday reality of those reading this book. As you know, school was a struggle, and I was a D stream boy having one seizure every 36 hrs, where learning was done on top of the side effects of medication. I was from time to time humiliated by teachers, and peers, that left scars that I carry to this day at age 43. Never was I praised by teachers and peers, and instead only criticised. I scraped passes, got my degree but I was bottom of my year at university and not allowed graduate membership of the Royal Society of Biology, as I got a 3rd Class Honours Degree, despite it being a passed degree; and then continued to experience the same experiences I had at university during my vocational training. I am left with social anxiety disorder, which according to 'wikipedia' I am affected to a degree that meets the criteria for a diagnosis of Post -Traumatic Stress Disorder if you are someone who questions logic i.e. is suicidal ideation many years later not "near death"? Social anxiety disorder meets the same diagnostic criteria, according to the Diagnostic Statistical Manual, as post-traumatic stress disorder but for two criteria, and they are; for someone to be diagnosed with post-traumatic stress disorder there has to have been a near death event at the time of trauma, and that the trauma has to have come from a one off event such as a road traffic collision. It is the case that with social anxiety disorder, the death can occur many years later in the form of a suicide where the trauma has been caused by many years of trauma. The final outcomes of the two conditions can be just as catastrophic, yet everyone has heard of post-traumatic stress disorder, yet only a very few people, in comparison, have heard of social anxiety disorder, which is ironic considering the prevalence of social anxiety disorder, both diagnosed and undiagnosed is far greater that that of post-traumatic stress disorder. Social anxiety disorder is the third most common mental health complaint after depression and anxiety, with a lifetime prevalence of 11%; and post-traumatic stress disorder with a lifetime prevalence of 7%, according to the 'National Institute for Care & Excellence (NICE)'.

At the time of first withdrawing from the family at these family events I had only held a low skilled job despite having an honours degree. My cousins on the other hand were both university graduates who got into accountancy at university, in an era where you needed very good grades, and after qualifying, got good jobs in London, and my sisters were both Strathclyde University graduates in law, and both became lawyers. My oldest sister had never failed an exam at school, had always been tin the A-stream, got 3A's and 2B's in her highers, received an unconditional offer for university before her final year at school, allowing her to enjoy her 6th year. Throughout my oldest sister's journey through her school years, her teachers never had a bad thing to say about her. Both sisters left university with 2:1 Honour Degrees in Law, and have been in good jobs ever since. My eldest sister was a prosecutor at the age of twenty four, and is now some successful lawyer living in a very wealthy Glasgow suburb; twenty three years into her law career, in some big law company, married with children; and I have learned that my eldest sister's son has been sent to the same school that she went to. I would never send my son to the school I went to. Just shows you how different our experiences were at school. It is for this reason that I needed more attention than the others, as their morale and self- esteem were much higher than mine, and our morale and self- esteem is a measure of the judgement we have of ourselves, which is very much shaped by the judgement others have of us. To give us all the same dose of something some of us needed more of than others was inadequate. It was too similar to the "one size fits all" model of practice of our authorities in society, and with my feelings of anti-authority I inevitably felt anti-family. Some of us live much more eventful lives than others and will therefore inevitably require more time than others to update relatives on what has been happening in our lives. To deny us the time to report back on events since the last time we met felt like a snub.

Attention is a need of all people. It tells you people care, it gives you a feeling of belonging, it makes you feel valued, and builds bonds between you and others, where healthy attention can repair the damage that others caused when making you centre of attention for the wrong reasons e.g. the clock face in French; as well as giving you one to one in private unhealthy attention such as during destructive criticism when receiving feedback.

We all get angry when we meet someone who can only talk about themselves, which demonstrates that we all need others to show an interest in us up to a point. Once you are beyond that point i.e. high morale and self-esteem, it then becomes narcissism i.e. attention seeking. Once the morale and self-esteem is at a level like the others, the extra attention can then be tapered off to a level of attention that everyone else is getting. To give everyone the same amount of attention where the attention is not personalised to meet an individual's needs, and is best described as being generic, is just "tick box" obligatory attention, with no real interest or concern. A sports coach wouldn't give one of his top performing athletes the same amount of attention as another one of his athletes whose diet and fitness levels are all over the place due to coming back after an injury.

I would describe my family as being very establishment in attitude towards its members. To give everyone the same amount of time and attention was not just tick box and obligatory attention but it was also a one size fits all approach to taking care of family members. This one size fits all culture is the very ethos of establishment i.e. authoritative bodies, such as social work and housing. As my family had the same ethos as establishment and I had grown up anti-establishment, my isolating myself to another room was also encouraged by the anti-establishment rebel within me. I saw family more as an authority that had rules dictating where we were to be on particular dates, what obligations we had to fulfil on these dates i.e. have a smile, be in a party state of mind, be enjoying the company, talking about some subjects but not others that mattered; than as a support network made up of caring compassionate relatives. It was a family that was very institutional in nature and was of the attitude that all people should smile and be in a particular way for the gratification of others; that I couldn't have cared less about, considering I only saw these people once every year for a few hours, where time spent with each relative on a one to one was like your 15 minutes with your G.P. and that was all you were entitled to so the others could get their 15 minutes. You couldn't get a more impersonal model of family. This model of family created the most meaningless, as well as disappointing relationships, and gave me more reason to have nothing to do with it than it gave me reason to be a part of it.

I believe that our family could have worked better for all of us if there had been more 1:1 time with uncle and nephew, aunt and niece, more invites up north and down south, more activities and past times shared between uncles/aunts with their nieces/nephews, and a grandmother who didn't have preferences over others, which just created a hierarchy in the family. I had a grandmother who always took the side of the eldest in the family where regardless of who was at fault it was the youngest who always got the blame. My grandmother was forever criticising me and telling me off and forever mentioning how my eldest cousin was a wonderful impressive young boy that his parents could be truly proud of. This just created a division between me and my cousin during my formative years that affected me far more than it affected him.

Some people reading this might think "Needy". The last thing I would call myself is Needy. I treat my depression with meditation and aerobic exercise without any help from family, friends, mental health professionals or the pharmaceutical industry. I have treated night time panic with slow breathing, brought on by feelings of being alone in a world that doesn't care; where I have no one to turn to, to help me fight these two monster conditions on top of my night time epilepsy. I use positive thinking to keep me going during times of feeling like my life is in free-fall; as I do not know where my life is going, as it is absent of goals due to absence of opportunities, and have no-one to speak to, to help ease the distress this causes other than my own self talk. I feel that I have lost twenty years of my life in terms of joy and what I could have done with them without these debilitating conditions, thus inspiring me to try and reclaim as many of these years back by going to the gym and exercising aerobically as well as making sure I eat a diet that is good for brain, mind and rest of body. I would describe myself as a very independent person who performs far better in any new role under self- directed learning, evidenced by the work I did when I was an advocate, which because I excelled at, made a number of authorities fear my charity enough to want to bad mouth it enough to have it closed if I had got funding. During this; over three years of being an advocate, I resolved many life issues for people that were life transforming and eliminated the power imbalance between lay person and establishment, and probably made a lot of people in the advocacy community itself feel very insecure. I have been twenty years socially isolated and coped without friends and family by getting by with nothing more than my own company as well as symptom self-management techniques such as meditation, exercise and positive thinking. I can do all the things that most people would not dare do through fear of other peoples' evaluations of them such as go to the pub on my own; as well as go to night clubs on my own, and sit on my own in restaurants on Saturday nights etc; and I am quite happy to admit to people that I have just met that I have no friends nor supportive family, and I get a buzz doing things on my own that most people would require to do with someone else holding their hand. The number of people who can't attend a new social club night without taking a friend with them! I would therefore describe myself very much as being an independent person, and a survivor; and therefore, the last thing I would describe myself as being is "Needy". You could say in response to me saying that I am not needy that I am biased, but my claims of not being needy can be and have been evidenced in this very paragraph.

I don't get jealous. I don't compare myself with others, as life is a journey, and no two people walk the same journey. We all walk journeys that are different lengths, have more hills than others, have more mountains than others, where the mountains have different gradients and altitudes to others. Some lives are therefore more demanding than others. A person's life can be anything from a "walk in the park", to a "walk through the Himalayas". Some of us will need more muscle, bigger hearts, higher red blood cell counts and bigger lungs than others. Some of us will need the odd mountain rescue from time to time, and it is too easy for those who have lived lives that are not too challenging to persecute those who use up a lot of resources on their journey through life, and I am afraid to say that my sisters have been guilty of this. My sisters think I am attention seeking, have been given too much attention from my parents in comparison to them, have been a challenging son that has just created chaos for my family, never stops complaining, aggressive and afflicted by challenging behaviour. Parents with a child with extra needs should explain to their children all about the "activities of daily living", going over with them where their sibling struggles, and why as well as what help will be required in helping their sibling meet these activities of daily living i.e. education, socialising, health and wellbeing etc and therefore, how this extra time given to their sibling will be spent, so that the other children are under no illusion that the extra time is preferential treatment over the others, and it also educates the other children on their siblings needs, making them better people and ensuring that there are no ill feelings between the siblings when they are older and that the sibling with the extra needs will not be denied a family due to fallouts created by frictions that go back to childhood brought on by the illusion that one child was given preferential treatment over another. It is because of my parents failing at doing this that I am in a position where unless I meet a partner I am now without family for the rest of my days. No one to advocate for me if I ever become ill to the point of needing looking after. My days as a disability advocate inform me of how vulnerable having no one to act as advocate, next of kin, someone to act as power of attorney or guardian etc makes a person; and it is therefore, for this reason that I stick religiously to a healthy lifestyle i.e. exercise, meditate, eat a healthy diet, watch my weight, look after my cognitive health through reading books/playing chess/doing sudoku, minimise alcohol intake, as well as sugar and salt etc, so that I will remain independent all my life and have no reliance on people like social work, who have already proven themselves to be untrustworthy through both my advocacy work as well as my experience of being put off the social work course in 2008.

I have not spoken to my sisters in three years. In the four and a half years of living away from home, in both the Midlands (2001-2003) and Slough (2009-2012), they never came to visit me once. The only times we have seen one another up until three years ago was once per week on a Sunday at the parents' home, and the meeting of them just felt like a chore because I knew that if our parents weren't here we would never see one another again. In 2015 I said to my father that my sisters and brother in laws could have gone a long way in helping me with my isolation by meeting with me for coffees and going for a lunch and introducing me to their friends, and I said to my Dad that it was a neglect as they knew I was suffering and were not interested in helping. When I said to my Dad in March 2015 that I did not want these people in my life because I grudged them so much, but at the same time, I needed them so much and was therefore very confused and asked him if he understood where I was coming from, he said, "No, I don't understand where you are coming from". That made me feel even more misunderstood, as well as trapped, and I ended up attacking my Dad. My Dad managed to escape by breaking free from the hold I had him in, and sprinted towards my front door and out the flat with me chasing him, and he phoned both the police and ambulance service because he thought I had lost all sanity as I had been on the phone to him earlier that day reporting symptoms of 'derealisation'. Immediately after my Dad escaping, I went for a walk, and when I came back to my flat I saw the ambulance as well as the police arrive at my flat. I was taken up to the Accident & Emergency department by the police, where they waited for the Community Mental health Team to come and see me. The police waited with me until I had been seen by medical staff and it had been determined whether or not my Dad was going to press charges against me for assaulting him. I spoke to the policeman before he offered my father the opportunity to press charges, and educated him on the hierarchy of needs; mentioning that love and belonging were a need, and that these things are not just needs during childhood; and that as we are provided with love and belonging during our formative years we are just as dependent on having these things in our adult years. I told him that I was angry and quite rightly so. The policeman said to me that he understood my complaint with family and appreciated the hierarchy of needs. Surprisingly, the policeman could even tell me the name given to the hierarchy of needs. After I made reference to the hierarchy of needs he said, "Maslow's Hierarchy of needs!. Yes, I have heard of it and appreciate what you are saying, but unfortunately the law does not and maybe should recognise this". There was a police woman supervising me as well, and she said to her colleague, "I am sorry, I am ignorant, you will have to tell me all about the hierarchy of needs. I've never heard of it". That is when the three of us started having quite an academic discussion on Maslow's hierarchy of needs and suddenly became two psychology lecturers with a psychology student. The nurse who came into the room to get a syringe for another patient found the experience quite surreal; to see and hear two people in police uniform holding me there like a prisoner, until my Dad was offered the prospect of charging me with assault, having a discussion on Maslow's hierarchy of needs. I think there might have been a bit of a disguised smile.

The time came where the policeman said to me that he had to go and see my Dad. I was told by the police officer that my Dad was in the waiting area and that he had to ask him if he would like to charge me with assault. I said, "Fine, it won't be the first time I've been arrested and charged over a matter relating to my health". The policeman left, and then five minutes later came back through the swing doors into the treatment area. The policeman said, "I have asked your father if he would like to press charges against you for carrying out an assault on him round at your home". When I heard him say this I thought to myself, "He is going to want to press charges. People would say that would be too much of an injustice, as well as a stab in the back, for a father to want to press charges against his own son, but with the injustices I have experienced to date, which I never saw coming before they did, I would not put it beyond the realms of possibility for this police officer to say: 'and your father wishes to press charges'". The police officer then said, "Your father does not wish to press charges against you, and therefore you can now wait here without our presence until the community mental health team come to see you." The police left and I felt I had been a very lucky guy, not because I had been a bad guy who had got away with doing something bad, but instead a guy living in a world that persecutes people with the needs that I have, and did not imprison me, when imprisonment would have been a desirable option for society, since I am seen as being a square peg, which society sees as being a nuisance, when allowed to enjoy the same liberties others are allowed to enjoy.

When the CMHT eventually came down to the Accident & Emergency, I told them I had no regrets doing what I did to my Dad, how I wished I had caught him, and he had been lucky to get away. I told them that my Dad should have shown more leadership between me and my sisters. The mental health nurse said, "Tim, you are very lucky. You could have been charged" in a way that was like, "and you deserved to be". I replied to this by asking, "Am I being held for sectioning?", and the CMHT nurse slowly shook his head saying, "No Tim, you are not being held for sectioning". I then
asked if I could be excused for five minutes, walked out the Accident & Emergency, and just walked home. My attitude and inner dialogue had me saying to myself, " If they think I am lucky sitting in an A & E having assaulted my father, then they have immediately failed at making good first impressions and winning my confidence in them being able to help me; and therefore, are not fit to be looking after me". I believe that it would have been professional for the mental health nurse to have been impartial over whether or not I had done the right or wrong thing going for my father, or at least kept his opinion to himself, as until he has been given a history of the case and carried out his assessment of me looking at the evidence, he could not have possibly had a view on whether my reaction to my father was understandable, proportionate or rationale. Let's face it there is a difference between assaulting your father and chasing him out your house as he was found out by you to be using your home behind your back to sleep with a woman behind your mother's back, and assaulting and chasing your father out your home as he bought you salt and vinegar crisps on his way round to yours when you had instructed him to buy you grilled steak flavour. This refusal to ask me questions over the history of me and my father's relationship; ask questions about events that led up to the assault; and ask me for my rationale for attacking my father before forming an opinion on whether I had been "Mr Lucky Guy", told me that the CMHT were judgemental and therefore not fit enough to be looking after me, especially when they come from an area of medicine that requires one to be holistic to not have unbalanced views that can hinder recovery and effectiveness of treatment plan implemented in the addressing of my mental health problems. I therefore saw the CMHT as being nothing more than procedure, and were there probably more for the gratification of the system, as it gave people jobs and allowed government to say they were investing X amount into mental health services. I certainly did not see it as a service that

was there to benefit me. I therefore decided that my "five minutes" was instead going to be a walk home.

As I was walking home; I realised as I was turning from Dumbarton Road onto Crow Road, that I was now feeling the beginnings of a warning to a seizure coming on. I suddenly thought to myself "I've been longer than seventeen hours without medication due to the wait for the Community Mental Health Team" and as I am thinking this, the transition came on; when the seizure becomes irreversible, and the next thing I knew was that I was walking around a retail park car park not knowing where I was, suffering from really bad amnesia at around 1am in the morning. There were cars in this retail park at 1am. I have been told that they are the cars of staff who work in the supermarket who stock the shelves and take deliveries throughout the night. Eventually I came round and found my way home. I was fortunate as it was a car park that I had been walking around in, and I had already been arrested back in 2001 for playing with door handles, getting into a car and looking through a man's CD collection. What's to say that it couldn't have happened again and that would have been the second incident in one day with the police. Fortunately for me, I came round and woke up the next morning in my bed.

CHAPTER 24

My mother had shown great interest in me from the year 1975 through to 2003. Unfortunately, in 2003 she bought two Scottish westie terriers and she was never to be seen again for the next fourteen years. Weeks could elapse without her phoning, months without her visiting my home; and if I phoned her with a problem, she would say, "Well why tell me?". An example of a problem was back in September 2012 when I moved back from Slough and I was looking for a job as a support worker. This used to be a guaranteed job due to my previous paid experience and voluntary work. Unfortunately, all care homes were now moving from morning/afternoon/night time shifts, which were all awake shifts, to shifts where the night shift was now a sleep over shift, as the employer could pay a cheaper hourly rate. As a consequence of this I could no longer get work as a support worker anywhere due to having night time seizures upon awakening in the middle of the night. It had the same effect on my life as being a professional, such as a doctor, who had been struck off by his professional body and lost his registration. A nice guaranteed £15,00-£20,000 post, that made a single guy with my living costs, a very wealthy guy, was an opportunity now demolished. This was a big blow for me to handle. It made me feel suicidal, and therefore I needed someone to talk to who could show me some empathy. I therefore phoned my mother and told her what a blow this lost opportunity was for me, and that I was finding it hard to cope. I felt angry, betrayed by the greed of the world, its lack of flexibility as well as its judgemental attitude; trapping me in a cycle of helplessness and hopelessness. It had me just lying on my couch having strong suicidal ideation and feeling that I needed an ally who I could have a real rant with, who would understand and empathise with me; and make me feel that I was not alone as they would be with me, supporting me until I eventually found a purpose again that was fulfilling and made me content. After my mother answered her phone and I explained to her how I was feeling, all she had to say was, "Well, it's the epilepsy" in a "What are you complaining about, and why are you telling me?" tone. It was cold and totally lacking in any empathy. I was needing somebody to have a good rant with to get this off my chest. I also needed someone to encourage me to hang in there and see another day through and not bring it all to an end. I was socially isolated and had no one to fulfil these two needs. I felt that no one cared. I had just learned that I had been taken advantage of by a lover because of my depression, socially isolated because of the social anxiety disorder and denied the security of guaranteed employment because of the epilepsy. This was a bomb of a cocktail to handle, and all I had was my Dad who showed an interest. This proved a major problem more than a help as, just like the old physics equation that states "Pressure=Force/Area", my Dad was the only "Area" (Shoulders) for the "Force" (the issues) to come down on, thus, increasing the "Pressure" to such a point that my Dad's "shoulder's" broke, causing our relationship to break up. If there had been supportive relationships in the family (Shoulders), the "Area" absorbing the" Force" would have been greater, and the "Pressure" less, preventing the breaking of any relationship. As a consequence of this broken relationship, my Dad was running me to the doctor one day in July 2016, due to me having difficulties with my literacy skills brought on by the depression, after I had been up all night feeling symptoms of rage towards the abandonment of me by family and my Dad doing nothing about it. I had a seizure at 4am that morning, and when I got into the passenger seat of my Dad's car, I grabbed him by the throat and pressed my house key hard into his face, telling him he was a useless father. The skin on his face started to break causing bleeding to occur. I was controlled enough to take the key away from his face, and we drove off.

When my Dad parked at the sea front car park in Helensburgh, after the pair of us being twenty minutes early for my doctor appointment that day in July 2016, we had an argument about the unsupportive nature of my family, where my Dad out of temper said in the car park outside the Helensburgh swimming pool, "You just make everyone ill. It's always Tim, Tim, Tim and you make us ill!". I responded to this by carrying out a judo shoulder throw on my Dad, and he landed on his head. His scalp split open and there was blood everywhere. The swimming pool staff arriving for work ran over and put towels around his head and called an ambulance. My Dad told the swimming pool staff that he had slipped while he was lying on the ground, while a lady put towels around his head. I stood there for five minutes not feeling any regret or concern, and made it obvious to everyone supporting my father that he did not slip by tutting and shaking my head, where I then just turned my back on him and walked away. By the time I was across Clyde Street, that ran parallel to the car park; making my way to the doctor's surgery, the ambulance for my Dad came past with its sirens blaring. I walked into the doctor's surgery, waited to be called in, where I planted myself in the patient seat, and told the General

Practitioner that I had just badly assaulted my father. I said I didn't care if he pressed charges and I went to prison. I told my General Practitioner that I would be happier in prison, as I would not be isolated; and I was certainly made a thug enough of, and angry enough, by both family neglect and social exclusion, to be there. My sisters now use these two incidents as reason to have nothing to do with me. I think that giving these two incidents as reason for having nothing to do with me is putting the cart in front of the horse. It was because they had nothing to do with me that I reacted on both occasions i.e. March 2015 and July 2016 the way that I did.

 For the next six months I meditated twice a day on most days, and my temper has never flared up again to the point of becoming violent. My meditation practice back in January 2017 did go back to a consistency along the lines of three consecutive days of two sessions a day, to four consecutive days of one a day, thus, resulting in mental wellbeing going through good days, but then having seriously bad days, where I would be on the phone exploding with my father on days where I was suffering from burnout brought on by social isolation and feelings of resentment towards family. I was suffering from suicidal ideation and had lost my fear of death, but did not want to die; but as already mentioned about suicide in a previous chapter, you feel yourself having to take your life because life has become impractical and not necessarily because you want to. It's like being a jogger who still wants to complete the full marathon but is finding himself with no choice but to stop running before finishing due to physical exhaustion. You can't live with burnout while having no support from friends and family to get through it. It's like being in the desert where you don't want to die but dehydration is going to make continuing the journey impractical. Yes, suicide can be a death against your will as much as cancer, stroke, heart attack etc. I saw myself being a suicide time bomb, and that family had the wire cutters to defuse it and were refusing to. This was filling me with pent up rage. I woke up in the middle of night thinking "my family are killing me and this death is so avoidable, and they will be at my funeral shaking everyone's hands looking like butter wouldn't melt in their mouths". I thought "they will be happy I am gone. If they take my life then they will have to come with me. I will be damned if I miss out on a life and they get on with their lives, and live happily ever after".

I had earlier in 2016 watched a news bulletin where a young man in his early 30's shot his mother, her new lover and his sister. I thought at the time of watching it that I knew exactly what caused that killing to occur, and that me and my family were heading that way, and I would be remembered by society as the "psychotic/loner epileptic son". I had been meditating inconsistently and only getting to the gym once a week maximum. I still believe the days of twice a day of meditating gave me enough respite from the depression to give me the stamina and endurance to get through the days of major depression which happened when my meditation practice dropped to once a day, which is why without the meditation I would be dead. According to research made reference to in a 2009 article titled: "Suicidality and Epilepsy: A complex relationship that remains misunderstood and underestimated", that can be found in the journal "Epilepsy Currents", 20.8% of people with epilepsy will attempt suicide. Those who have ended their lives have not wanted to die, but have had to die, because life has become too impractical for them; and this is why it is so important to never say, "He's not suicidal. If he wanted to kill himself he would have done it" as the "not doing it" is the part of him that is wanting to live, but wanting to live is not the difference between taking your life or not taking it, and it is instead the practicality score of someone's life that is the difference between taking their life or choosing to live, which when becomes too low i.e. impractical, will cause a person to take their life. The runup to the suicide is terrifying for the person, as just imagine what it must be like to kill yourself at the same time as not wanting to kill yourself. This can bring on "out of body feelings" due to the ambiguity of the two messages. It is beyond 10/10 fear when no one understands you, nor is anyone listening to you. Society calls someone a coward if they take their life, but society does this to those with mental health problems. It causes the mental health problems in those affected by them, and then tries to blame those affected by mental health problems as being the reason behind why they have the mental health conditions by inventing incredibly stigmatising condition like "Personality Disorder"; especially so in cases of people with conditions that affect the brain such as epilepsy, therefore it's no surprise that society would even accuse a person's suicide as being because of the type of person they were by calling them a "coward". Psychiatry just sweeps society's failings under the carpet. When I worked at the Epilepsy Society and the psychiatrist was telling me how to deal with my key client's challenging behaviour, my key client Paul shouted, "Fuck off!, Fuck Off!, Fuck Off!" and punched the psychiatrist, making me feel brilliant! Psychiatry sweeps under the carpet: "He's got epilepsy and therefore gets denied educational and vocational opportunities that makes him angry and suicidal", by creating theories such as: "He's got epilepsy, giving him something called Personality Disorder, that makes him angry and suicidal." Psychiatry stitches up symptoms caused by political failings, as symptoms caused by brain.

In February 2017 my mother's two westie terriers were now both passed away and she was now back to coming along to meet ups that I had with my Dad. My mother started to have a presence in my life again on the night of my 42nd birthday. She maintained this presence up until January 2018, however, she is back to having two new westie terriers and has not been seen since. I have still had anxiety over who will be here to fend for me when my father is not here, however, I feel that day has come when I see how ineffectual he's been at fending for me with family.

I have had great difficulties respecting my father in recent years. I have not been a bad brother, as I have never mentally or physically compromised my sisters. They have turned out very well. They are both married and have children. My older sister has two boys, and my younger sister has one boy and another on the way at present. They are both law graduates, and my eldest sister has been a lawyer since the age of 22, and is now 44 years of age, and my youngest sister was a lawyer since the age of 22 up until recent. My father informed me that she no longer does this but has recently been given a job that is well paid and proportionate with her level of education. I don't know what that job is as I was not listening at the time of being told. Both of my sisters have a large ring of friends and are, therefore, well socially connected. They have both turned out well, and have never lived with essential unmet needs, as if they had, they wouldn't have turned out as well as they have. There is, therefore, no evidence of damage done to them by anyone, and therefore, I do not know where I have sinned so badly, that has made it so worthy of them abandoning me, and refusing to have anything to do with me. The very fact that my father defends their decision to not support their brother with his mental health needs, has made me feel very let down, and has me see my father as being a bit of a walk over. I therefore blame my father's lack of ability to act as my advocate, for this lack of obligation felt by the sisters to help their brother meet his mental health needs, and enable him to become socially connected. I also blame my mother for acting as a bad role model to my sisters by becoming more concerned about her dogs' needs than her son's. It is for this reason that recently when I have been in the company of my father, I have become impatient with him, felt feelings of grudge; and found myself diving into a bad mood. This has caused me to have a recent clash with my parents over something that is a symptom of my social isolation. I very recently booked onto a course called "Business Start Up" as I want to start my own organisation teaching people alternative therapy. This course is part of a Scottish Government Initiative to encourage people in Scotland to become self- employed. I booked for this course on the internet and picked where I was going to study it. I picked Lochgilphead, in Argyll and Bute, which is the local authority area, where my home town of Helensburgh is located. I believed this place to be just 7 miles up the road to find out when sitting having a coffee in a café one day with my parents that this place was 74 miles away. Remember, I gravitate into a bad mood when I am with my father. When I found out that Lochgilphead was 74 miles away I thought to myself "I have been living in this local authority area for two years. I should know where Lochgilphead is. That should be common knowledge that it is not close by, and the only reason it is not common knowledge with me is because I have been isolated and not had anyone to have meaningful conversations with, where the names and locations of these towns are shared; nor have I had any meaningful reason to research the local area because I have had no one to enjoy it with". This information coming to light just made me feel even more resentful towards the two people I was sitting at the same table with, and I went ballistic on the pair of them because of how much I blame family for not helping me out of my isolation. I told the pair of them that it was hopeless repeating the same thoughts and opinions that I have shared with them on so many occasions, and therefore, decided to just leave the pair of them standing there out on the pavement outside the café. My mother didn't appear in the slightest bit bothered. I walked away and felt very calm and tranquil. I had told my mother what I thought of her in a way that allowed me to draw a line under our relationship, as well as my father. I told her that when her arthritis deteriorated to a level where she would need the support of friends and family, she would realise how important family is, and how much she had failed as a mother in showing any concern for her son, and not bothering about the huge fracture that existed between me and my sisters in the days when I was informing them of how much mental pain I was in. I told her that I would have made a better son than these two sisters will make daughters, in the days she has ahead of her as a woman with a deteriorating condition. I reminded her that my younger sister had stopped speaking to my older sister for a while, as she felt my older sister to be so cold and uncaring when she phoned her up looking for emotional support, when she accidentally knocked a man and his child off their bike at a roundabout. I told her about the time my younger sister had reported on the night of my arrest during a complex partial epileptic seizure, how my eldest sister could only speak as a lawyer, and not as a sister of a brother who had been wrongfully arrested during a seizure. I told my mother that she could expect the same coldness from my older sister, when she is relying upon her daughter in the future to take care of her, if my mother were to outlive my Dad. I also told my mother that she would regret throwing away a son who was a former support worker, disability advocate as well as a person with an empathy for someone suffering from a long- term disability. I have not spoken to them since and have no desire to be acquainted with any of them and I am looking at ways in   turning this negative into a major positive.

I went out for an evening in Glasgow on the 20th January 2018 after saying my final goodbye to my parents and drawing a line under my relationship with them. I went into a pub and met two men who I had a number of drinks with. I was onto my fifth pint of lager and it was now about 10.30pm. I came back from the toilet and sat down at the table with the two gentleman and one left to get his last train home, but myself and the other stayed for a couple of more drinks. I was starting to enjoy my booze. The guy I was with was enjoying his booze just a bit too much as well. He stood up from the table when the bar started playing the Deacon Blue song "Dignity" and he started punching the air above him. Unfortunately, he enjoyed punching the air above him just a bit too much and accidentally put his fist through the air vent causing all this filth to come pouring out of the ceiling. He started trying to repair it by standing on a chair and I said, "You better sit down as you are confessing to every customer and doorman that you're the vandal". It was hilarious though, and cheered me up a good bit. It was then that the humour was suddenly replaced with a strong feeling of concern. While I was sitting there with the remaining gentleman, I suddenly felt the world I was in getting fainter, and the world I go into during a seizure getting greater. The world I was in, and which you are in as you read this book, was going from 10 to 9 to 8 to 7 to 6 to 5... while at the same time the world I go into during the seizure was going from 1 to 2 to 3 to 4 to 5.... The seizure comes on under the influence of alcohol in a similar way to how it does under the influence of Monosodium Glutamate. As long as your medication is in your system, there is no warning, and instead you immediately experience onset of transition. The transition is much slower, where at first you don't actually know if the onset is happening, or if you are imagining you are about to have a seizure; and as well as this, it is the real world going, and the seizure world coming, that brings on the fear and anxiety; unlike a sober seizure where you have the warning that climbs from 1 to 6, and then sudden increase to 10, to full development of seizure, where the onset of fear and anxiety is first experienced in the climb from 1 to 10 during the warning. It was during this alcohol induced epileptiform brain wave activity that the real world and the seizure world were switching interchangeably, where the real world was going from 10,9,8 back to 8,9,10; at the same time as the seizure world was going from 1,2, 3 back to 3,2,1. At the time of the seizure world being a 3 for the fourth or fifth time I said to the gentleman I was with that I better go and get my last train. I was feeling fearful and very vulnerable, and the pub around me felt more and more like the inside of a chapel in another land, in another time, in another place. As I got up, the world around me went back to being 100% real world and I immediately took my night time drug treatment, which would take around an hour to an hour and a half to get into my system. I started visualising in my mind world maps, where I started to label all the major cities and tell myself a little bit about each city in terms of population, landmarks, history etc. Fortunately, there was no more threatening experiences to be had on the way back home and I got back safely without taking a seizure.

I find the visualising of maps of the world; which I then mentally label with all the world's cities quoting their populations and landmarks, helps prevent a seizure from coming on, when I feel the developing of a warning, especially a warning that has been brought on by the anxiety of having a seizure in a place where I feel vulnerable to having one. It is also said that we all have autistic traits in us, and that we all have our little irrational meaningless obsessions, without meeting the diagnosis of having a learning disability. As a child and adolescent, I always had an obsession for cities of the world and their populations and surface areas. Call me "Sad" but I am sure many reading this book can relate with this, and can identify something that they have a daft obsession with. One of my so-called relatives has an obsession with public transport systems of the world, and knows all the lines of all the metro systems of the different cities. There might be something genetic in it. This obsession with cities has given me a passion for cities, and it is as though this passion is what can also prevent the beginning of the process behind having a seizure. It's ironic that a trait that is seen as a symptom in someone with a learning disability can defuse a seizure. This visualising of maps is what I use when I get that feeling just before a warning to a seizure. It is the anxiety of losing familiarity with my surroundings, and being taken off to another time and place, as well as all the potential consequences of a seizure, that brings on the warning at a time when I feel vulnerable to a seizure e.g. awakening, after having warning that just subsided, missed dose, ingested MSG, sleep deprivation, places with large gatherings such as lectures/trains etc. Very often it is the anxiety of having a seizure that brings on the warning, which then develops into seizure. In the days when I had day time attacks I found that the visualising of maps of world and cities etc, at a time where I feared having a seizure e.g. out on my own in pub, or on crowded train; provided for my mind a zone where my mind felt confident, as it was a zone where I felt very knowledgeable and at home in, due to me having a passion for everything found in this zone, and I felt like I was in a sanctuary which was shielding me from the anxiety of having a seizure, thus, preventing any warning from developing the second you suspected/imagined the beginnings of a warning that could in itself bring on a warning. If you get the maps of the world/cities/populations in before the warning becomes properly established then this technique can be used to prevent a seizure. If, however, the warning gets in before you get the opportunity to thinks maps/cities/landmarks/ populations, you then require mental arithmetic to try and prevent the warning progressing to the point of no return, which is the seconds before onset of psycho-hallucination.

After coming out of the pub that evening that I was in with the guy I had earlier met, I headed to Glasgow Queen Street where I sat on platform 8 of Queen Street Train Station waiting for my train, where I was now confident that I would not have a seizure as it was now half an hour ago since my last semi-onset of a seizure. I found myself thinking "Thank God for the diamox blocking my sodium ion channels". The diamox is a drug that acts when you are about to have a seizure. It unfortunately isn't as effective upon awakening as it is when you are awake as your seizure threshold is much lower upon awakening. I found myself thinking to myself that the epilepsy was a very clever condition and so was the drug treatment. I thought to myself what an amazing universe the brain is and what little we know about it. I thought if I had had a seizure in that pub I would have been in a terrifying world, borne from a psycho-hallucination, where the experience of being in that other gothic world, flooded with people, would have been as real to me as the experience of being in London walking through a crowded Trafalgar Square. That experience in the pub also acted as a reminder of how you just don't mess with it, in terms of being inconsistent with medication, drinking alcohol to excess, or allowing yourself to go sleep deprived.

 Living with epilepsy requires a very disciplined life, and I believe that you develop many good quality personality traits because of the disciplined life you have to live. I believe that it is the discipline acquired from living with epilepsy that has given me the discipline to exercise in the gym, walk on average 3 miles per day, follow a calorie controlled diet, drink minimally if at all, meditate twice daily and has cut out a journey for me that has made me so unique that I am not scared to be a non-conformist which has opened up my creativity. It's true what a poster at the epilepsy connections charity has written on it, and that is "You will never discover your true potential trying to be normal". It could be said that because of the personality traits gained from living and coping with epilepsy I do not rely on psychiatrists and anti-depressant/tranquiliser medication to control my anxiety and depression. No disrespect to psychology but I have not needed them either. I believe that the challenges thrown at me has made me a very independent person. It is because of the nature of the condition and all the positives that have come out of the negatives that I sat there on platform 8 of Glasgow Queen Street train station, after my near seizure in the bar, thinking to myself "I have too much respect for you i.e. the epilepsy, to live a life without you". I thought to myself "You are a vicious bastard, but one I have too much respect for to waken up tomorrow and never meet eye to eye with again". I thought to myself "In a perverse way, I would actually miss you if you were to never make an appearance again." It is for this reason that I don't want to be completely seizure free and would prefer to continue having the one seizure every ten to twelve nights as that is a completely different ordeal to live with than having one every 36 hours that could happen at anytime and anyplace and require a drug regime that has the most notorious side effects. I would never think like this during the onset of a seizure. Give me a button to press that would stop a seizure at the time of onset and it would be pressed 100% of the time causing me to never have a seizure again, as every seizure is terrifying, and there would never be an onset where I would never press the button. The onset to that 1 in 12 night seizure would make me cast my vote in exactly the same way the onset to any of the seizures I used to have every 36 hrs would have had me cast my vote during the days of living with uncontrolled epilepsy, however, in between seizures I am of the opinion that I would prefer to continue living with one seizure every ten to twelve days. I actually waken up the next day thinking to myself "Yes! I had a seizure last night, and it absolutely scared the living shit out of me, and it was a terrifying experience, but I'm glad I had it". I mark these seizures in my diary and flick through my diary thinking to myself "Isn't it great that, that black mark appears every ten to twelve days". I was seen by a neurologist called Dr Gallagher for the first time in fifteen years back in 2015 for a review of my drug treatment, and I actually said to him, "I'm absolutely fine being on the medication combination that I am on, so leave it alone". I went on to further say, "It's become nothing more than a glamorised bad dream experienced every twelve nights". My neurologist raised his eyebrows to this statement, then looked at the medical student; and said, "Okay Mr Bone, we will just draw a line under that conclusion". I know it sounds very ambiguous but life is full of irony and I would say that over the years I have developed a relationship with my epilepsy that is ironic in nature. I feel that I am too curious about epilepsy, especially with the symptoms that I get, and therefore, there are too many unanswered questions that need answering before I would wave goodbye to it, such as: "Why do I go into another world as convincingly real as walking through Times Square New York?", "If a seizure is brought on by a disturbance in electrical activity where all electrical activity becomes disorganised, and no two seizures would look the same on an electroencephalogram, then why are my symptoms so consistent?". I think to myself "The brain is an amazing organ, and a complex partial epileptic seizure is a reminder of how amazing an organ the brain is". I have become so fed up with this world that I see the seizure world as an opportunity for a bit of escapism, even though at the time of the seizure, you feel like you are jumping from a very hot bath into a frying pan. These questions and appreciations have made epilepsy an obsession for the scientist within me i.e. molecular biologist, and the symptoms are so frighteningly and disturbingly impressive that the artist within me has become obsessed with it; and like any obsession, detachment from it is difficult, and therefore, has you wishing a 99.8% cure but 0.2% shortcoming of a cure.

It is now January 2018 at the time of writing, and as already mentioned, I have been meditating religiously for 45 minutes both morning and night since 28th

August 2017, as well as getting back to the gym three times per week. Having practiced consistent meditation practice for the last five going on six months, I am now feeling no symptoms of depression, and I am moving on with the future as well as not letting things and people from the past rob me of the present, that would only deny me my future. I have decided to draw a line under my relationship with my family. It is the healthiest option if I am to remain of sane mind. No one has been listening and it is these cries for help falling on deaf ears that just results in a symptom cycle of: deaf ears, increased anger, increased depression/anxiety, more deaf ears, more anger, more depression/anxiety, more deaf ears, more anger, more depression/anxiety etc, leading to the development of a depression/anxiety vicious symptom cycle that I rely upon consistent meditation practice to keep under control. This depression/anxiety symptom cycle was causing me to become, what the layman would call, a "psychopath", and leading to me wakening up in the middle of the night with overwhelming feelings of isolation, helplessness, hopelessness, feelings of claustrophobia; that could be best described as being shoved in a coffin with my family sitting on the lid, bringing on feelings of claustrophobia, mental suffocation and suicidal ideation, as I was starting to see suicide as the only practical way in coping, thus, bringing on symptoms of panic attacks, where I found myself having to slow breathe through the nose, counting to ten while breathing in as well as while breathing out when I started to feel depersonalisation and derealisation; which are two symptoms in themselves of a complex partial epileptic seizure. Unfortunately, these panic attack onsets have brought on night time seizures, due to a warning manifesting in me before the breathing defused the attack, which despite that "affection" for that one in twelve night time seizure I make reference to, I hate experiencing as it brings on so much distress and anxiety, and there is no feeling as isolating as the feeling of you slipping into a complex partial seizure on top of the isolation brought on by family abandonment and being without social connections. I blame a lot of my lack of social connections on the replacing of face to face interaction by things like social media. These factors make the whole onset of a seizure the more psychologically disturbing where you feel yourself slipping into a world of unfamiliarity, convincing as daylight is day, feeling the presence of other people moving in on you, that brings on feelings of being threatened and extreme vulnerability, to then experience blackout and then amnesia where there is little information about yourself to come back to you to navigate you back to recovery. It is the case that if you are unemployed, where you have nothing arranged to do or anyone to meet every day of your life, then you have no answers to stumble across to answer the questions you find yourself needing to answer in order for you to navigate your way out of the amnesia. You just purely rely on the amnesia lifting which you don't know will eventually happen as you have no knowledge about yourself having epilepsy. There is nothing about yesterday to come back to you as you no longer have a memory from yesterday to spontaneously appear in your mind; you have no memory of having done anything with anyone on a recent day as you have no social connections; you have no memory of any conversation that you had with someone that spontaneously comes back to you as you've not spoken to anyone in days; you have no memory of what you have on today to try and bring back to yourself as you have nothing on today; you have nothing in your diary that you can recollect happening on a previous day that would help you navigate yourself towards present date and day of week; you have no memory of a thought that you might have had yesterday about today to guide you towards where you are to be and when you are to be there; you have no work commitment that you spontaneously remember being given as you are between jobs as the advocacy charity that you ran had to close as it was a small fish swimming amongst sharks in the form of much larger charities, and you have to just wait until the good old temporal lobes have recovered which is when the brainstorm has passed and everything has settled.

CHAPTER 25

When I was fourteen, I was sexually groomed by a scout master when staying the night at his home. I told my parents about this abuse and my mother raised it with the local procurator fiscal at a party she was at, as my family were friends with this procurator fiscal. For those who are not acquainted with the Scottish legal system a procurator fiscal is a lawyer that works for the local prosecution service, playing the same role that a District Attorney fulfils in a country like the United States of America. The procurator fiscal offered the opportunity, in response to what my mother told him, to have the local police investigate this scout master. As you would expect from a family without a concern for a son being slowly killed by isolation, depression, anxiety and seizures they told this procurator fiscal not to bother instigating a police investigation into this scout master's behaviour, who many people he knew through the scouts, could talk about an experience they had had with him. Members of the local guide group could talk about having been pinched by him while helping them up ladders. This scout master was called "Dirty Ron" by everyone. When I was on a camping trip in the Scottish highlands with the scouts in 1987 this scoutmaster insisted that every boy was to wear shorts for a two week period despite the weather being cold as well as wet and ground being marshy. This scoutmaster said before we all left that trousers were banned! As well as this he used to put boys over his lap and sing a song spanking their rear end like a drum to the beat while we all clapped our hands. We were young and naïve and paedophilia was a term that had not had anywhere near the amount of coverage, if any at all, in 1987, in comparison to the amount of coverage it gets today. I doubt this scoutmaster is alive today, as he was either in his middle sixties, possibly seventies during this era; which was over thirty years ago.

As I have been sexually exploited, I can compare it with the abuse that I receive from my family. I can say that never did the abuse caused by the scout master ever affect me to the point of wanting to take my life. The abuse my parents and family have treated me with has made me want and feel the need to take my life. All I can say is that society has a huge fixation on sexual abuse and a much lesser fixation on domestic abuse. Never does society discuss or address abandonment or neglect, whichever of the two you wish to call it. That is an abuse that kills as it involves someone's essential needs not being met by those who have the resources to meet these needs, and instead point blankly refuse to help that person meet these essential needs for their own convenience and gratification. To deny needed attention and help in meeting essential unmet needs of a family member, which the other family members have the skills, the knowledge and resources to be able to help meet, which if allowed to continue to be unmet could result in the cost of a life in the family, is as bad as locking someone in a cell and refusing to hydrate them or feed them and just watch them waste away until death. A neglect that many people would naively say is minor, which results in a death due to pushing someone to taking their own life, is as bad as a major neglect that results in a death caused by forced starvation and dehydration. People have to stop judging a book by its cover. The taking of a life, is as bad as the taking of a life, regardless of whether it is a quick death or a slow painful death. In fact, it is the slow painful death which is the less humane, yet seeing someone put a bullet in someone's head looks so much more violent than locking someone out of family and watching them slowly waste away over a number of months.

My meditation practice has saved my life. During these meditation sessions I have had images of me with a gun in my mouth pulling the trigger, that my anger and rage as well as disappointment with the world and its people had started to engage with. It is during these engagements that the part of me that wants to cope and survive tells me to stop and focus on my breathing and let these thoughts pass through my mind like dark clouds in a sky. These meditation sessions have got rid of the suicidal ideation as well as suicidal feelings. It has been the "chemotherapy" for this "tumour of the mind", and without it I would be ashes. I could only have my family back in my life if they confessed to their sins and showed remorse for what they did or I should say did not do. You could say there's the abuse that "Did" and there's the other type of abuse that "Didn't". As my family show no desire to confess, nor show remorse, I cannot have them back in my life. I had been trying to make them see their sins so that they would start to show a commitment towards helping me through this pain as well as confess and show remorse, so that I could start accepting their help. This is what was driving me crazy and I have decided to let go, just like the old meditation principle instructs, and focus on the present, letting go of the past, and look forward to meeting new people and forming new relationships, instead of reflecting and commiserating to the point of madness over old relationships.

One thing that has played a large role in me being able to accept this identity of the isolated individual in a world that doesn't care has been the reading of my espionage books. I read books by an author called Mark Greaney, who has a character called "Gentry" in his books; who is a former CIA Officer who could not fit in at the CIA because he saw how ineffectual their operations were as well as being a man with an ethos that was incompatible with the ethos of the CIA. The CIA ethos in these books is very much about political gain, whereas Gentry's ethos is that of social justice. Gentry lives on the run from the CIA, as he has gone against the grain of their establishment, who now want him dead, and he now operates as a private assassin working on cases where the elimination of a particular person e.g. head of state is done in the name of social justice, even though social justice might not be the motive behind the person he is carrying out the assassination for. Gentry's experiences take him from one country to the next where he remains on the run from the CIA and he spends no two nights in the same residence. This man has no friends, no family and has no home; and lives with a constant feeling of not belonging. I see many parallels between my life and Gentry's life and they are that we are both square pegs of society. We are both without friends and family and a sense of belonging in the community. Our ethos's, views and beliefs are contrary to those of the societies that we are from. We are both prepared to do things our own way and not the way of others if their ways are seen as being less effective, entirely self- defeating or purposeless. We are both not scared to make ourselves unpopular and do what we see as being the right thing to do. For example, Gentry made himself very unpopular with the CIA through doing things his own way, I made myself very unpopular with the alliance that oversees advocacy services when running my advocacy charity as I had my way in providing advocacy that they did not like. Gentry went against the grain of the CIA in the name of social justice. I went against the grain of the alliance overlooking advocacy services in the name of social justice. The CIA want Gentry dead because he went against the grain, whereas the alliance of advocacy services wanted my organisation wiped off the map of advocacy services as well as my own name because I went against their grain. Gentry most probably has a hatred for authority as it abuses its power and takes advantage of the unlevel playing field that exists between itself and the vulnerable. I hate authority as it is the bully that is the large guy picking on the small guy, but recognise that I can at least put authority in its place and be victorious by targeting authority at the foot soldier level if not at the establishment level, in the same way that Gentry attacks the CIA by not trying to bring down the CIA but by instead choosing to rival individuals within the CIA.

Gentry has to be very fit to rival the strength and fitness levels of his rivals. I have to keep very fit to rival epilepsy, anxiety and depression. I also have to keep very fit as there is no one in this world who will fend for me or look after me if I become ill and can no longer fend for myself. I also have to keep very fit to protect myself from the damage anger and stress can inflict on your cardiovascular as well as nervous system.

Gentry's rivals have nearly killed him on many an occasion. My rivals i.e. anxiety, depression, epilepsy and society, have nearly killed me on a number of occasions. Gentry as well as myself are both living in a world where our views, beliefs, opinions are entirely at odds with the views, beliefs and opinions of the society that we live in; and we are both highly pragmatic individuals who have great difficulty living in a highly unpragmatic world causing us to experience frustration, fall out and isolation from those in charge and their followers i.e. the vast majority of the population, for the correct reasons; remembering that the vast majority of people are just sheep.

Many authors of these espionage books that involve the exposing of corruption of power within authority, such as the CIA, or within the political cabinet of a country's government i.e. President, Defence secretary, Foreign Secretary, Home secretary etc, have been in roles e.g. journalism, military, politics etc where they have learned about the corruption that goes on within government and government run departments and the kinds of people that work within these authorities e.g. the black sheep. When reading these books, I can therefore be sure that people like Gentry exist in reality. I even believe that many of the authors base their characters very much on being people they see as being like themselves which is further evidence of there being people like Gentry in reality. As many of them were journalists, they obviously liked working for themselves and not a boss or someone who has authority over them, hence the fact they are now an author. This has given me a feeling of belonging as well as a feeling of pride in being one of society's black sheep, and has made me aware of the fact that what makes me different to most are strengths, and that society's difficulties with me have often been down to me being a good person. These books have had the same effect on me as attending a support group would have had on my mental and physical wellbeing. When I have woken up in the middle of the night overcome by feelings of isolation as well as rage towards the world, I have been able to tell myself that I am not on my own and that there are people like Gentry wakening up feeling exactly the same thing if not worse e.g. wakening up homeless in the streets, and I suddenly experience a feeling of belonging that helps me cope with the feeling of isolation. I walk through the city of Glasgow, and I see homeless people who have one leg missing and I think to myself "Probably a former military soldier who since getting his leg blown off has been seen as having nothing more to offer the military, thus, nothing to offer society as the only work he would have done if physically capable enough to do so would have been skilled manual or unskilled manual work, therefore rendering him as nothing to offer, other than be a drain on the welfare system, resulting in society ignoring him, which is why he is homeless with a beggar cup in his hand". It was only the day before writing this passage that I learned that Glasgow City Council are going to fine people for begging in the street. This had me think "Yes, authority like you sit back and watch others cause them to end up in the very situation that they find themselves in, and then you criminalise them for doing nothing more than trying to cope with the situation that others have put them in". It really is the "pot calling the kettle black", and it just fills you with a rage if you are not meditating or doing some other cognitive technique that can defuse as well as prevent rage. What this country needs is a good riot! I have recently heard myself, saying to myself, that the fairest society that would give people little reason to be angry would be one where there was no law enforcement; no obligation to be a good civilian; there was no such thing as money/trading; nothing was expected of anyone by anyone, and it was pure anarchy where it was perfectly acceptable for a person to give another person a good belt in the gob for saying something disrespectful to them. In such a society there would be no authority-civilian relationship; society would be grass and trees as well as eco-systems and we would be respectful towards one another through fear of repercussions; we would keep fit and do cardio training as it would be a survival of the fittest life and we would grow up with survival skills e.g. hunting, defence, home building etc, making us much better people to one another, as well as more interesting people, who were genuine, as no one would be scared to have as well as share an opinion, view, belief with others, as there would be no such thing as conformity, as a survival of the fittest society would make us independent minded as opposed to oppressed individuals. A fair society would be an "every man for himself society", which would be the fairest by far. A society where we walk around with spears as opposed to mobile phones. I would like you to think hard about this and form an opinion on the matter, and if you agree with what I am saying then please spread the word. I ask you be genuine as my biggest complaint about people is that they are not genuine, or the majority at least are not genuine, but this need not continue to remain to be the case in any one person. People conform through fear of being rejected, or having something taken away. In such a society there would be no such thing as "Approval" as it would be every man for himself, and there would be nothing that you could have taken away, as if someone takes from you, then you just take from someone else.

Scotland is a left- wing country with many resources, with the capabilities to grow its economy, and be a prosperous place for a person like me i.e. not academic nor vocational, to live. Due to right wing policies of Westminster shaping the size of the Scottish bloc, and successive British Governments taking more than its fair share of Scotland's wealth, it is the case that Scotland has had very limited resources to grow and provide opportunities for the mainstream population. It is difficult enough to get a job being a member of the mainstream (neither academic, nor vocational) because of this, therefore when you add on top of this the discriminatory effects living with epilepsy, depression and anxiety have on employment opportunities it is even harder for disadvantaged people living in Scotland to live a life where they can bring their potential to fruition. The Equality Act 2010 is inadequate for disability and it again is legislation that was introduced by a British Government that could be described as being the old right- wing conservative party. Scotland has no control over employment law and therefore cannot introduce legislation that would address the inadequacies of the Equality Act 2010, which I believe it would if it had control over such laws. These inadequate laws as well as inability of Scotland to grow its economy has contributed hugely to my social exclusion, which social isolation has been a huge ingredient off due to lack of employment prospects as well as all people I have met over the years who have looked like being prospective friends moving south to London or Manchester. I therefore do grudge my Scottish peers for being so cowardly and voting unionist. I don't think the Scottish nationalists put enough emphasis on the relationship between unionism and social isolation. I have not had the benefit of being able to remain in touch with friends I had at school and university, as none of them have stayed in Scotland, and instead have all flocked south of the border or to other shores. This requires you to be born again, and go back to being age four which was the age you first met friends but you can't go back to age four at the age of forty three.

I have started a "Meetup" group in Glasgow and we go bowling and play pool. The group is picking up in numbers. It now has forty three members and was started on the 20th December 2017 and is now as I write ten weeks old. My meditation practice is now giving me much more mind control when facing my performance anxiety and intrusive thinking that used to mess up my eye ball coordination skills. I had avoided pool and bowling for the last twelve years, and I am glad to say that my meditation practice has conquered my performance anxiety to the point where neither performance anxiety nor intrusive thinking affect my performance and I have been winning games of pool against seasoned pool players. When I went to play ten pin bowling on my first night, my meditation kept me calm all day and enabled me to show up for the game and play. I started to become anxious in the final hour before we played as, unlike the pool, there is an audience to contend with, but I started doing lots of Positive Affirmations saying things to myself like, "My name is Tim Bone and I won tonight's ten pin bowling", "My name is Tim Bone and I had a fantastic night at the bowling tonight", "My name is Tim Bone and I won so many strikes tonight". As I continued repeating the positive affirmations, the nerves went and were replaced with confidence enabling me to win the ten- pin bowling. Remember, make your positive affirmation present tense and use a positive word!! More on this later!

I now write this paragraph of the book on the 15th March 2018 and I have had to close my meetup up group as I again for the diary have more evidence to add that evidences my claim that people are not genuine. For those who are not aware of what meetup is, it is a company that offers an online service that allows you to set up a society where you are given your own online page that allows you to advertise social events that people can book a place for attending. What happens is people join your group, and they can book to come to an event on your society's page. I had arranged pool nights, card game nights, ten pin bowling nights, curry nights and bar nights; and the attendance was poor. There were only two or three people who would book per event, and it would always be the case that one or two would either cancel last minute or just not show up. With every night at the pool we have only had one of forty five members attend, and fortunately I have a former client from my advocacy days, called Alistair, who attends as well. Alistair is very sociable and is therefore a guaranteed attendance. Therefore, there has always been three (myself, Alistair and one of the forty five hopeless hopefuls) in attendance out of forty five members. This is sadly a good turn- out rate when many other clubs that have been around a few years have 2000 members and only get eight people booking to their events, therefore meaning, maybe only five or six attend their events. I couldn't keep this club going as I did believe that the numbers of people joining yet not booking for events was illogical. I felt that people joining, not booking/cancelling or just not showing was typical of all the human traits that I have had too much exposure to. I was convinced that the growth of this club, looking at the illogical behaviour of my members and the members of other groups, was going to involve having to expose myself to the human traits that I have too often in the past found disappointing, disheartening and frustrating and that I just could not take any more of it. Running the group was exacerbating my depression and causing me to just hate people. I sent an e-mail around telling everyone that due to the poor turn out, and seeing too much "All gob" i.e. joining, but "No Action" i.e. booking and attending events, I was fed up and must have been of a people confidence level above theirs, and that because of this I obviously had expectations of them that were too high, and therefore the club would be better off run by someone whose people confidence score was the same as theirs, therefore I just shut the club down. I am afraid to say it but there is a massive failing in our society, and that is people are not raised to be able to form relationships with people at a conscious level as they are too self-conscious and fear other peoples' judgements of them, and therefore they can only form relationships at a subconscious level which happens when two people spend much time together due to a common purpose such as sharing the same job role, being pupils/students at the same school/college etc, coming across one another often enough walking their dogs or in the local shops if they live in a little town etc. Put two people in a situation where they get together purely for the purpose of becoming friends and they discover in the vast majority of cases that this is a skill that they do not have or they do but they are too plagued by insecurity to use it. I have found out from reading about other peoples' experiences of social anxiety disorder, that after public speaking, the next worst fear of those belonging to the mainstream population is being introduced to someone they don't know and having to hold a conversation. I do not have this issue. I find the ability to speak to anyone, anywhere and at anytime, is instinctive; and therefore I do feel that my isolation is down to society's failure to develop individuals into confident, knowledgeable, free of the fear of other peoples' judgement beings; and that this has held back my ability to grow a new circle of friends causing me to close down my meetup group. I walk around the street grudging other people for this confident front on the surface, but deep insecurity on the inside, that the majority of people are affected by. My grudge for people the other day was so strong that I deliberately raced up the stairs of platform nine of Queen Street station, in the centre of Glasgow, as fast as I could, hoping to make a collision with someone walking around the corner to knock them out my way so that they would go flying and I could shout out loud, "Fuck Off Person!!!!".

As the closing of this group put an end to the prospects of making future relationships, I found myself relapsing with a rage towards family as the success of the meetup was going to play a huge part in being able to let go of past relationships. I have managed to get this rage under control with my continued meditation, but the closing of the meetup group had set me back. I now intend to meet friends using facebook. Wikihow instructs you to just friend locals, get a bit of dialogue going through facebook and then suggest meeting in person. I intend to do this in order to get games of pool, cards and more. Let's just hope for the best! Did I not say that trying to make a friend past a certain age at a conscious level is like trying to break an eight digit security code, and if you do make a friend the formulated life of school, moving onto job/further education, job, getting married & having family, and then retirement that the vast majority live (many through social expectation) prevents any time to do anything with friends out-with that formula. The formulated life is a real "ball & chain" to both those living it and those not living it. Getting access to opportunities to make friends requires you to break the barriers of this formula which can be described as trying to break that eight digit code. This formula makes many people so boring as it denies them opportunities to new experiences thus denying them the acquisition of new knowledge, skills, views, beliefs and opinions as well as developing new passions for particular topics. The formula makes life so boring when life could be so, so much more interesting. It's what a director of my former advocacy charity once shared on her facebook page, and that was an article from a magazine titled "All of us will die, but few of us will live".

CHAPTER 26

Up until 2012 I was an individual plagued by social anxiety disorder where I avoided all performance settings. These performance settings were vocational, academic, social in nature, as well as settings that involved carrying out certain independent living skills. As already mentioned, this was due to the scarring effects of my education as well as the scarring of my mind on the sports field. Sport is a part of the curriculum in our schools that I believe damages a lot of people, and causes a whole lot of future crippling effects on one's ability to function in the world as an independent adult. This is especially the case when competition is a natural human streak, and is a way in proving oneself to others in a world plagued by insecurity, where people tend to like making themselves feel bigger by making others feel smaller, and guess what! They turn to competition in every life setting e.g. job, size of house, model of car, vanity, level of education etc as a tool in achieving this.

It is because of all these scarring effects that, when my friend Alan filled in my driving application form for me, I had great fears about being able to perform in lessons and show myself up in front of the driving instructor as well as other road users and pedestrians. I worried that I would be the worst student the instructor had ever seen. I remember lying in bed the night before my first lesson and worrying about this. It was then that I was also teaching an Expert Patient programme in Slough and I remembered the term "Visualisation". I also remembered a friend once saying to me, "We bring the worst luck in our lives upon ourselves". I researched visualisation as a cognitive technique for improving confidence. I learned that Visualisation works in two ways. One way is to not focus on any negative thoughts that have negative imagery or contain a negative message in them and instead picture in your mind yourself performing well at the lesson you fear attending, and hearing your inner dialogue telling yourself you did really well at today's lesson, before you have even attended today's lesson. You are to picture yourself sitting in the car being told by your driving instructor that you are doing really well and hear his or her voice saying this to you. You should picture his or her facial expression, hear what they are saying in a praising tone and see yourself feeling really good about yourself. You should even take a few seconds to put yourself in your own body within this image and see the world through your own eyes as you will during the driving lesson and create in your mind the feeling of reward and satisfaction. You should see you and your instructor sitting in the car at the end of your lesson, being told by him or her how well you have done and how they look forward to seeing you at the next lesson. You should have these thoughts throughout the day leading up to your lesson. If any thoughts that are negative in nature enter your mind, such as seeing you and your instructor in the car with you looking terrible and them shaking their head, you are to pause that thought and see it blow up in your mind and immediately replace it with a positive thought like the ones I have just described. This technique can be used in the run up to any performance situation that you have fears about. Yes, even meeting new people and socialising.

After spending a day visualising these thoughts in my mind, I attended my lesson feeling really confident and did not suffer from performance anxiety. I got in the car and I could drive and perform well at the lesson. At the end of the lesson I had turned what was fantasy into reality and I found myself enjoying my lessons and learning to drive. This is why I would say to anyone affected by performance anxiety when learning to drive that you should arrange for your lesson to be in the evening or at the earliest late afternoon so you have the benefit of the whole day visualising your lesson going really well.

Visualisation is also seen as a religious tool by some people as it is a technique that people use as a means of employing the "Law of Attraction" into your life where it is believed by some that by visualising yourself succeeding you will attract into your life the necessary people, resources and opportunities to make that success a reality. Some people swear by using visualisation, in this way. You will remember me quoting earlier in this chapter what my friend said to me: "We bring upon ourselves the worst luck in our lives". Well the same is true with the opposite of this statement. We can bring upon ourselves the best luck in our lives. Some people claim that this technique works by sending positive energy into the universe where you ask the universe for something positive to happen, and that the universe will use the energy in a way that brings about changes that deliver upon that request. I was sceptical at first about this theory, however, I am science educated being a graduate in molecular biology and it is true that everything around us is energy. Epilepsy is energy; light is energy; sound is energy; the electric current that goes through the filament of your light bulb is energy; the dog sitting on the carpet is energy i.e. potential energy; a moving car is energy i.e. kinetic energy; you speaking is energy i.e. sound energy; you reading this book is energy i.e. your eyes moving and focussing is kinetic energy, the creation of an image on your retina and the transmitting of the information to the brain via the optic nerve is electrical energy, the brain making sense of this information i.e processing and storing in memory is the kinetic energy of neurotransmitter molecules.

If we look at something totally unrelated such as a building across the road to wherever it is you are reading this book at this present moment. Take a look at that building. It is sitting there stationary i.e. potential energy; it is made up of bricks that are made up of Aluminium Oxide and Silicon Dioxide (Chemists can correct me on this). These compounds are made up of Aluminium, Oxygen and Silicon atoms. Atoms have nucleus's in the centre that have positive charge, and electrons that exist in shells surrounding the nucleus that have negative charge. The atom stays together by forces of attraction between the positively charged nucleus and the negatively charged electrons, therefore they are held together by forces that are made of electronegative energy; and the aluminium, silicon and oxygen atoms are held together by the giving of negatively charged electrons to create atoms of different charges that have an attracting effect on each other causing them to form a bond which is also formed from electronegative energy. The same atomic theory can be said for all the other substances that that building is made out of, from the bricks to the slates on the roof; the carpet to the flexes of the cables of the electrics, which have electrical energy flowing through them. What this tells you is that this building is made from energy, and the same could be said for every stationary, moving, living, non-living item on this planet and that this energy results in a product e.g. the creation of a home, the getting from A to B by train, the taste of your coffee, every chemical reaction you can think off. If everything around us including ourselves is made of energy then there is no reason why our thoughts are not also made of energy and therefore I do believe that there may be a lot of truth in the law of attraction where our thoughts send positive energy into the universe that sends back to us a product called positive results which are energy.

 As I see the theory of the Law of Attraction attracting positive results into one's life being a very credible theory, I decided when learning to drive back in 2012 that I would only allow images of positive outcomes to enter my mind whenever I had thoughts associated with learning to drive. I always made a point of seeing images in my mind of passing my test and the instructor shaking my hand and saying, "Well done. You passed your test". For some reason I always saw the examiner being a woman. Don't ask me why as I do not know. That was the first image and lasting image that my mind created. Never did I see myself failing my test. Throughout the period of time that I was learning to drive, any near appearance of such a thought about failing the test was exploded and immediately replaced with "Well done. You have passed your test", where the instructor had a smile and in my mind I could feel the shaking of her hand, and my instructor in the back putting his hand on my shoulder and saying, "Yes, Well done and on first attempt as well". When it came to the day of the test, I just fixated my mind on this image all the way to the driving centre, and guess what! The examiner was a woman, and when I sat my test, I will never forget the lady telling me to just pull up aside the kerb on my left; and when I stopped the car and put the handbrake on, put the gear stick into neutral and switched of the engine she said, "Well done you've passed". Visualisation has alongside exercise, thought blocking and meditation been one of the biggest discoveries in my life in terms of mental health symptom management. Visualisation is a tool that belongs to a set of tools called "Positive Thinking", and learning to drive taught me how guilty I was in the past of "Negative Thinking"; which involved negative forecasting which had brought upon myself so much bad luck in the past. My friend Alan always said to me that you will learn a lot about yourself through learning to drive. Learning to drive makes you learn a lot about your own psychology if a lot of it is out of place, just as meditation has done, and it is interesting that driving is a meditative experience, as it keeps you fixated in the present moment and has this same effect.

After passing my test I was anxious about driving a car that was not dual controlled, and was also very anxious about driving unfamiliar routes. I saw the driving of each unfamiliar route as being driving out of the comfort zone. I knew the highway code, I had just passed my test but I did not know how much my fluency on the roads in Slough had been down to me being very familiar with these roads and that driving unfamiliar roads would be a very different story. These two things combined, made me anxious about driving a car independently of any instructor beside me to put on the brake. This was especially the case as someone who had suffered from performance anxiety. I decided that I was going to start driving as soon as possible after my test, as I knew that the longer I left it, the harder it would become to make that transition from person who has passed test to independent road driver. The first thing I made sure of was not to tell other road users that I had just passed my test. I would not put a green "Passed sign" on my car. If a driver is seen to not indicate, people think "Driver who didn't indicate". If a driver with a green "P" is seen not to indicate, people think "A driver who shouldn't have been allowed to pass his test". I knew how important it was not to hear words of discouragement from others in my early days as a driver, therefore I refused to put this badge on my car. I think people that do put this badge on their car are potentially doing themselves a disservice. I wanted to be treated and thought of in the same way as any other road user. I could just imagine an emotionally unintelligent person in a car park saying something like "Stalling your car! Back to school for you!".

 I therefore decided to drive my first unfamiliar route on my own to a town called Motherwell from Glasgow. Motherwell is a town about fifteen miles away from where I was living in Glasgow at the time. I prepared for this drive by visualising driving a car in my mind a week in advance, morning and night for twenty minutes, feeling myself driving the car along an invented route in my mind; seeing through my own eyes in my mind what I would see in reality while getting into my car and driving an unfamiliar route. In my visualisation I felt myself opening the door of a car and feeling the car handle on my fingertips. I got in the car and felt myself sinking into the seat and shutting the door and hearing the door close. I felt the seat belt being pulled by my hands and being clicked into place. I felt my foot on the clutch and the turning of the ignition and the feel and sound of the engine coming on. I felt myself putting the gear stick into reverse and elevating the clutch to the bite and felt the bite in my mind. I looked around and did my observations in my mind, felt myself putting my foot on the gas, releasing the hand brake and the feeling of the car slowly going backwards, looking out the back window as I reversed out of the parking space as well as looking all around me to make sure I stayed a clear distance from the cars to my right and left. I felt myself turning the wheel with both hands and seeing out the front window as the car became aligned with the road out of the parking lot. I felt myself putting the car into first gear going through all the motions of breaking, clutch and forward motion of the gear stick and then felt the bite of the clutch, the pressure on the accelerator, and off I was, feeling myself moving forward, and seeing from the driving seat myself approaching the give way at the exit of the parking lot. I felt myself breaking, again going through all the motions and crossing two lanes of traffic as I pulled out onto the road taking a right turn after seeing some cars pass by from my right as well as left before doing so. I imagined the colours of these cars and noticed the speeds. I even pictured in my mind the registration numbers of these cars. I then started to drive straight down a road that I had made up in my mind with shops and pedestrians down one side and street lamps as well as parked cars on both sides of the road, with red sandstone tenements going down each side of the road. I stopped at give ways, did right and left turns, approached roundabouts, felt my fingers on the indicators, felt myself going through all the motions of gear changes and as well as seeing cars ahead; approaching from my right and left, looking in my side mirrors for coming off at roundabouts and doing left turns. I joined slipped roads, looking in my side mirrors while joining dual carriageway and motorways, and kept creating in my mind new roads with new features, different scenery and drove like this in my mind for twenty minutes finishing my visualisation pulling into a car park in Motherwell, going through all the motions of parking and turning off the ignition, unclipping the belt and thinking "I did it!", and going for a coffee to celebrate. Throughout this visualisation I imagined myself feeling confident, competent and not having a single anxiety in the world. Just before the visualisation I asked myself, "The last time you felt confident what did it feel like?" and I thought about the feeling of confidence, and used what I remembered confidence to feel like to recreate feeling confident in my mind when doing these twenty minute drives in my mind. On the day I drove to Motherwell, the drive went as perfectly as it did during my visualisation. I felt confident prior to the drive, remained confident throughout the drive and had discovered the art of what is called "Mental Rehearsal". Mental rehearsal is as effective as real- life experience in building confidence and ability, as the mind cannot tell the difference between doing something in fantasy and doing the same thing in reality. Freud was both correct and incorrect when he said that the only way to conquer your phobias was to face them. What he did not say was that the facing of your phobia did not need to be faced in reality and could be as equally faced in fantasy.

I was told by my driving instructor that as many as half of the people who pass their test don't drive as they fear competency on the roads when left alone in a non-dual controlled car. If you fit that description then this is a tool for you that won't just get you from A to B by car, but will also open up a whole load of employment opportunities and suddenly make your world incomparably more accessible as well as so much more incomparably larger, as it is a tool that can be used to unleash a whole load of potential, as it is transferable to so many different settings. Visualisation, or mental rehearsal, whichever term you prefer to use, can be used for combatting your fear of public speaking, asking out a member of the opposite sex, learning a new hands on vocational skill, attending a social event on your own, building confidence for job interviews etc

Another technique that belongs to the positive thinking set of mind tools is a technique referred to as "Positive Affirmations". Positive affirmations are statements that you say to yourself that are said in the first person, have a positive word in them that is making reference to the achieving of the desired goal e.g. succeeded, achieved etc and make reference to the desired goal. I had learned about positive affirmations from teaching the 'Expert Patient Programme' where again these work in two ways. One way is through the already mentioned "Law of Attraction" that many, including myself, believe in; despite having its critics, and the other way it works is that it gives you a "can do" attitude as well as ethos; creating a mindset where you see, create and utilise opportunities as well as find yourself subconsciously making the most of these opportunities, thus, carving a path towards succeeding at whatever your aim or goal is. As already mentioned, the mind can't tell the difference between fantasy and reality, therefore if the mind hears yourself saying that you have already achieved the very goal that you are working towards achieving, the mind will believe this goal to have already been achieved; thus, giving you the confidence of someone who has achieved this goal, while you go about the achieving of this goal.

After ending Fairway Advocacy in September 2017, I looked back on the over three years of its existence and thought of it as being a major success, and continue to do so to this day as during its short life it had had a life transforming effect on so many peoples' lives and my charity had moved mountains for many. My charity did not fail. My charity was closed due to my charity existing in a world that cannot prioritise spending, where success is too often down to who you know and not what you know; in a world where people get jealous, feel insecure about themselves and take their bitterness over not being rich and famous out on those who look like becoming big and successful with time. The closing of the charity was also because we live in a world where we put quantity before quality. The funders think "Epilepsy Connections, huge charity therefore we will make a priority when designating funding", and then think "Fairway Advocacy, one man band, funding to be pulled". What they should have thought was, "Fairway Advocacy transformed the lives of 120 people, unlike Epilepsy Connections, who most people with epilepsy living in the Glasgow area have never heard of!!!, so let's give Fairway the funding instead". As far as I'm concerned, Epilepsy Connections may as well be called "Cocoa Pops Connections". They are there purely for their own self- serving purpose, as with their funding they rent out the first floor of an office block right in the centre of the 15th biggest financial centre in Europe. I feel that charities like Epilepsy Connections just take advantage of those with epilepsy co-existing with learning disability to create jobs with fancy job titles, allowing those who hold these positions to boast about being socio-economic one and two to their friends and relatives at parties and family get togethers. These positions are held by people who are all about ego. They get defensive as well as aggressive when they meet someone who might know more than they as a result of having an experience that they know they will never be able to rival. They especially get jealous or feel threatened by anyone who is seen to know more than they; and have the skills, knowledge as well as experience to make a bigger difference than they; this is especially so when that person who is seen as being a threat is a man. I would associate these disability charities as being more concerned with gender inequality than disability inequality where woman are represented amongst the workforce more than those with disability. These woman numbers are also very disproportionate where for every one man there is around seven women. Look at some of these charities websites and the "about us" page has a staff team photograph where there are up to twelve females and one very lonely looking man in the photograph.

When I started Fairway Advocacy, I worried that I would not get clients or I would not successfully resolve any cases. This was a real anxiety and it kept me up one night in March of 2014. I decided while standing in the kitchen that I was going to use visualisation as well as positive affirmations to attract into my life success at getting clients as well as resolve cases. I decided to visualise by lying on my bed for forty five minutes and created a scenario in my mind such as a meeting between myself, a client, a housing officer as well as an anti-social neighbour. I would picture in my mind as though I was experiencing it for real, so I was visualising the scenario in my mind as though I was seeing it through my own eyes as opposed to looking down on myself as a fly on a wall. I would feel myself shaking the hand of my client and the housing officer, I would picture the room and all the details such as pictures on wall and the smell of the air freshener. I would feel myself pulling out a seat and sitting down at a table which the antisocial neighbour was sitting at. I imagined the hair colour of the neighbour, the clothes they were wearing, the voice they spoke with etc. In my mind I introduced myself and spoke about the problem my client was having and felt myself putting a diary on the table making reference to a chronology of all anti-social behaviour. I saw the dates, the times, the occurrences etc The meeting would end with the housing officer telling the neighbour that they would be receiving an official caution of eviction in the post in a few days, and that everyone was in agreement round the table with a consensus in the form of a devised terms and conditions that the neighbour had to satisfy, that we were all happy with. I would visualise leaving the centre with my client and him thanking me so much outside the housing association office where I would feel him shaking my hand and me giving him my card to give me a phone if the trouble started again and receiving a signed mandate from him allowing me to make phone calls to his housing officer on his behalf whenever he wished to log a complaint. I would then open my eyes and I was back to lying on my bed in my room.

These visualisations were accompanied with me doing positive affirmations throughout the day which involved creating and saying to myself a statement about the achieving of a goal by myself that was present tense so that my mind believed that the result had already been achieved. These positive affirmations were unique to my goals which were to make a success of Fairway Advocacy. The positive affirmations that I used to make a success of Fairway Advocacy were:

"My Name is Tim Bone and Fairway Advocacy is the biggest achievement of my life" (mental image of me standing outside Fairway Advocacy)

"My Name is Tim Bone and I have achieved a huge number of resolutions for Fairway Advocacy's clients" (mental image of me scrolling through Fairway Advocacy's archive of results)

"My Name is Tim Bone and I have received a huge congratulations from the most influential of people for making a real success of Fairway Advocacy" (mental image of me walking up onto a stage and having my hand shaken by a cabinet politician)

"My name is Tim Bone and I have grown and developed Fairway Advocacy into the most successful advocacy organisation" (mental image of me standing inside Fairway Advocacy with all my staff walking around me)

As can be seen all these positive affirmations are personal i.e. My name is Tim Bone; present tense i.e. said as though the goal is something I can say I have already achieved in the present moment; and have a positive word in them e.g. "Achieve". This is the structure that all positive affirmations should conform to. Each one of these positive affirmations also has a picture attached to it that I see in my mind as I hear the positive affirmation being said in my mind. The image is optional however one should still do as "seeing is believing"!

It was through the use of these visualisation exercises that I gave myself to do in my bedroom lying on my bed with my eyes closed; as well as the positive affirmations that I did throughout the day, that my confidence and self- belief multiplied by many times, and I attracted into my life three and a half years' worth of clients and results that amounted to a total of 120 successful resolutions doing a 15hr week. This project had the making of a charity that was going to grow, but unfortunately, I had to close it for reasons related to Fairway Advocacy being a "small fish swimming amongst sharks". One thing you have to realise about visualisation i.e. mental rehearsal and the law of attraction, is that your goals have to be realistic. My goal was a double-barrelled goal. I wanted resolutions but I also wanted to become a big advocacy charity walking all over the authorities winning cases for clients at a time of government cuts to services i.e. British government cuts, and other advocacy charities having a vested interest in allying with the government due to the receiving of statutory (Government) funding under the Mental Health (Care & Treatment) Act due to lack of available funding for charities. This created one realistic goal, but also, one unrealistic goal. The realistic goal was the achieving of resolutions, the unrealistic goal was the project surviving the long term and growing when swimming among what I would call the sharks i.e. statutory funded advocacy charities, the other neurological charities that would always be prioritised funding over an organisation like Fairway Advocacy, and people like the Scottish Independent Advocacy Alliance who would bad mouth Fairway Advocacy. It looked increasingly likely that the SIAA were not going to renew our membership for reasons that I would have to share with the funders that would certainly have affected our already very small chances of getting further funding.

As you can see, I achieved the resolutions but did not achieve the long- term growth and development of the project. What conclusion can we draw from this? The conclusion that can be drawn is that visualisation and positive affirmations bring success by building confidence; inspiring and motivating you, cultivating an optimistic "can do" mentality as well as recruiting the law of attraction, but goals have to be realistic in order to come to fruition. You also have to be a believer in the law of attraction in order for the law of attraction to take effect. You can't be saying, "I have achieved" at the front of your mind, but also saying, "I won't achieve" at the back of your mind. You've got to be 100% mentally occupied with the "I have achieved" ethos. As far as you are concerned there is no alternative to succeeding. You don't even accommodate the prospect of an opposite to success happening. As far as you are concerned there is no such thing as failure and that there is only one outcome, and that outcome is Success!!. It is vital that if any thoughts of failure or bad outcome enter your mind, you immediately explode that thought and replace it with a triumphant thought that can be in the form of inner dialogue or mental image. It is also necessary for you to be able to appreciate that law of attraction can work in two ways. These two ways are one step forward followed by more steps forward; but also, the odd step backwards that creates opportunities, that result in taking more steps forwards. It is important when you experience one of these steps back that you keep believing in law of attraction and recognise this as a step back that will result in many more steps forward, by keeping a positive mental attitude by continuing to do your positive affirmations as well as visualisations.

CHAPTER 27

As already mentioned back in July 2016 my depression caused for me problems with literacy and numeracy as I had difficulties processing the words that I was reading. The depression was making it impossible for me to process information. As I have said with reading you take the information in (Concentration), you put it all together so that it makes sense (Processing) and then you retain the knowledge that you have processed (Memory). My processing was so impaired by my depression that I could concentrate but I was not making any sense of what I was reading. I worried that I had some sort of dementia and this on top of having an insight into the problems being cognitively impaired can cause frightened me, and caused great anxiety for me, that resulted in anxiety polluting my concentration so I was no longer concentrating either. The crippling effects the depression had on my reading made me paranoid about other cognitive faculties, such as listening and being able to process what people were saying to me as well as remembering what people were telling me. This resulted in me becoming anxious when people spoke to me due to being terrified over my cognition; which affected my concentration, and therefore could impair my ability to follow phone calls and watch the television. It didn't affect me so much when speaking to people in person, but I became very distressed watching the news and not being able to follow what was going on in the world.

This fear when listening to people, and the disabling effects that it had on my communication skills as well as literacy skills, went through its ups and downs. These disabling effects lifted when consistently meditating; however, they came back if I went three days with only getting one meditation practice in per day.

A large part of what caused the anxiety about having some cognitively deteriorating condition was scare stories that I had been reading on the internet, as well as in the odd newspaper article, where I was being told that social isolation can bring on early stage dementia. The literacy issues came on before the scare stories, but the problems with listening and following people speaking came on after the scare stories. It was because of these fears over cognition, brought on by affected literacy, that my Dad took me to the G.P. surgery on that morning in July 2016, where I ended up carrying out a judo throw on him in the Helensburgh swimming pool car park, causing him to experience a blow to his head off the ground that hospitalised him in the Paisley Royal Alexander, Accident & Emergency Department. I left my father in the car park as others came to help him, where they waited with him until the ambulance arrived. I left the car park and attended my G.P. appointment, as has already been mentioned in an earlier chapter. I was offered a referral to the Community Mental Health Team but decided a few weeks later, after receiving my letter from the Community Mental Health Team with a date for an out-patient appointment, that I would not attend for three reasons. These reasons being that I did not feel it appropriate to have my scars treated by the very society that had inflicted them. I also believed that it would just cause the issues I went to the doctor with to become more crippling, as psychiatry can't be described as being empowering; and also because the psychiatrist would most likely put my issues down to something that can't be helped by saying it is part of my personality, especially with a history of epilepsy, thus, destroying my confidence in myself being able to conquer the issues that I was presenting with. I also recognised that I was a meditator, and when meditating consistently I was not affected by these cognitive issues, and that the distress caused by affected literacy, that had caused me to refer myself to the G.P., had occurred over a period of time where I had not been consistently meditating. The rage that caused me to carry out a judo throw on my father had happened on a morning of a day where I had not done my morning meditation nor had I been consistent with my meditation in the days leading up to that appointment. I was certain, and I still am certain, that psychiatry was not the answer, nor were cognitive tests to reassure me that I was cognitively fine, and instead what was needed was   the practice of consistent morning and night meditation. This conclusion proved correct, as for the next six months I was a consistent meditator and all cognitive issues either disappeared, or at least improved dramatically, and continued to improve until January 2017, when my meditation practice became inconsistent again. As a consequence of the meditation practice becoming inconsistent, cognitive symptoms as well as other symptoms of anxiety and depression went through periods of remission and relapse, but in August 2017, I had decided that I was finally going to commit myself to long term consistent meditation, and be as consistent with my meditation as I am with my anticonvulsants. I had told myself that it can't be consistent for a number of weeks and then inconsistent for a further number of weeks. I told myself, that was being just as inconsistent as twice a day for three days, followed by once per day for four days. Since August 2017, and the time of writing i.e. 30th March 2018, I have been a consistent morning and night meditator, and have had no periods of inconsistency.

As well as consistently meditating, I am also consistently getting to the gym two days/week, where I am doing two half marathons a week in terms of calorie expenditure in the gym. I now have a resting pulse rate of forty- four, and I am now having meditation sessions where I am in the thought free zone for up to the full forty- five minutes during the best of my meditation sessions. My mind is totally within the space of my breaths, and not focussing on past or future thoughts. It is my idea of what it must be like to be in a part of the universe where there are no planets or life form for millions of light years. In the gym, I am taking a meditative approach to exercising for an hour on the cross trainer by only focussing on getting to the end of the present minute, and not allowing myself to think of time done and time still to do. This, I have noticed, has increased my pain threshold, and has enabled me to go for longer periods on the cardiovascular equipment. I have noticed myself experiencing feelings of euphoria during the day; and wakening up with euphoria, feelings of reward, motivation, as well as confidence. This will be a combined effect of both the meditation and the exercise, however, each on their own is capable of giving you the same feel good factor, evidenced by periods of only getting to the gym before I took up meditation, as well as evidenced by periods of only meditation, when gym attendance has dropped. All I can say is, "Who needs anti-depressants!". I put an exclamation mark after that previous question, as it is a rhetorical question. It is more a statement to the anti-depressant industry, that I will let no one profit from mental health problems affecting me, that have been inflicted upon me by the very society that prescribes these pills. My interpretation of mental health is that it has become an industry like Christmas, as well as package holidays to the Mediterranean. Two things make me a meditator and athlete. One is, I will not allow anyone to profit from misery inflicted upon me by others, who will have inflicted misery themselves on others during their time, as we have all been on the receiving end of it, or we have been joining in giving it. The other reason is that I am an anti-authority person, and will not keep alive an industry that authority has created. I see meditation and exercise as the "water and carbon dioxide foam", the authority, as well as drug companies, as the "Fire", and the majority of the mainstream population as being the fuel that keeps that fire burning. Those in the mainstream, who are not the "fuel" for that "fire", are the proper left- wing socialists who campaign and show an interest in all human rights i.e. the human rights activists such as 'Campaign 38'. Too many people calling themselves left wing because they are bitter about not being rich, when their neighbour is rich, but couldn't care less about any other human right related issues. This is not left wing. This is bitter. It is in fact a very right-wing thing, to be only interested in wealth inequality! I have joined an organisation called "Campaign 38" who circulate campaigns to e-mail addresses asking for the support of the e-mail account holder to support their campaign, which will one day be over a   poverty related issue, the next day will be concerning a disability discrimination related issue, the next day an issue concerning the inhumane treatment of people in prison, and many more left wing issues. It is people like they who are the minority of the mainstream who are not the "fuel". Speak about inequality in wealth with the rest of the population and they are all ears, however, talk about disabled people being on the receiving end of inhuman treatment, or the welfare state's abandonment of former military personnel injured in war, and they are not interested, which is why it is allowed to continue. I would say that these people are bitter right-wingers, who are never suspected of being right wing as a result of their accent and post code, just demonstrating the judgmental attitude of the human race, where everyone believes to be a right winger you have to be wealthy, privileged, educated and posh, which in itself is evidence of bitterness and judgementalism, which is both divisive and right wing. It's like what Nelson Mandela said, and that was, "you measure how left wing a society is by how it treats its most vulnerable", and the answer as to how we treat our most vulnerable in Britain is "SHOCKING!!!". Political Parties either have a policy that penalises disability, or they don't have a policy. The "left" only addresses the areas that win the votes and allows people to take out their jealousy e.g. distribution of wealth, and gender inequality. That's not to say that these areas are not big legitimate areas, but they cast way too large a shadow over the other areas. Every bus driver would tell you he's left wing despite so many grudgingly give a person with a disability card his ticket with the most unfriendly facial expression and body language. I've seen this as a support worker and a disability advocate when taking clients on buses to meetings and social events where their disability card gives them free travel due to being on out of work benefits. I've even come across disability social workers, who would claim to be left-wing, throwing someone with epilepsy out of their office and putting an end to their education!!!, then down to the polling station to vote for the "left", despite only a few hours ago carrying out a worser human rights violation than cutting the foot soldier's pay to increase the pay of those at the top.

CHAPTER 28

On the 21st November 2017 I had taught a session on 'Mindfulness' to a group of people affected by epilepsy at a charity in Glasgow. The first thing we discussed was a slide that was titled ***"To take or not to take?"***. That is the question!". This slide informed everyone that to determine whether anti-depressants were the answer for their depression, or if they would be better taking the mindfulness route, it was important that their decision was a well-informed one and that they knew all the facts. It had come to my attention during my research that one of the things that would be crucial for someone to know in order to be able to make an informed decision would be that the anti-depressant industry has been funding a large number of clinical trials. This is a fact that I had read in the scientific journal "Scientific American" dated 2015. Professor Irving Kirsch, a psychologst who studies the placebo effect i.e. the imagined effect, found that sugar pills were just as effective as anti-depressants in the treatment of depressive symptoms. Irving Kirsch also mentions that the anti-depressant industry claim from clinical trials that these drugs increase the happy mood neurotransmitter called Serotonin but what they don't make reference to in their claims is the number of studies that have shown no increase in serotonin levels using these drugs. Irving Kirsch also claims that many medical professionals believe that placebo pills should be prescribed first as
they are just as effective as anti-depressants. According to the Citizens Commission on Human Rights UK website, Professor Irving Kirsch quotes in a University of Hull study that anti-depressants are "No better than placebo", where placebo was nothing more than sugar pills. This quote was quoted on a page on the CCHRUK site titled "The massive cost to the NHS for antidepressant drugs that don't work" and has as its first paragraph:

"The profit-driven psychiatric industry is making a killing from selling anti-depressant drugs in the UK"

Many of the drug trials are therefore biased, and there are reputable psychologists carrying out placebo studies that demonstrate they are no more effective than placebo, and as well as that they cost a lot of money. I will let you come to your own conclusions on these drugs. My conclusion is that they are a fraud and that I will stick with meditation, exercise and increasingly diet thank you very much; which is empowering, adds lost years onto your life, allowing you to maintain your independence thus preventing others from exploiting your helplessness as well as enhancing quality of life. I want to be an old man aged 86 swinging a golf club on the first tee, and not an old man having his porridge fed to him in a nursing home where I am left to sit there all day vegetating in a chair vocalising, "Goo, Goo-Gah-Gah" with a carer putting in my care notes that I had done lots of things today, which I did not do, simply to satisfy the Care Inspectorate; putting in my drug Kardex that I had received my morning anti-convulsants even though my carer had failed to give me my morning medication, causing me to have had four seizures that day in the chair I am vegetating in. I know this happens as I have worked in these places!

As I write this chapter in the book, in the month of January 2019, I have learned that my former client, that I advocated for when Fairway Advocacy was functioning, has been hospitalised in a mental health ward due to a breakdown brought on by living in isolation as well as the stress and anxiety that comes with lack of available family support in a person with moderate learning disability. Alistair has been admitted into hospital as he had attempted to take his own life with a knife. The last I heard of Alistair was that he has been drugged up to the eyeballs on strong medication, and his friend who has been enquiring about him has told me that Alistair is so drugged up that he can't recognise anyone, he becomes very distressed when visited and that he will be in hospital for the long term. When I was made aware of this I couldn't help think "Yeh, and there will now be a social worker saying to Alistair's housing association over the phone, "You can give that two bedroom house to the Baxters now'". I don't mean to be cynical but I did read about cases like this when I was running Fairway Advocacy. It was before Fairway's intervention, that a council in the Glasgow area were not prepared to give a client of mine, with Multiple Sclerosis, a chair lift to get her from her lounge to the toilet, even though they knew that she lay there incontinent on the lounge floor on a regular basis. The council had been denying this woman a chairlift for months. Anyone who can do this with no conscience, as their boss has told them to do this, is capable of worsening a person's state of mind to an extent that, on the surface, makes the giving of that person's home to someone else look perfectly legitimate i.e. "They had gone mad. They were depressed and not coping living on their own home". Totally criminal!!, if you ask me. The housing association very often refuses to deal with anti-social neighbour complaints of those with learning disability, allowing neighbours to bully them to the point where they have a breakdown, and then, they find themselves in hospital as a result of having tried to take their own life, freeing up a home by creating for social work/housing association an argument for putting that person in residential care by claiming that not being able to cope in the community was the reason for that person's breakdown.

When those with learning disability report harassment by others, all they receive as a response is "Have you got any witnesses?". The famous get out clause!! I have recently noticed that council websites now demand that you use an online complaint form to report an antisocial neighbour, unlike the old days when you just gave them a phone call. This change in way of reporting an anti-social neighbour to the environmental protection services typically disadvantages those with learning disability who have limited literacy skills in many cases. If you read the text messages from some of these people you often have to phone them to get a verbal interpretation for clarification.

CHAPTER 29

As already mentioned, symptom self- management began in 1993 when I used 'Distraction' for symptoms of Obsessive Compulsive Disorder, and then again for the second time back in 1998 when I took up cardiovascular exercise to combat new symptoms of obsessive compulsive disorder as well as prevent moderate depression escalating into major depression, thus, instead reducing moderate depression to light/moderate depression. I also, as already mentioned, used mental arithmetic for defusing warnings developing into seizures, as well as thought blocking and meditation for anger management. It could be said that through living with epilepsy, anxiety and depression, I have developed a lot of life skills and quality traits of personality. 'Discipline', has been one personality trait e.g. getting to the gym; 'determination and perseverance' have been other traits e.g. meditation, positive thinking and getting back up on my feet after each knock; 'stamina and endurance' e.g. having to live with depression, anxiety, frequent seizures, living in an overly critical society, having an unsupportive family and no friends, living with ill emotion towards the world and its people and finding healthy ways in coping e.g. exercise, meditation, positive thinking. I have also grown up outspoken, assertive, unpretentious, and independent minded; free of the pressures of social expectation, the opinions as well as thoughts of others; opening up a new world with many more opportunities than the world most people settle for through living up to society's expectations. I have learned life knowledge such as the grip capitalism has on the throats of the mainstream i.e. have you got the newest version? The lead weight that conformity is to the ankle of most civilians, limiting self- exploration and development of individuality and fulfilling of potential.

Most of the personal development began back in 2003 when I volunteered to teach the Expert Patient Programme (EPP), which led to the training officer job at Disability Information Greater Glasgow, which then led to me becoming a rescue medication trainer in 2008 at Epilepsy Scotland before moving down to the Epilepsy Society in 2009, where I was allowed to become a rescue medication trainer, as well as a support worker, where I taught the administration of rectal diazepam and buccal midazolam to support staff for two years. Unfortunately, when my manager failed me for my drug training in the residential unit that I worked in as a support worker, I was no longer invited to train other support staff the administration of rescue medication.

This failing of drug training was a real blow to me. No one talks about sexual discrimination against men, especially where the discrimination could cost lives due to a shortage of drug trained staff. I was told that there had been an evening where the night shift were men and women but none of the drug trained women were on shift meaning that there was no one on the unit drug trained. I was made aware that a resident had gone into status epilepticus and there was no one to administer rescue medication and that this involved phoning around the other houses for a drug trained member of staff to come over to administer the buccal midazolam. It is essential for rescue drug treatment to   be administered immediately when someone experiences status epilepticus, due to the risk of Sudden Unexpected Death in Epilepsy, also known as 'SUDEP' in the medical community. If SUDEP had happened, I am sure the talk in the staff room would have been, "If only the manager had drug trained the men". The problem with gender discrimination is that it can cause a lot of collateral damage, especially in a care setting. If you ask me, what my manager did was endanger life through the slandering and destroying of the future career prospects of support workers at the Epilepsy Society who so happened to be men. Section 22 of the "Mental Health Act" says that if you are a risk to others or yourself due to your mental health status then a 'Compulsory Treatment Order' which could involve sectioning will be granted if you practice your unconditional right under the Patient Rights Act to not cooperate in the receiving of mental health treatment. I would say that this section of the Mental Health Act makes reference to someone like my manageress as she had a "chip on the shoulder" i.e. Major Insecurity, that was causing her to keep men at the bottom of the workplace hierarchy that was endangering the lives of the residents in her unit. There was obviously a problem with morale and self-esteem that was causing my manageress to behave in a way that was endangering life of residents, as it was creating scenarios where there were no drug trained staff on shifts where residents were experiencing status epilepticus. The mental health community should be creating moral and self-esteem pills that they should be forcing women like this manager into taking so that she will drug train the men, thus, safeguarding the lives of those these men provide care for.

I then decided that with the ill treatment I had received from society, especially with the experience of the sexist boss setting me up as being too unsafe to administer medication, which resulted in me being deemed too unsafe to train those to administer rescue medication, I was going to bounce back and not be floored, by using the life skills I had, and work for myself thus only being accountable to myself. This is what gave me the ability to successfully run an advocacy charity for over three years, which I closed due to lack of available funding to apply for, but also as the impression was given to me that someone was very unhappy that they had not been a part of our success, and had a vested interest in seeing us off the scene to protect egos and remain in their eyes the big wigs. These people were also receiving government funding to provide services which gave them a vested interest in siding with the government run authorities that my advocacy charity was successfully winning cases against. I was a small fish swimming amongst sharks who had the powers and clout to create a situation for me that could have caused a scandal tarring my name if I continued to take on the cases I was taking on as an advocate and practice a style of advocacy that won good results for the client and created a loss for the bully boy authority. Social work were making their complaints in August 2017, and the people who oversee advocacy were starting to side with the complaints, when all I had been guilty of doing was fulfilling the role of an advocate. I saw this as the beginning of the end of my charity and possibly the beginning of the end of my name, by creating for me another major injustice that I would have to live with. There was nothing to stop a female winning favour with the social work department by referring herself to my service and then accusing me of sexually harassing her, or even worse sexually assaulting her, bringing an immediate end to not just the charity but also me being able to work in any paid or voluntary role where I would be working with vulnerable adults. I would have not put it past the social work department trying such a stunt with me when I saw how they behaved back in 2008, when they learned about my epilepsy at the time of me being a social work student on placement. What social work did in 2008 told me that these people would feel no shame or remorse playing a stunt that could see an innocent person in prison for a few years, living with a criminal record, and his name on the sex offenders register. Yes, that is how low I think of these people, and if there are any social workers who feel offended reading this, I would say to them take your complaint to your colleagues and don't raise it with me. If you don't like the image I have of you, and the things I have to say about you, then you have to ask why I have these images and opinions of you, as they have not come from nowhere. I take responsibility for the impression I give of myself to others, which is why I behave respectfully towards others, and consider others when making decisions that won't just affect me but could have a knock- on effect on them. In my eyes, I don't see why social work should be an exception to this rule, and I am sure that the other readers don't believe that social work should be an exception to this rule either. Social work have given me no reason to be impressed by them, but have given me every reason to think very little of them, and always be expecting the worst intentions from them, and it should be your priority to change what people like me think of your profession by addressing the behaviour coming from the profession, instead of labelling me cynical and paranoid. The years 2008, and 2014-2017, are full of behaviours from social work that would take a child out of social work's care and put that child into care! Forgot, Social work is the highest authority therefore that can't happen. For those reading, who may think this is harsh, you will learn later what those in social care are prepared to do to see you off the scene in a future chapter!

In response to the siding of the 'Scottish Independent Advocacy Alliance' with the 'Health & Social Care Partnerships', that are government authorities; the complaints the SIAA were making to the directors of my charity and the reliance of a reference from the SIAA if funding could be found for Fairway Advocacy to apply for, I decided to close my advocacy charity. I bounced back from this with the idea of writing a book, and as a result of my experience of self- management, being a self-management trainer on the Expert Patient Programme, as well as delivering my own self-management course, I was invited in September 2017 to become a symptom management trainer for the "Epilepsy Futures Course", at an epilepsy charity, where I teach those attending life skills that will help them overcome the barriers created for them by their epilepsy, society and unmet mental health needs.

From the learning of life skills and self-management skills through living with epilepsy, anxiety and depression, I plan on becoming a symptom management trainer; training others the techniques that can be employed in the treating of depression and anxiety as an alternative to drug treatment. I know I am on route to this as it would be a venture created solely by myself with no help or advice, nor being told by anyone how to start and succeed at this venture. Life has proven when people stay out the equation and I am left to my own devices, I succeed and excel; however, when people poke their nose in my personal development by playing role of teacher, mentor, manager, etc the carpet is pulled from under my feet. It appears to be the case that I build the sand castles and others just come along and knock them down. I need to make castles out of stronger stuff which is why I seek a future taking the road towards self-employment, where I am free of any type of regulation by others.

The frightening thing is having epilepsy has given me more than society has had to offer. In fact, society has given me nothing. I couldn't care less who was in power in government, so long as they don't privatise the NHS, as I do get my anti-convulsants off the NHS. As a consequence of having epilepsy I have developed life knowledge and life skills that make me self-employable. I believe that this is a good example of self- empowerment, but at the same time a terrible reflection on our society that illness can enhance you more than society can. This means to some of us society is our biggest ill. My conditions should be labelled as epilepsy, anxiety, depression and society. The irony is, society is the parent that gave birth to two of these conditions. This has given me an empathy for the gang lords who run our criminal underworld. It could be said that they have profited and built big business, and become chief of big empire, living the life of luxury, living of the millions made out of other peoples' misery, but that success came from circumstances caused by society's abandonment and exclusion of these people, resulting in angry civilians feeling they owe society no good civilian and looking to take out their rage on society by breaking every rule in the book and becoming society's biggest ill since society was their biggest ill during childhood, adolescence and early adulthood and beyond. They are an example of how society's cruel treatment of some can backfire on society, and maybe lessons could be learned that unfortunately will never be learned. It also explains why maybe one in fifty people in prison have epilepsy. I wonder how many of the remaining forty-nine in fifty have other forms of disability? What can be said is that there are many people with high functioning learning disability in prison who make up their percentage of that one in forty nine. Crime and politics are just as closely tied as disability and politics, inevitably resulting in disability and crime crossing paths. Psychiatry would say this was evidence of people with epilepsy and other disability having 'Anti-Social Personality Disorder', or some other 'Personality Disorder' type, when it is nothing of the sort. It is called society treating a person like muck! Unfortunately none of this relationship between politics, disability and crime is covered in any of the medical text books, and anyone who has progressed in life by following a level playing field, such as a medical student who would pass his exams so long as he revised for them; will have no knowledge or experience that teaches them that so long as one's personality is consistent with the terrain that their life path has followed then they have no psychiatric condition. Personalities are shaped by peoples' life courses and psychiatry recognises none of this. It is after all rumoured that President Nixon's equivalent of a home secretary requested the invention of personality disorder to label those who protested against the social injustices in American society during his time in power. As has already been mentioned, psychiatry believes that the world is a level playing field for everyone and that you "make your bed and lie on it"; "what you get out, is what you put in"; "others treat you, the way you treat others"; "No pain, no gain" etc and therefore any complaints made by you and ill emotion can only stem from some sort of irrational state of mind rendering you mentally ill. That's the thinking of someone who believes we live in the perfect world. The belief of living in such a world is as much a false illusion as the seizure world during a complex partial seizure is. You could accuse the psychiatric profession as being a bunch of doctors experiencing a seizure that never lifts and that every conclusion i.e. diagnosis that they make is a diagnosis being made by someone whose cognitively impaired as their interpretation of the world around them is completely inaccurate and untrue. It must be a great life to be someone whose only injustice in the world has been their exam paper being harder than the year's before, where the education system and employment opportunities has allowed you a role in society that pays £80,000 per annum salary as well as providing you with the opportunity to run a private practice on top of this £80,000 per annum salary where your next question to your spouse will be "Will it be Delhi this year or Beijing?". These people are the least able of forming non-biased open- minded conclusions looking at others' behavioural reactions towards society's treatment of them.

THE FUNCTIONALITY CONTINUUM

After having read this far through the book you will have decided on whether you are a member of the fraction of the population that is anti this plague that infests the lives of those with epilepsy, or if you are a member of the fraction of the population that spreads the plague. I would hope that you have either remained anti the plague or have been converted into becoming anti- plague.

If you are truly left wing or centre right, but not extreme right; then I would hope the next time you meet someone with epilepsy or any other neurological condition, you would be non-judgemental of them and treat them as equals, as to treat them the opposite way leads to a lifetime of issues that can result in a fatality in those less equipped to cope. Such behaviour of the mainstream towards people with epilepsy, in the knowledge that this behaviour will cause mental health issues and possibly a fatality, is on a par with torture, in the knowledge that torture can cause death. The mental torture as well as fatalities that western society is responsible for in those with complex partial epilepsy, has and continues to make me feel that western society commemorating armistice day should be seen as double standards by those affected by complex partial epilepsy. It is because of western society being guilty of double standards, evidenced by my own experiences living in western society, that I cannot bring myself to commemorating 'Armistice Day'. Most people are capable of cooperating in mass genocide if the order to kill is given by an authoritative figure. This was proven in an experiment carried out by a psychologist called Milgram, at Yale University in 1963. Milgram's experiment involved taking a sample of men from a cross section of society and ordering them to administer imitation electric shocks to a human which the participants believed to be real electric shocks. These shocks increased from zero volts right up to 450 volts, where two thirds of participants would keep administering increases in electric shocks when ordered to do so up until the 300 volt mark and the remaining third were prepared to keep administering shocks right up to the 450 volt mark. Milgram concluded from this that most humans are prepared to kill someone if the order is given from an authoritative figure. I therefore see the vast majority of the public as being a potential Nazi as well as a potential Hitler right hand man when this was the defence that Hitler's right hand men used when they were tried for their war crimes i.e. "I was acting under orders". This theory proven by Milgram would certainly explain how colleagues/mentors have managed with a free conscience to participate in the constructive dismissal of myself from jobs and courses. In my last job, where evidence was constructed to put me in a position where I either resigned or got sacked, one of the participating members of staff had been a man who I had been getting on with really well for the previous few days until I was asked to accompany him to a client's home, where he asked me on route what the address was, which I said I did not know as I believed him to have the address. This colleague suddenly turned nasty and shouted at me, "Isn't that very stupid? Going to a client's home and not taking with you the address" in the most hostile way. This guy had gone from good friend to aggressive bully in a matter of a few working hours under the instruction of someone from above. While these moments of unexplained hostility was coming from those outside the office, others in the office were fiddling with rotas under the orders of authority…………….. More on this later.

Last Armistice Day I thought to myself that every discriminator, judgemental person, bully, person who just stands back and watches the discrimination, non-genuine person who disappoints, person who back stabs and therefore can't trust, greedy person, selfish person; and every person obsessed with wealth, power and status (the three things being the roots of all wars) will be wearing a poppy today. What double standards. What I can say is that living with epilepsy, anxiety and depression has made me the opposite of all these things and has made me a less dangerous individual; yet I am probably more likely of spending some of my years behind bars than any of these people. It is also because of these other peoples' behaviours and their inability to stand firm against authority, that people like me have the relationship difficulties that we have and find ourselves having to wear the label of "Personality Disorder", thus, evidencing society and her people to be the cause of so much ill health. It is also because of all these people you find wearing poppies on Armistice Day that 1 in 7 people with my type of epilepsy will be pushed into attempting to take their own lives. The truth is this country's people are as dangerously right wing and capable of ruthless treatment of vulnerable people as race hatred groups are of those who belong to different ethnic minorities.

I want to emphasise the strengths of the minds and brains of people with epilepsy, as we only focus on the weaknesses. Every epilepsy charity I visit only provides services for those with learning disability who have needs that cannot be met in mainstream society. This creates the illusion amongst the mainstream that epilepsy is a condition, which all people who suffer from are also affected by learning disability. This image of epilepsy seriously compromises those with epilepsy without learning disability, living in this judgemental world.

It is the case that 40% of people with epilepsy have a learning disability, which can be anything from mild to severe. When I worked at the Epilepsy Society, the residents I looked after had poorly controlled epilepsy, co-existing with moderate to severe learning disability. What we are not told anything about is the other 60% of people with epilepsy in terms of their cognition.

I have now been meditating morning and night since December 2013, but I only started meditating consistently morning and night since September 2017. During my time as a meditator I have had afternoons where I have sat on the couch that I meditate on, analysed my behaviour and looked at the rationales behind both my behaviours and decisions that I make, and noticed patterns in my behaviour that evidence many things about myself as a person, allowing me to understand myself better. My meditation practice also has me look at the behaviours of others that I have noticed in   my forty three years of being a civilian living in British society in academic, vocational, commercial, social etc settings; and have noticed the rationales behind their behaviours, the decisions that they make, as well as patterns in behaviours, thus, being able to draw conclusions about the mainstream population. I have also been able to do the same psychoanalysis of those with severe to high functioning learning disability. It is from these afternoons of psychoanalysing the world, as well as myself, that I have been able to find a number of theories that explains me, the mainstream population and those with learning disability that might explain my isolation and incompatibilities that have existed between myself and mainstream society. These are theories that maybe psychiatrists would say are evidence of a 'Personality Disorder'. I disagree with what the psychiatrists would conclude from these theories, and instead see these theories as evidence of strengths and qualities the world is scared of other people having as well as being evidence of having undergone a lot of personal development.

These theories, are theories that I made no deliberate attempt to create. They are theories that just naturally surfaced in my mind during three of my depressive days, where I have found myself getting up at 10.00am and going through to the lounge to sit on my couch all day, and still find myself in my vest and boxer shorts at 4pm that same afternoon. The fruition of these theories I believe to be "spiritual awakenings", that one who meditates experiences when they get to a milestone in the progress they are making through their meditation practice. They do say that before a spiritual awakening your symptoms can temporarily worsen which would explain why I have had these awakenings on depressive days. As already mentioned, meditation makes you a human psychologist who has done their training at the "University of Living with Anxiety and Depression".

One thing that came to my attention while I was sitting on my couch a couple of years ago while I was asking myself why I couldn't make any friends and didn't have a single relationship in the world other than with my father, was the fact that all meetup groups I had been attending either had people show up with a friend, as they did not like turning up for the first time on their own, or they came alone but they had already become a regular. I had also met people at meetups who had come on their own who confessed to me that they had to have a few drinks to get tipsy before coming that evening. I then asked myself, "Where are most people's friends from?". After asking this question I remembered my aunt saying that there are only two times people meet new friends for life after school and they are university/higher education or outside the school gates picking up your children. I then disagreed with this to myself as there are people who still have friends that they work in the same workplace with, play sport with, are members of the same club or society as, or some other type of institution. It then came to me. That was the problem. The vast majority of people in our society can only meet people through being members of an "institution". Institution is required to get people meeting, crossing paths with one another often enough on a regular basis, before becoming confident enough to let their guard down and form relationships with one another, which includes the formation of friendships. I realised that I had not been a member of an institution that I belonged in nor provided for opportunities to meet up with others beyond the "gates" of that institution since July 1997, when I was at Glasgow University. Since July 1997, I was either a member of an institution where my peers were too financially hard up to have any time to socialise, or an institution where the staff had a judgemental attitude towards me because of my epilepsy or felt threatened by me as a result of having more knowledge/ability than them in an area they saw as being their expertise. I also avoided some institutions such as sport teams due to my performance anxiety, thus, barring me from forming new friendships through the playing of games and sports. It also came to my awareness that I could instinctively generate conversation with anyone in any place due to a high level of social confidence acquired from living a very unique life which had given me a very high "sense of self"; where I had developed views, beliefs, opinions etc that I was eager to share with people, thus, allowing me to overcome the confidence barriers that most people are affected by when meeting new people for the first time outside of an institution setting. I came to realise that I don't need institution to form new friendships with people, but these prospective new friends do require institution to form friendships with me, resulting in the isolation of myself. This is an example of where a strength can appear like a weakness, and explains why someone with my social skills can't form a friendship but can arrange a meeting with Occupational Therapy and convince them into reversing their decision on adapting a person's bathroom; or successfully mediate with an anti-social neighbour who has been bullying a client of mine affected by learning disability. People think social skills are communication skills that get you the approval of others, which is why they would draw conclusions about your social skills by the number of friendships you have, but the truth is there are many different types of social skills such as assertiveness, having a presence, debating, initiation and maintenance of conversation with strangers, good articulation, ability to empathise, ability to mediate, ability to educate/inform, ability to lie and manipulate, peer pressure resistance, insightfulness and intuition and I'm sure you can think of other.

After discovering this theory over the reliance on institution most people have in forming new friendships, it came to my attention that the reasons for this reliance is because our culture does not encourage the developing of friendship formation skills independent of institution as a result of having us in nursery, followed by school and workplace/institute of higher education. This confining us to an institutional way of living is further encouraged by segregating us into families, clique of existing friends, membership of recreational clubs and societies; being experienced alongside the previous mentioned institutions that shape you into a contributing member of society or exclude you i.e. nursery/school/workplace/institute of higher education. Recreational clubs and societies could also be described as being forms of institution. This made me realise that we live in a society where peoples' friendship formation skills development is never encouraged and that school, workplace, college etc disempower people from a young age, resulting in them effectively growing up institutionalised in this area of their personal development; meaning socially excluded people like myself, who institution rejects; thus "throwing us out into the wild" where we inevitably go on to develop skills others don't develop, end up living in social isolation. Social exclusion has effectively empowered us in areas others fail to grow and develop. It is an example of the upright guy in an upside- down world, who looks upside down to everyone else. "Personality Disorder" is an excellent example of how psychiatrists label this upright guy as upside down, due to them being advocates of this upside- down world. People like me, for example, will not have friends because we are rejected by institution. As a result of this we have no one to speak to so we will go out to a pub and stand at the bar, in our early twenties, and be forced to talk to someone we don't know, who then may have a friend come back from the toilet and you get speaking to the pair of them for the rest of the night, where you at first are pushing yourself out of your comfort zone and you find the discomfort zone gradually becoming more and more the comfort zone. As a result of this, by the time you are in your thirties, you can talk to anyone and everyone at any time or place, and you get labelled antisocial and attention seeking as you are so well practiced at generating conversation out of anything with anyone, resulting in the unintentional drawing of attention to yourself through being the driving force behind all conversation in groups made up of new people, where everyone takes offence in their own subtle way, resulting in a mental health professional telling you that you have a personality disorder or a learning disability; as they think you are guilty of not respecting a boundary or you don't know the boundary is there. They say, metaphorically speaking, that you are likely of inviting yourself into the house of someone you've just met, sitting down before being invited to take a seat, followed by putting your feet on their table either because you are disrespectful of house rules or you are just clueless. Whichever one of the two you are, it is the same consequences i.e. you get thrown out of the house!! Some of our social skills are in the outsized department and that this is not a disability as these very well developed social skills (overdeveloped when compared to the vast majority) have many transferable benefits such as being able to manage an advocacy service for those with neurological disability for over three years all on my own winning 120 cases.

Another theory of mind also came to surface a number of months later, when I was sitting on my couch having one of my days where I would come in from my bedroom and sit on my couch at 10.00am, would still be sitting there at 4pm thinking "Shit, this has been a damn awful day" and feeling terrible about having wasted a day. I was also reflecting on why I had wasted a day, which was because of social exclusion, and it made me hate the world ferociously. I wanted to go on a killing spree, and then kill myself. I was just sitting there thinking what is wrong about this world, and suddenly it came to me when criticising the world and its people that there are two major flaws in most people.

Just sitting there in my lounge, I pondered my relationship with the world as well as psychoanalysed what had brought on my misfortunes and other bad experiences with the world, making me come to realise that my relationship with the world has been one where a "black" has been paired with a "white". Society can be described as being the "white", and you are the "black". The black is your personal self i.e. the part of you that came into this world; and the world is the white, which is the society that you live and work in and unfortunately compare and contrast yourself with others in. The white is where we develop our major insecurities, thus, making us want to fit in and be like everyone else, that inevitably diminishes our black, robbing us of our individuality. We all have different black/white ratios, and the more personal you are i.e. the more that there is that makes you the person you are, and less like everyone else, the more "black" you have in that ratio.

The white sets the rules and regulations that you have to abide to every day, and your existence can be defined by how well your black merges with the white. Some of us have a black and white like bedfellows, and others have a black and white like Britain's armed forces relationship with Nazi Germany. People may think that's an exaggeration, but tell that to the families of those with epilepsy and other hidden disability who have committed suicide due to the incompatibility between one's black with the white. Remember 1 in 7 with complex partial seizures will attempt suicide in their lifetime due to an ill relationship their black has with the white. Living with some hidden disabilities e.g. epilepsy, autism, anxiety etc has you living with more chance of losing your life at a young age in British society as a result of others' intolerance and ill treatment towards you than there was chance of losing life during second world war of a young British troop.

The less black you have, the closer you are to blending with the white of society to produce a lovely very light grey. This very light grey is what our society sees as "ideal grey". The more like this very light grey your "shade of grey" is, when your black blends with the white, the more favoured and loved you are by society. You also don't score very high on "sense of self" being very light grey, and it is therefore for this reason that you tend to conform and be like the rest i.e. the mainstream.

The more issues and problems that you have had to live with that have been unique to you, the more personalised your life course has been, therefore, the more black there is to your character, making your relationship with society a very dark shade of grey. The darker the shade of grey that you are, the more incompatible with the world you will be, as you will be more removed from being very light grey, which is the shade of grey that society worships. The more alone you are in the world with your problems; the bigger your black becomes as you develop knowledge, skills, beliefs, values and principles that others don't develop; making you a much larger black and, thus, a much darker shade of grey than the very light grey people. You will therefore likely grow up feeling more of an individual than a member of society, which if combined with high IQ will result in your behaviours, views and beliefs being shaped by logic as opposed to what makes you popular, thus, making you a non-conformist as well as someone who is at odds with people and society, resulting in your social exclusion; causing you to possibly find yourself growing up assertive, outspoken, calling a spade a spade, making a career out of a talent, and not being scared to put anyone in their place, as you will grow up non-judgemental. This large amount of black creates incompatibilities between you and society that can also end up in you becoming self-employed as you have great difficulties abiding to boundaries and plans created by those above you if they have flaws or are lacking in logic, making it difficult for you to work for a boss. Unfortunately, these incompatibilities can also result in trips to prison, suicide, homelessness etc.

As I have had an isolated life that has given me a high sense of self combined with having a high IQ, I have grown up non-conformist, and like all non-conformists I see myself living in a society not made up of different social stratifications i.e. high court judge down to binman; but instead made up of conformists and non-conformists. I basically see everyone as belonging to one of two groups of people, and socio-economic class means nothing. People like me therefore do not differentiate between a 'chief executive' telling us to "get down and do ten press-ups" and one of our peers telling us to do the same; meaning that wherever you work you will have fallouts with bosses and peers when things don't add up or could be done more effectively, creating difficulties for you such as trying to hold down a job, being victimised at work, getting a good reference to find another job etc; resulting in you being diagnosed with a 'Personality Disorder', where you eventually find yourself ending up having to claim a benefit such as Universal Credit. Some of us, due to our life experiences are just too unpretentious and mature for this infantile behaviour of being a sheep (employee) or acting like a spoilt child (employer), who must not be seen by their own egos to be taking advice from anyone they see as being beneath them, and insist on winning every argument and always getting their own way.

This 'non-conformity' and principle of mutual respect is as strong a belief to people who are very dark shades of grey as 'Allah' is to a Muslim, as conformity would mean conforming to a system that has abused you your entire life; and you also have far too many skills, knowledge and potential to be working for anyone else as a result of your very personalised life experiences. Your personalised life has empowered you to the point of not being able to work for an employer who is essentially a type of institution. In a perverse kind of way; living with epilepsy, depression and anxiety has been very empowering, and has empowered me to the point where I cannot belong to an institution following rules, regulations and codes of conduct that I do not believe in, and instead do much better being a one man band evidenced by three very successful years running my own advocacy charity called Fairway Advocacy. It is for this reason that I believe many entrepreneurs are people who have had very personalised lives, and probably have had their own set of unique problems that they have not told the population about. Some entrepreneurs/celebrities do admit to lifelong depression and anxiety; however, what I would like to know is how many of them have epilepsy, or any other chronic hidden disability that they do not disclose, through the fear that the stigma of having could affect their celebrity status.

The more towards ideal grey you are, the more judgemental you will be, due to lack of personal development resulting from living a life that has lacked so much in the way of personalised life experience. The personal development of an ideal grey person has been a very generic one as their life could be described as the "Prescribed Life" which is school, job/higher education, then job, retirement, death; bringing up children and grandchildren on route, with minimal time for making new friends. As you would expect, the word "Generic" would go with the word "Judgemental". Those who have had a generic personal development will have fewer beliefs, views, values etc and therefore will sing from the same hymn sheet of those in charge i.e. authority, and therefore will choose to just go with the grain regardless of who is above them, which again is why I don't wear a poppy on armistice day as nine out of ten people will shoot when told to shoot at whatever they are being told to shoot at; therefore, nine out of ten people would shoot an innocent person for being a certain religion if ordered to do so by an authoritative figure that would make the killing legal. I've seen this in workplaces where colleagues are your friends until someone above them tells them to participate in a constructive dismissal of you and they do just that. This as equally applies to colleagues who have been your friend, as well as played you at squash and met with you for drinks for as long as fourteen years.

Beneath light grey are the population of people with moderate to severe learning disability. They are very black simply because they have not developed life skills, life knowledge nor engaged in new experiences. This lack of personal development is not down to lack of exposure like it is with the mainstream population. These people are put through very personalised "deep end" experiences every day, often as a result of abandonment and judgementalism, putting pressure on them to develop skills that unfortunately they have great difficulty doing because of neurodevelopmental issues that took place in the womb, or because of the expression of genes that code for certain learning disabilities. Those with **very severe** learning disability are therefore, also very dark shades of grey, like the non-conformist, which is why being a non-conformist with problematic behaviour could have you believed to be someone with a learning disability. Those with learning disability therefore, very often face social exclusion. As already mentioned, the white also sets the rules and regulations i.e. the boundaries, and as those with learning disability, due to neurodevelopmental issues as well as genetics, have difficulties understanding these boundaries, they often cross the boundaries without realising they are doing so, and get into trouble, making themselves unpopular and creating for themselves issues very similar to those who are a very dark shade of grey non-confomist i.e. issues borne from an incompatibility with the white. This would explain why Alistair and I have become good friends. His dark shade of grey obviously hit it off with my dark shade of grey. It might also explain why people with learning disability, who I have never met before have just come and sat down at my table in coffee shops and started talking to me while their carer has been waiting for their coffees. Do the learning disabled dark shades of grey see the non-conformist i.e. high IQ/critical-reflective thinker/high sense of self dark shade of grey as being their ally. Do learning disabled people have that instinctive ability to detect a chemistry that attracts them to my table?

What makes me a very dark shade of grey is that I have lived with social anxiety disorder, of the performance type, that has caused me to be side lined at school and given bad treatment from pupils, teachers, higher education educators as well as employers. This has caused within me to have to do a lot of sticking up for myself, defending my dignity, cope with living with mental scars; making me a very assertive, outspoken, fed up person that takes no nonsense of anyone. It's caused social isolation due to me not being able to join societies/clubs that involve an element of performing and not being interested in anything else that the clubs/societies in British society engage in. This has resulted in depression and anxiety, resulting in me having an anti-bully ethos, an anti-top down ethos, an anti-inequality in human rights ethos as well as developed me into an anti-authority person. I have developed skills in coping, problem solving and speaking up for myself, which can be evidenced from the successful running of my advocacy charity for 3.5 years. I have also developed views and beliefs through my unique travels that I feel passionate about; and as these beliefs, views and values, which I have a lot of confidence in, define me as a person; I have a lot of confidence in myself, apart from when I am in certain performance settings. As I have a lot of confidence when it comes to the expression of my views, beliefs and values; I am contemplating joining a debating society, as this is all about arguing views and beliefs using logic as I am also a very logical person. People who have survived lives that have nearly killed them are logical as well as pragmatic people. When you are trying to save your life; you have to be truthful, rational, resourceful, non-pretentious, and independent minded with others as well as with yourself.

I have also lived with epilepsy resulting in incredible amounts of discrimination that has also given me the traits that I have described myself as having as a result of living with the social anxiety disorder. I have learned meditation, aerobic exercise, distraction, positive thinking, thought blocking, slow breathing for panic, as a means of combatting the anxiety and depressive disorders experienced as a result of all the trauma I have had to live with. I have therefore managed to turn all these bad experiences on their head, by making living with them an empowering experience, resulting in the development of skills and expert knowledge, that has given me a strong mental backbone, that I would never wish to waste by working for a person who would just take you for granted and treat you like dirt because you were born with epilepsy, and developed social anxiety disorder because of evil children and teachers at an all- boys school, that has only been further engrained in me by future generations in this intolerant world called 'Society'. It is my experience, due to the issues that I have had to live with, that people could be described as bigots and   disability's equivalent of racists. In a nutshell, most people living in our society have very little in the way of having a "Black" as a result of the lack of personal development they have undergone due to the prescribed life that the institutional ethos of our society has encouraged. This institutionalised way of living is a major reason behind peoples' ignorance, and I see this as being the first of the two major flaws. The prescribed way of life gives those a comfort zone to live in that causes them to stagnate. As a result, the mainstream rely on media as their only source of lifelong learning, which is why they are so ignorant of anything that is not related to their academic/vocational training or their job.

The other flaw that came to me during my psychoanalysing of my experience of the world, and people, was that people only see the effects of the primary shot that they are about to play i.e. primary damage. They don't see the secondary shot that results from the primary damage that they have just caused, nor do they see the neighbouring shot that their first primary shot makes. They therefore have no knowledge or awareness of "secondary damage" nor do they have any knowledge or awareness of "collateral damage". For example, the time I was put off my social work course, the primary damage those behind my dismissal from the course saw was me being upset over no longer being on the course; however, the secondary damage was for me to live with a lack of closure that would fill me with a depression that I would have to live with for the next three years, which if I had not been able to work on mental health grounds, I would never get a job again, as I would have it on my CV that I went a period without employment as a result of mental health issues, causing me to live a purposeless life, resulting possibly in self destructive behaviour such as alcohol addiction or worse e.g. suicide. This illustrates how people cannot see beyond the shot they are about to play. Such a primary shot carried out by social work could have resulted in a further four or five shots happening, one after the other, with the damage escalating in severity, in terms of impact it would have on one's life, also recruiting more people affected by their bigoted action. It is also the case that the stress of me living without closure could have caused a lot of emotional distress, not just for me, but also for family which could have in my case resulted in my father; especially when he held a post working in the public sector, having many work related difficulties in terms of work relationships with social workers resulting in him blowing a fuse at work and losing his job. This illustrates how people cannot see the collateral damage i.e. the primary shot's unintended neighbouring shot, and its further shots. Many of the other experiences I have been through, evidence the same lack of awareness or knowledge of the primary shot's neighbouring shot and the further knock on shots that the primary shot and neighbouring shot causes to happen. This evidences in people a lack of initiative, intuition as well as insight.

I also became aware that not all people in my life had been so blind to these things i.e. neighbouring shots, secondary shots and the knock on shots these secondary shots result in; and therefore, I could evidence that this initiative and intuition exists on a continuum, and that some people have more of it than others. I then said to myself, "maybe these people don't give a shit, and that it's not that they lack initiative nor intuition" but then the meditator in me said, "But this lack of intuition and initiative can be evidenced in the decisions that they make every day concerning their own lives" This evidence of lack of initiative and intuition can be read in the examples that come later in this chapter.

I then asked myself, "Is initiative and intuition a measure of intelligence?", and the answer that came to me was, "No". What came to me was "If initiative and intuition are intelligence, then how come you see very intelligent people behave in ways that evidence lack of initiative and intuition, and you also have come across people with lower intellect who evidence signs of higher initiative and intuition", and as an example I thought to myself "Yes, the degree educated person that asks for change of £20 note to someone in Central station, then gets followed and mugged; when the person with the lower intellect can piece together: asking a man for change of £20 is telling man I have money + Man desperate for money= Man mugs me" . This told me that on this continuum, initiative and intuition can be scored from Very Low to Very High

I then realised after analysing many of my own life experiences that I score high in initiative and intuition, as well as intellect. I also realised that most people score lower average to higher average on initiative and intuition, and that this lower average to higher average is in fact not very high at all. Just because something is average does not make it a reputable score. Becoming aware of this I suddenly realised why we live in such an ignorant world, that I am actually a very special person that should never allow people to destroy me, I should instead think much more highly of myself and that my expectations of other people have been way too high over the years. This finding on that day, the 13th December 2017, made me realise that this was science, and not to be taken personally, and it was to my credit that I could exist on this continuum at the place I belong on it, living in the world I live in, and still be alive today, and that every day alive was another credential to my name. It also made me aware that I am not on my own, and that there are many others like me. I then suddenly felt the lifting of the major depressive episode.

This continuum that initiative and intuition scores exist on is a continuum that I have called the "Functionality Continuum", that came to my awareness during a spiritual awakening resulting from consistent meditation practice. It is a theory that is full of self-praise, which I learned from the "black mixing with the white theory". It is a theory that also makes you realise that self-praise is something no person should feel awkward about giving themselves, and that we have been led to believe by western society that it's arrogant and obnoxious to say good things about ourselves, and that self-hatred is advocated more than self-praise purely for the sake of keeping people as ideal very light grey as possible. The less you like yourself the more you will follow other people, inhibiting the developing of views and beliefs that may not be in industry's interests for one to develop. Anyone noticing one's self- praise who thinks the words "arrogant" or "obnoxious" is unfortunately guilty of this western thinking.

The 'Functionality Continuum' theory goes like this:

At one end of the Functionality continuum i.e. the left, you have "Low Functionality" and at the other end you have "High Functionality". This is a continuum that all people have a place on and the name for combined initiative and intuition is the **"Ability to Apply Intellect to Practice"**

THE FUNCTIONALITY SPECTRUM

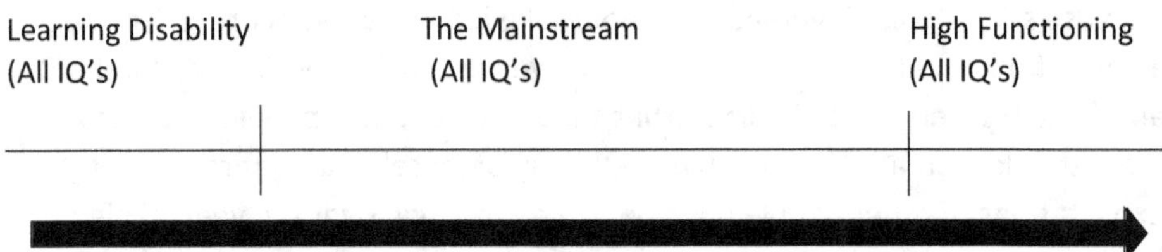

ABILITY TO APPLY INTELLECT TO PRACTICE

There are two traits that define Functionality i.e. **Intelligence (IQ)** and **Ability to apply Intellect to Practice (AItP)**. Ability to apply intellect to practice is basically your ability to use your intellect to navigate yourself around everyday scenarios that occur. It is this ability to apply intellect to practice that allows you to cope with the unexpected. Ability to apply intellect to practice is our problem solving skills, our Initiative, our insight, ability to risk assess, ability to make wise decisions, put in place preventative measures, work out that someone is lying, find a solution to a problem, understand metaphoric talk, counter peoples' arguments such as we do when we are debating, cope with the unknown and unexpected, make a wise well informed decision when determining your political orientation e.g. are you a unionist/nationalist or a Brexit or In- Europe supporter, being an outside box thinker who can join up the dots, and many more.

These two traits that define functionality are scored on the following scales:

IQ: Low to High

Ability to Apply Intellect to Practice: Very Low to Very High

There are three types of people who are all a combination of one of each of the following two variables i.e. IQ and Ability to apply Intellect to practice (AItP)

LEARNING DISABILITY

IQ: Low, Average, High

AItP: Very Low, Low, Below Average

MAINSTREAM

IQ: Low, Average, High

AItP: Lower Average, average, higher average

HIGH FUNCTIONING

IQ: Low, Average, High

AItP: above average, high, very high

Therefore, any member of the learning disabled population, the mainstream, or the high functioning are one of a possible nine different combinations of the two variables: IQ and Ability to apply Intellect to Practice.

A Learning disabled person could have high IQ but below average Ability to Apply Intellect to Practice (AITP), which is the case with many analytical science academics. As their AITP is below average, they do not like the unexpected. They like predictability and knowing what's coming next, meaning they tend to have expertises in subjects such as maths, physics, engineering, chemistry etc, which are sciences full of equations that will never change. It is the same mathematical formula building a bridge in Los Angeles as it is in Glasgow, but It's not the same "formula" being a journalist in Los Angeles as it is in Glasgow, nor are any two days the same for journalists, but the formulas remain the same whatever day of the week it is for a physicist.

By spending their lives applying formulas they need not concern themselves over getting themselves out of any unexpected trouble or scenarios that they have never been in before, which requires the application of intellect to practice. This theory is consistent with what my old university friend called Cameron said to me, "Dr Lawrence knows everything about oncogenes, but nothing about anything else".

A learning disabled person, like my friend Alistair, who has average IQ, but a Low AltP, will use the same formula at talking to a stranger, as he will a friend. Alistair can't adapt to different types of people. I leave him for 5 minutes in Costa Coffee while I go to the toilet and by the time I arrive back I hear him saying to all the staff behind the counter, "Aye, It's a party at a caravan in Wemyss Bay and you're all invited!!" nodding his head at each of the four members of staff, one by one, and he's being deadly serious even though they are all in hysterics which he can't see; as picking up social cues such as body language and facial expression also comes down to ability to apply intellect to practice. A person with moderate ability to apply intellect to practice would respond to Alistair by saying, "You can't say that to people you don't know! They don't know you for Christ's sake!! They won't trust you. They would be too scared to stay in your caravan just in case they woke up and you had a knife at their throat!"

When I serve breakfast to a learning disabled client at the Epilepsy Society, who has low IQ and very low AltP; he grabs the plate from me and shouts, "Fuck off!!! and get out my room!!!", throwing the plate of breakfast at me; as the team leader is always the one who gives him his breakfast in the morning, but because the team leader is at a meeting and I am giving him his breakfast, which is not part of the usual routine i.e. formula, I am on the receiving end of a psychotic explosion, as he can't cope with this unexpected situation. You can see from this that people with learning disability have a reliance, or at least a very strong fondness for routine as it protects them from having to cope with the unexpectedness of the world.

People with moderate AltP are like bulls in a china shop with their eyes closed. It is because of their only moderate AltP that they are forever designing systems that are one size fits all. A good example of this is something that I have had to handle while I have been writing this very part of the book. I swear on my Grand Dad's grave that this happened while editing the grammar in this part of the book in the Costa Coffee in Sauchiehall Street on the 14th October 2019. What had happened was a women with a baby in a pram, came in at 10.00am, which was a time when the café was not busy, and there were many empty seats at vacant tables, with no one sitting at the tables beside these vacant tables, yet despite this, she chose to sit down right beside me when I was editing this chapter, where the lady could see that I had a laptop, and it should have been obvious to her that I was working and that she should have thought "Maybe my baby will start crying, and this will stop the man beside me from being able to do his work, possibly causing him to get angry.". Instead of thinking this thought and coming to the wise conclusion that she should find another table to sit at with neighbouring vacant tables, her family of four others arrive, and her daughter, who looks sixteen years of age, and therefore should know better, starts rocking the pram backwards and forwards where the baby starts to let out a few screams. I say to the family, "Did you have to choose a seat beside my seat when you could see that I was working?". The lady started telling me that I   was out of order and that this was a café as well as a public place. I told her it was exactly that and not a kindergarten. I said, "You know that a baby cries, you also know that a man is interrupted from doing his work by babies crying, you can see that I am working, and you can't put these things together and come to the conclusion that you better pick another seat?". The lady and her family   got mad and the daughter stood up, growled and said, "You're a wanker!!", with the woman responding by complaining to the manager; who responded by taking my side as I am a regular, and I explained the logic to the manager so she could conclude that this woman and her family were out of order.

What this experience of mine in the coffee shop evidences, is that the majority of people have a one size fits all attitude due to their low ability to apply intellect to practice which is frighteningly average, maybe higher average. This lady thinks that because it's okay to sit at a table beside men talking about football with her baby then it is okay for her to sit down beside anyone else, even a grieving mother back from the hospital talking about bad news regarding her son with her friend. This one size fits all attitude unfortunately exists within every system that makes up the infrastructure of our society; whether it be health, education, social care, law and order, mortgages and loans etc. This is what drives the people who do not fit this one size fits all society crazy and fills them full of rage and anger management issues. This one size fits all attitude and model of operation of the entire infrastructure of our society causes in those with high AItP major depressive disorder, burnout, relationship difficulties; including family breakdown as well as anxiety disorders. This one size fits all ethos also damages our NHS, creates a failing education system for many, a failing welfare and benefits system and a highly ineffectual justice system that creates many injustices for many honourable people etc; and all the just mentioned only paints a part of the picture!!

I see a lot of this moderate ability to apply intellect to practice going on around me the whole time amongst the mainstream population. An example of a situation where the majority of the mainstream population demonstrate an AItP that could be described as low even though it is average, is where their immediate reaction to seeing someone stop at green lights and put their hand brake on would be to blast the horn and shout, "Baw Bag" i.e. West coast Scotland slang for "scrotum". Never would they think "This person might have stopped because they are experiencing chest pain or feel themselves becoming hypoglycaemic"; nor would they therefore think "I better get out my car and see if he is okay". This mainstream person is more likely to sit there and continue blowing his horn even after coming back from an in- house training day on diabetes. I see a lot of this type of behaviour all around me, where there are a number of reasons as to why something might have happened and all people can do is freak because what they are seeing does not comply with what they are used to seeing i.e. routine; nor do they have the ability to apply knowledge to everyday real life encounters to see what other things might be responsible for what they are seeing and react appropriately, which evidences a shortfall in insight, initiative as well as problem solving skills. This lack of insightful behaviour and failure to think up a way to resolve the matter is evidence of average AItP having quite a low score. The person blowing their horn knows about heart attacks and hypoglycaemia. This person even knows about the biology of heart attacks and diabetes. This person also knows that you can't drive experiencing these two things, yet they cannot put the pieces together to see that this might be the reason as to why this car in front of them has come to a stand-still and someone better get out and check if this person is okay. This example demonstrates that what is moderate AItP in the average person is actually still quite low. This is certainly an observation made by anyone who belongs to the far right of the functionality spectrum where AItP is high to very high. This is why the high functioning are susceptible to conditions like depression, as they see all the flaws and ignorance in humanity, the damage humanity is responsible for; and have to live with the frustrations caused by the behaviours and attitudes of others, that are shaped by the ignorance of others. As a result of this, depression is likely most prevalent at the far right of the functionality continuum especially when it is the far right of the functionality continuum where misanthropy will be very prevalent. Those to the far left of the continuum i.e. learning disabled also get depression as they are often victims due to their very low AItP causing them to have a very limited number of responses and interpretations of everyday situations created by the ignorance of the mainstream; making them vulnerable, causing them to get picked on and bullied with no understanding as to why they are being targeted, thus, resulting in the development of anxiety and depressive disorders.

Ability to apply intellect to practice teaches us boundaries e.g. knowing not to talk about a one night stand in a best man speech, and those who score very low will cross boundaries that anger the mainstream; and those to the far right of the continuum will see the mainstream cross boundaries that the mainstream aren't aware of themselves crossing. This will annoy those to the far right of the continuum, causing emotions such as anger/rage/despair, resulting in the developing of depressive disorders. I sometimes believe depression is a condition that only affects intelligent people with high AItP as well as those with low to very low AItP as they are the ones' who experience an incompatibility between themselves and the society they live in as a result of differing behaviours and attitudes. The mainstream don't experience this incompatibility as they don't see the cracks like the far right do, nor do they behave in ways or have outlooks that are incompatible with the world they live in; instead they conform and suffer from insecurity, low morale and self-esteem as well as stress with burnout, but not depression. Stress with burnout as well as low morale and self-esteem is called "Depression" to sweep under the rug the real reasons as to why people suffer from burnout and have low self-esteem. These real reasons being so society can get away with: industry paying low wages; working people overtime; people being pressured into having the most up to date version of one of society's most recent inventions; the encouraging of people to use alcohol as an alternative to remedying low confidence; the labelling of self-praise as arrogance; the discouraging of the developing of views and beliefs that deviate from what authority want your views and beliefs to be; the developing of self-loathing that begins in infancy that's responsible for the creation of societal expectation that benefits many industries; the living in a culture of put down and belittlement for the benefit of creating "don't answer me back" hierarchies that make people vulnerable and easily exploited; a culture of snobbery and judgementalism, where how seriously a complaint of yours will be taken is determined by what you do for a living; a selfish culture that believes in doing noisy home renovation in its flat without telling any of its neighbours, and many, many more.

Those who are high functioning suffer from depression; that has also been dressed up as a clinical condition to possibly discredit our views, beliefs and opinions; so that this world can shut people like me up, and stop people like me starting a revolution. This has already been discussed when criticising the theory of personality disorder.

Conditions such as bipolar disorder and many anxiety disorders are exempt from this theory as there is the possibility that these are neurological and not psychological/environmental in origin. Both psychological and neurological mental health conditions cross paths as they both affect the mind, meaning mind techniques can be used for remedial purposes for either type e.g. meditation, visualisation, distraction, aerobic exercise, positive thinking etc as they all address the mechanics of your thinking as well as affect your neurotransmitter levels. Your thinking affects your feelings, and your feelings are created by the neurotransmitters produced by the blood brain barrier. An example of this is meditation keeps your mind present, thus, preventing future and past thinking, therefore preventing feelings of anxiety and depression; however, meditation also encourages the production of "Dopamine" which is the "reward and motivation neurotransmitter" produce by the blood brain barrier. Aerobic exercise and diet are also very effective ways in increasing dopamine levels. Aerobic exercise, meditation and diet also increase the neurotransmitter "Serotonin" which is the good mood neurotransmitter.

Another example of evidence of moderate ability to apply intellect to practice being a low score is when builders across from my flat had left out overnight a huge metallic structure on the landing before my landing. This was a structure which, if I had left my house during a night time seizure, or if someone had another condition making them very confused causing them to leave the house, could have had me or that someone else fall down the stairs and break our necks. I dare say that fatal accident enquiries come across these acts of neglect the whole time, and having been through everything I've been through in my life, I dare say, there is a huge amount of coverup. Again, there was no insight used when determining an appropriate place to put this metallic structure. I therefore believe this lack of insight as being more evidence of the mainstream scoring unimpressively on ability to apply intellect to practice, which is a dangerously low score. They know that there are conditions that make people confused and go wandering. They can see a big metallic object on a landing getting in the way of access up and down the stair case, but they are incapable of putting the two together and seeing a very unfavourable outcome, thus, preventing them from finding a better place to put the metal object to prevent such a potential unfavourable outcome from happening. This makes you feel that people are a blind folded bull in a china shop, especially when they are behaving this way in an area with a large elderly population where anyone could have a stroke, early dementia or a complex partial seizure that can all cause momentary confusion leading to person leaving home in a confused state in middle of night.

They say that those with learning disability are easily manipulated as a consequence of not being able to apply intellect to practice. This is true but I also see it amongst the mainstream population how easily manipulated mainstream people are by big business as a consequence of those who own big business very often, if not always, being people who have very high AItP. As a consequence of having relatively low ability to apply intellect to practice, those people belonging to the mainstream often cannot see the drawbacks in buying certain things nor the potential future problems such a purchase could create, and can only see the advertised advantages of making such a purchase. As a consequence of this they cannot way up the pros and cons of buying something and therefore cannot make a well- informed decision on "to buy, or not to buy", causing them to make very unwise decisions regarding the spending of their money. I see evidence all around me of people making unwise purchases and getting themselves into unnecessary debt, buying things they cannot afford as well as not being able to priority spend, thus, becoming overcome by luxury spending. An example   of this average AItP when it comes to spending amongst the mainstream population is when I got speaking to a man at a bus stop back in 1999 on a Sunday morning in Glasgow. As part of the conversation I asked this man what he did at the weekend and got as an answer that he had gone out for a few drinks and then a nightclub. I was then asked if I was going away this summer and told him that I was thinking about going to New York. In response to this the man told me that I was a very lucky guy and that I must have been very rich and how much he envied me as he would love to have my kind of money. I responded to this by telling him that he drinks ten pints which equates to £40 gone already. I reminded him that he then spends £10 on nightclub entry and then buys a kebab that costs £5, and when he gets a taxi back to Dalmuir he spends £15, meaning that a night out in Glasgow comes to £70 per night and he does this every week of the year, meaning that he spends £3,640 per year on just drinking and getting a sore head. This man responded to this by saying that he didn't go out every week and it was in fact once every two weeks. I replied by saying that this was still £1,820 per annum and that a return flight to New York was £354, a bed and breakfast was £30 per night making it £300 for ten days, bringing the total to £654. I told him that the subway trains were a flat rate of 50 pence, a plate of food was £5 and that the portions were huge. I also informed him that the shopping as well as the sights were dirt cheap. I then asked him if he felt that if he spent his £1,820 more wisely, he could probably afford two holidays per year to New York and never mind just one; or even better, New York for one of the two holidays per year and Chicago for the other one. This I see is another example of how the mainstream's score on applying intellect to practice is quite low. They have the IQ to do arithmetic, but they do not know how to use it to put things into perspective, thus, compromising wise decision making; especially when it comes to money, alcohol, driving, diet/exercise and many, many more. The human race is a very vulnerable species as a result of its ignorance and naivety. The human race is poor at "joining up the dots" and as a result of this cannot enjoy the liberties it gets to enjoy responsibly. This is a classic symptom of those with learning disability; however, this is a symptom that is also evident amongst the mainstream to those who are high functioning, which is why high functioning people become frustrated and angry as well as depressed as they would describe the world as being "a fool's world full of fools". A misanthropic website that I had been browsing summed up the human race in one sentence and that was "The success of capitalism is the gullibility and stupidity of human beings!!"

Another example of the mainstream's AltP scoring relatively low, was when I was in nurse training, where I was always getting it in the neck for underperforming as a consequence of my performance anxiety i.e. social anxiety disorder. This is a clinical condition that you would think the nurses would have questioned to see whether or not I was affected by. They were old school nurses, they would have had their lectures from psychiatrists and psychologists when they were trained in the hospitals, therefore, they would have been in possession of this knowledge, yet it never occurred to them that this mental health problem might have been present. I am surprised I was never asked if I was suffering from anxiety or depression. I could not report my performance anxiety as I was not aware at the time that, that was what I had, and that it was a recognisable mental health condition that treatment was available for. This is evidence of the nurses not being able to apply their intellect to practice to get to the roots of the problem. They could only see lack of ability as being the reason, and therefore, the solution was to bully me into giving up the course. Someone with a high value of being able to apply intellect to practice would have got it out of me that I suffered from performance anxiety, would have advised that I get an appointment with my G.P., and would have had the course content adapted to meet my needs, thus, demonstrating good problem solving skills.

Another example of the majority of the mainstream scoring relatively low on AItP would be in their ability to instinctively bring up subjects to talk about with people they have just met for the first time. I have been informed that most people don't like talking to people they don't know as they fear running out of things to talk about. This is partly because they don't know how to bring up subject matter in a way that makes it relevant to the current discussion, ensuring a constant flow of conversation. This again I believe to be down to only having a relatively low score for AItP. As well as having a modest scoring AItP, they have a love for the comfort zone, which is another term for a "**zone of routine**", where their love for this comfort zone is very similar to the love someone with learning disability has for routine, where they acquire no new knowledge nor do they acquire any new experiences to grow and develop their knowledge or skills reservoir. They basically stagnate. It is a symptom of the institutionalised prescribed way of living, discussed at the beginning of this chapter when discussing the first theory of mind that came to surface. This is why the mainstream are still going to the same holiday destinations at the age of 45, as they were at the age of fifteen. Tenerife, Magaluf, Crete, Rhodes etc; are they not just the same place but in different locations? Ask a person with high AItP where they are going for their holidays and they will say, "Off to New York this year, after me and the wife going to Beijing last year". They want to see North America after seeing the orient. Whereas mainstream people with relatively low AItP want to see Tenerife after seeing Magaluf! The more a person scores on ability to apply intellect to practice, the less their love for the zone of routine, as they are more able of coping with the unexpected; making them more adaptable and open to new experience, which is why; how they spend their free time in terms of past time activities today, is not how they spent it 30 years ago, nor are the places they go to on holiday 30 years ago the same places they go to today. If we look at the latter i.e. things people do in their free time, it is this lack of openness to new experience, due to only average AltP, that is the reason behind why people in their 50's are still getting drunk at the weekends, like they did when they were sixteen years of age.

Another example of the majority scoring relatively low in applying intellect to practice is the drunks on the day before Christmas Eve getting on the train to Helensburgh Central from Glasgow Queen Street after their night out in the town, singing their heads off on the first carriage, stamping their feet and clapping their hands. I ask myself, "where are the police?". It could be the case that there could be a far right of the continuum (high AltP) person sitting on this train, who suffers from a major depressive disorder, who suffers from irritability as well as rage as a symptom of their depression, and is not going to have the tolerance for this noise and anti-social behaviour; resulting in a fight that could become very explosive and someone could be head injured, disfigured or even killed. I bet it has not crossed the minds of the majority of police that a susceptibility to experiencing fits of rage and irritability due to a depressive disorder could cause someone with depression to feel that these guys are crossing his boundary and result in all hell breaking lose, resulting in someone getting a head injury or a stabbing; as just like the person with learning disability (below average to very low AltP) "stands on the toes" of the mainstream, the mainstream stand on the toes of the high functioning person i.e. high AltP . This person on the train with both high AltP and depression was myself; and if it were not for the fact that I was meditating, all hell could have broken loose, and I have already been arrested once for having a seizure in public; therefore, the last thing I need is to be arrested or killed for having a depressive episode in public

Those with high AltP have to stand back and just watch the institutions that make up our society fail and consistently let people down because of the people who design and run them only having average AltP. Those with high AltP can see what's wrong with the system, what the people who design them are doing wrong, what is absent, what the future holds for such a system etc, and we therefore live in a constant state of frustration and anger, which is why we end up suffering from depressive disorders. They do say that higher IQ people are much more prone to developing depressive disorders, but according to this theory that I became aware of during a depressive day, sitting on my couch, those with high IQ and high AltP are even more prone to these depressive and anxiety disorders. This would be consistent with the fact that according to the Royal College of Psychiatrists 5% of the population are living with a personality disorder at any one time, according to a story found on the BBC News website dated 20th January 2018, titled "Personality Disorder Patients Let down by system". This figure of 5% is the same percentage of people with an IQ of 125. It is the case that people with high IQ question logic, and don't just take anything that they are told for granted. Those with high IQ will always question the legitimacy of what they are being told. It is for this reason that those with high IQ see how non-sensical the world is and therefore choose either not to abide to its code of conduct, or do so, grudgingly. This can cause those with high IQ to often be at odds with society and its people, causing relationship difficulties, resulting in them being diagnosed as being awkward people who can't get along with people, resulting in them being labelled with a personality disorder. The psycho-emotional problems that those at odds with society will have to live with, will inevitably result in conditions like depression and anxiety. Those who score high on AltP and IQ will see the non-sensical nature of our world with even greater transparency.

You can therefore have high IQ but not be very good at using it. You can be low IQ but be fantastic at using it. This is why an average IQ street criminal can con a way above average IQ Procurator Fiscal into believing he was innocent, and get away with a crime; or have a high IQ boss being made a fool off by an employee with average IQ, who is trying to make something look like someone else's fault. It's also why we have had very high IQ unionists with only average AltP, be conned by Westminster into believing Scotland should be in the union, and average IQ Nationalists with very high AltP know that Scotland is being ripped off being a part of the Union. It has been nationalists with high AltP that have been able of putting together very sound arguments for independence. I sometimes believe that unionists can't apply intellect to practice as they never have an argument for being in the union, other than just insult nationalists. It is of course the case that there are nationalists who have both high IQ, and high AltP.

 Boris Johnson, if what every anti-brexit person says about leaving Europe is correct, could possibly be high IQ with below average AltP. That would be saying that Boris Johnson has high functioning learning disability. Like I said I am not a psychologist so I will refrain from saying he has a learning disability but one can't deny that he does have an issue with understanding boundaries evidenced by some of the things that he says on television during interviews such as making reference to women wearing burkas looking like letterboxes.

One thing I know about myself is that I have an IQ of 125 minimum. I know this as it is the case that I have an Honours degree in one of the traditional academic subjects i.e. Molecular Biology, from a reputable university i.e. Glasgow University. The university is not important, it is the subject of the degree that matters. It is a fact that to become a graduate in a traditional academic subject required you to have a minimum IQ of 125, and that this was the minimum IQ required of someone to get into university before the 1990's epidemic of inventing university courses for the purpose of inventing more university places by Tony Blair's government, so that he could get 50% of the population educated to graduate level. It is also obvious from my observations as well as my reactions to these observations, the criticisms I have of the world and its people; the arguments and rationales I give for having the values, beliefs and principles that I hold, that I score high on initiative and intuition i.e. ability to apply intellect to practice. It is also obvious from how frustrated I get over how broken society is, what future time bombs are ticking away in society and what is needed to happen but is not happening to repair society; that I score high in problem solving as well as insight. It is also evident that I score high on IQ and AItP as a result of having run an advocacy charity, where I resolved 120 cases for those with neurological disability against social work, housing, healthcare, employee/employer conflicts etc. It is for this reason that I would put myself within the high IQ population, within the high functioning part of the functionality spectrum; despite all my teachers calling me "thick" as well as previous employers and educators making me out to be too neurologically impaired as a result of living with epilepsy. It evidences how judgemental our society is.

 I believe that scoring high on these two traits (IQ & AItP) has probably played a part in isolating me from the rest of society. If you were to map these variables out on a graph (see graph below) where along the X axis you have IQ and along the Y axis you have ability to apply intellect to practice, and you were to plot 100 people from a cross section of society on this graph where the learning disabled, mainstream as well as high functioning minority are represented; the mainstream would be around the centre spanning the whole IQ range. The learning disabled would be below the mainstream spanning the whole IQ range whereas the high functioning would be above the mainstream spanning the whole IQ range. Those scoring very high on both application of intellect to practice and Intelligence, make up a small percentage of the high functioning minority. It is within this "minority of a minority" that I reside, and I would be plotted towards the furthest end of the bar representing the high functioning on the graph. There would of course be others in this "minority of the minority"; however, they are few and far between, and I therefore see this as being another reason for my social isolation. People who reside on the same part of this graph that I reside on like large talk e.g. conversations about politics or any other big subject as opposed to talking about things like "Celebrity come Dancing"; prefer being on Wikipedia learning about science and how things work, as opposed to being on Facebook sharing pictures of Garfield with all their friends, giving it lots of loves; searching for as well as writing blogs on Quora titled "Why do I hate people so much!!". I put exclamation marks in that quote and not a question mark as it is more a statement than it is a question.

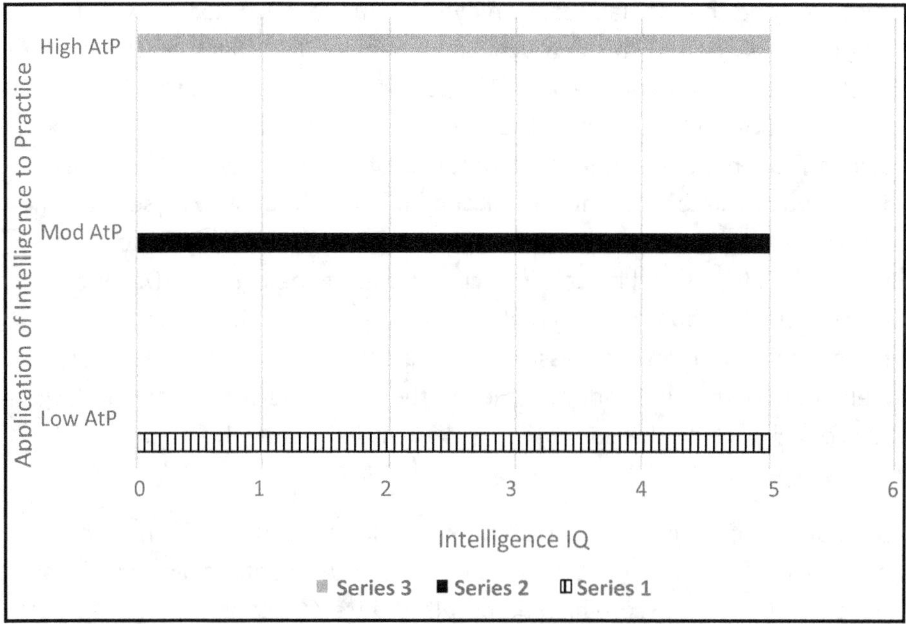

Does this analysis of myself and others, as well as the observations made about myself when compared with others make me arrogant?. Guess what, I don't care!!. If readers are saying that I should instead be saying bad things about myself and putting myself down then shame on you! You are guilty of a western thinking already mentioned that has been programmed into the mainstream population's minds for the purpose of stunting the development of individuality and creating an ideal light grey population that can be manipulated, pressured and exploited.

I do believe that scoring high on these two traits puts me in a minority of a minority population, that my friends from school and university also belong in, that has caused all my school friends and university friends to have left Scotland to other lands with better career prospects, leaving me in Scotland without friends. This unfortunately is the effect that I believe the brain drain has had on people who score high on these two traits living in Scotland. For a few weeks I had become friends with the gentleman that I got drinking with the night I went out in Glasgow on the day I had that bust up with my parents over me not knowing where Lochghilhead was due to my social isolation. That's right, the guy that knocked the air vent out of the ceiling while dancing. He is an educated guy who is my age and has high hopes and aspirations. His name was "Lars" and he sent me a text message to inform me that he was glad to meet me and that he had really enjoyed all our get togethers as well as telling me he wished to stay in touch, and whenever he is back in Scotland he will tell me so that we can meet up. The text message also said that he was going to be moving to London in the next few days to start a new job having previously told me in a coffee shop, that in Scotland there are only jobs at the bottom and at the top with nothing in the middle. I thought to myself reading this text that I would be very saddened to see him go, and thought to myself "Brain Drain". It's played its part in socially isolating me big time. Despite Glasgow being my home city, I know nobody here, yet know so many in London. There are many addresses I could knock on the door of if I locked myself out my home in London; however, there is no person I know in Glasgow who I could knock on the door off if I locked myself out my home on a cold winter's night.

I feel that having no opportunity to meet people who score high on both IQ and AltP stops me from meeting people of the same mentality as myself. I also believe that because I score high on both these traits, people when they meet me think I am of a totally different mindset than them and don't see me as a prospective friend. There is no doubt that my isolation has been caused by factors that belong to one of three domains. These domains being Psychology, Politics and Sociology. All our fortunes in life are determined by a combination of variables that stem from each of these domains. Remember what I said, "High **A**bility to **A**pply **I**ntellect to **P**ractice".

They say that all people with high IQ like speaking about large talk; which is discussing subjects that involve giving opinions, views, beliefs, questioning logic and involve problem solving. They say that the lower your IQ the more love you have for small talk, which is about discussing celebrity and gossip. This book is about a large talk subject, and the very fact that you bought this book and have got this far through it is evidence that you like large talk, and therefore, are most likely of high IQ. As far as applying intellect to practice is concerned, I do not know where you score on that. I don't know if most high IQ people score high on application of intellect to practice. The reason I cannot make a conclusion like this is because I have not met and got to know enough intelligent people in my life to date. As a result of this only you can judge if you are a high scorer in this area or not; however, I believe that if you would describe yourself as intuitive, open minded and non-judgemental then you see more shades of grey than most people, meaning that you score high in AItP, as ability to apply intellect to practice is a measure of how black and white one sees the world. The lower your AItP, the more black and white you see the world as being; making you more susceptible to bad decision making, drawing inaccurate conclusions, making unfair judgements; which a large proportion of people at the centre of a person's discriminative and prejudicial treatment are guilty of, and giving bad advice. This is why I could have never used psychiatry as a resource for meeting my mental health needs as the strong odds are I see more shades of grey than the psychiatrist would see, so how could he help me?. The psychiatrist could only frustrate me. Despite me having every respect for the science of psychology, I could only expect the same with the psychologist in terms of numbers of shades of grey that they would see; which I believe would be more than the psychiatrist, as the psychiatrist just treats a patient's emotions with drugs that are typical of someone seeing the number of shades of grey that they do; however, the psychologist does in fact study the different shades of grey for the purpose of learning as much about them as they can.

It is the case that people who see all shades of grey see what is broken in our society, and what is needed to put it right. They see the cracks and the gaps that everyone else does not see, that causes so many of society's ills e.g. war, crime, addiction, family breakdown etc. They so often find themselves at odds with so many people and can experience a lot of fall outs due to disagreements they have with others, where they are adamant about being right because their opinion on matters are far more evidenced than everyone else's. This can result in those who score high in AltP becoming very outspoken, and making a lot of enemies. This can also result in people bottling up their frustrations, and becoming incredibly stressed out to the point of one day exploding, becoming burned out, or driving a car off the road and onto the pavement killing pedestrians. They find this to be an extremely frustrating experience as well as an exhausting one to live with. This moderate (lower average to upper average) ability to apply intellect to practice amongst the mainstream is why we have so many "one size fits all systems". They say that it is more difficult being happy being a person who sees all shades of grey; and for those that do, it is very common for them to become depressed, as they see themselves surrounded by a world full of failings, doing everything wrong, and how much simpler it would be if everyone thought a bit more like them, thus putting everything right. The frightening thing is though, that wherever you are on this functionality continuum, is not a measure of your morality. Morality exists on another continuum, and there are unfortunately many high IQ/high AltP bad people, who just take total advantage of all the numpties (Scottish word for "idiot"). They run all the big companies in the major industries, taking advantage of peoples' naivety, and they are laughing. They are the reason behind the inequality of wealth and poor worker's rights; and play a major part in bringing about the end of the world. Those scoring high on IQ and AltP, with either high morality or low morality, do share common traits though and they are: they are fed up with people, angry, feel rage, feel they live in a world surrounded by fools, find people disappointing, hate authority, aren't scared to compromise certain people and many more.

Those with low morality, scoring high on both IQ and AltP, are therefore the drug dealers, the arms dealers, the money launderers, the fat cat business owners, the dictators and other psychotic politicians. Those who score high on both IQ and AltP as well as morality, are the green peace campaigners, the rioters, human rights activists, pro-constitutional changers, some entrepreneurs, trade union representatives, legal aid lawyers (if any still exist), disability advocates, politicians who mean well etc. Maybe we are too moral when you look at who our opponents are.

All successful entrepreneurs i.e. small business owners right through to large nationwide companies are probably High IQ and high Ability to Apply Intellect to Practice.

As much as I hate to say it, Tony Blair probably was a high scorer in both IQ and AItP. He fooled the country into opening up universities, providing courses that he encouraged the invention of by opening up access to universities for all people with no one doing the maths (excuse the pun!) i.e. where are we going to find the jobs for these graduates, how many graduates will there be per job application; meaning how many people will be left with dashed hopes and huge debts, and what will the effects of the "lost generation" going to be on our mental health services. The "lost generation" being something that Charles Kennedy had warned us about. Blair will have also used his very high AItP to get away with his war crimes. George Bush probably didn't have very high IQ but certainly had high AItP, which is why he has also got away with his war crimes. Blair also managed to dress the Labour party up as a left- wing party, when in fact, he had resurrected the old tory party under a labour flag, and under the noses of Labour's members. Blair was even quoted as saying, "I don't think that everything Thatcher did was wrong", and still managed to convince his party and their supporters that he was the man to be leading the labour party.

I don't wish to sound boastful about myself when giving myself the self-praise that you have read, but everything I say comes from conclusions made by the things about self and others that I have observed, which find themselves compatible with this theory of mind that just appeared while sitting on my couch psychoanalysing and making sense of the world as well as myself and other people, on the 13th December 2017. It's amazing, truly amazing, what you learn about the world and people just focussing on your breathing. They say when you meditate you will start to understand yourself more mentally. I do find myself asking that if 40% of people born with epilepsy are in the learning disability zone of the functionality continuum, does that mean that maybe the remaining 60% born with epilepsy are in the high functioning zone of the continuum.

I can only imagine that people who score high on both IQ and AItP make the good entrepreneurs due to having the initiative and intuition to generate wealth, especially when many of these people are those who are at odds with society and people, and became self-employed so that they could remove themselves from workplaces and people, whose naivety and ignorance frustrates them; which stops them from being able to work in teams as well as work for employers. It's no surprise when you read about Duncan Bannatyne on Wikipedia that he got thrown out of the army for punching a sergeant giving him orders. God save the queen?? My Arse, I Hate Authority!!, Bang!!!!!!

CHAPTER 31

WHEN EPILEPSY IS TOO MUCH OF AN ATTRIBUTE!!

I do believe that the next experience you are going to read about, which involves a setup to be followed by a dismissal, had happened as a result of me knowing too much on a subject area which, those who treated me so unforgivingly, believed no one working for them should have more knowledge on than them. This hasn't just been my own experience. My father when in Canada spoke to a man who had been diagnosed with 'post- traumatic stress disorder', which he had developed through military action. This man shared with my father that he gave talks to health and social care staff on living with post- traumatic stress disorder on behalf of a mental health charity, until he proved with time to be the most effective person to be giving these talks. The praise his talks were given by those attending made the staff of the mental health charity feel inferior over a period of time, and as a result of this he was never invited back to give another talk ever again. This I believe is the very reason behind my constructive dismissal as an 'Epilepsy Futures' trainer, especially when all those attending were people living with hard to control epilepsy.

The world is full of irony and there has been so much irony in my life that I think you could convert this book into a real carry on movie. This book was at first proof read by a person who had been "friends" with me for fifteen years and worked at an epilepsy charity in Glasgow called 'Epilepsy Connections'.

This person had invited me to teach a life skills course to his charity's clients in November 2017, and I taught those with epilepsy, accompanied with mild to moderate learning disability, about the strategies one can use to tackle depression and anxiety, which are as prevalent in those with epilepsy, as much as epilepsy in itself is. This course taught those attending over a number of seven sessions about 'Meditation', 'Exercise', 'Distraction', 'Visualisation', 'Positive Thinking', 'Defusing the Inner Critic', 'Investing in Future Health'. As you would expect I got on very well with those attending. I had an empathy with the clients, and the clients I noticed always warmed to me when we were in the company of one another. My sessions created much interaction and sharing of experiences where clients felt they could be open because I was open with them about myself. I noticed during the sessions that the full time member of staff of epilepsy connections, who was the course coordinator, was always looking withdrawn, never spoke to the clients but for the minimal amount of discussion that we all had during the coffee breaks and lunch breaks; and that his facial expressions and body language were exhibiting signs of despair; and looking like he was experiencing some sort of withdrawal symptoms where he was on the doorstep of death. In terms of my relationship with him I just got on with him and was curious as to why he was always looking so depressed. When we met, he always had a bright red face and gave me a very awkward look. There was no fluency in our discussion, it was just saying, "hello", bit of small talk about the weather, offering of a coffee and biscuit; and asking what I was teaching today, and then him doing a u-turn, me scratching my head thinking what's wrong??, returns with coffee, clients arriving, him sitting at back, me teaching, teaching session coming to end, me packing up and reading evaluations, then shaking hands with this full time member of staff and saying with a smile, "See you next week" and being ushered out the door.

When I first started doing voluntary work for this charity in 2003, the befriending coordinator, Sam Whitmore, always said to me that I should have his job as I knew far more than he did when we were having a coffee sitting in Starbucks not too long after I withdrew from the nurse training course due to the bullying as a result of my performance anxiety. What Sam had said to me about myself being better placed to do his job was always said with good spirit. I couldn't help think that maybe this was what this new member of staff felt towards me for the same reasons. I knew that this member of staff had 'seasonal affective disorder', but I believed there was more to his behaviour than this as the behaviour continued into the light months. I felt that my knowledge was having a negative effect on his pride and ego, and this made me feel vulnerable when I received an e-mail from him one day telling me that I would be taking the clients on my own to the Mitchell Library, in Glasgow, to do a computing session with them on a bank holiday Monday, all on my own without him or any other member of the charity's staff coming with me. I thought to myself this was not right and that I should not be taking the clients out on my own as this broke all policies on health and safety. First of all, I was not criminally disclosed, I had not done the charities basic first aid training, I knew nothing about the clients epilepsy in terms of any triggers; the seizure management protocol i.e the type of seizure, the usual duration of the seizure, how long I should wait between onset of seizure and calling an ambulance if seizure does not subside, the frequency of seizures, if rescue medication were required and if so I had not done the charity's rescue medication training. I also felt that this put the charity in a very vulnerable position legally in terms of the charity being sued if anyone had a seizure and died due to gaps in the trainer's knowledge of the management of a client's epilepsy. I worried that if I took these clients out on my own I would be getting a phone call the next day from the Executive Director of this charity lying to me that the course coordinator had been sacked and telling me that I had been unprofessional and should never have taken the clients out on my own resulting in me being dismissed as a consultant trainer. I wouldn't put it past anyone playing a stunt like this after having had experiences like the one I had in social work training as well as at the Epilepsy Society. I therefore immediately felt that with the course coordinator's possible vested interest in seeing me gone, combined with the previous dirty treatment I had received by people in positions of trust, as well as the Executive Director of Epilepsy Connections; who was also in my opinion a feminist who I always felt took a disliking towards me being friends with Sam Whitmore, and the fact that this arrangement broke all health & safety guidelines, was a possible attempt at constructively dismissing me. I responded to this by phoning the course coordinator and telling him that I was very vulnerable to becoming untrusting of people due to the treatment from others in the past, and that his e-mail to me had me feel very vulnerable due to the instructions being given to me going over the head of all rules and regulations. I also informed the course coordinator that any future repeats of the past could push me to taking my own life as I had a zero tolerance towards the world's evidenced intolerance of me. The course coordinator said that he was sorry that he had made me feel this way and that he understood my feelings in a very unsympathetic, very matter of fact, emotionally unaffected way. The course coordinator said, "I'm very sorry to hear that Tim", "I'm very sorry you've been through all these experiences and you feel this way". It was said as though he was reading these words to me from a book. I then received a phone call from Sam Whitmore who was the befriending coordinator back in 2003 who now had a much bigger role in the charity and he told me that the course coordinator was very upset and when I explained what I had said and why I said it he replied by saying, " I was going to make you apologise, but now I don't need to". In response to my phone call, Sam Whitmore came with me to the Mitchell library on that bank holiday weekend instead of me going alone.

After the session at the Mitchell Library, I was sitting with Sam in the café where he told me that he had been told that there had been great working difficulties between me and the coordinator. I responded by saying that I was not aware of any difficulties. I mentioned that I did notice he looked very distressed, but I also informed Sam that this never affected me from being able to do my job; and me and the coordinator had still managed to maintain a work relationship that if could not be described as friendly could at least be described as neutral, and that I was not aware of any rivalry or unfriendly dialogue that had taken place. Sam said to me that I he had received comments from Peter and that they were not complimentary in nature. Sam did not disclose what these comments were and told me that I should never have felt the distress that I felt the other day as I knew all the knowledge on epilepsy management that was required to take this class on my own even though it was in breach of all health & safety. The session at the library ended with just me and Sam standing outside Charing Cross train station with Sam saying, "Tim, you're a very valued member of the team! So!", and then shook my hand saying to me with a cheesy smile, "Don't fuck this up!!". Sam then said, "See you later", and while he walked towards Bath Street and I stayed at Charing Cross station, he turned round again and shouted to me, "I mean it! Don't fuck it up!!", pointing at me with a creep's smile on his face.

At a later date I received an e-mail from the course coordinator asking me if I had thought about adjusting some of the content of the course so that it was pitched at a level that both mild and moderate learning disability could follow. I responded to this e-mail by telling the coordinator that we should meet to discuss the adaptations for the next intake as he had already met the next intake and he therefore was better placed to adapt the content of the course than I was. I then received an e-mail from Sam telling me that we ought to meet to discuss the adaptations to the course. When Sam and myself met in a café in Glasgow he looked at the course content on my laptop and said that this was a good course and had great content. I have no idea why they had me meet with Sam and not the course coordinator. Sam then said to me just after discussing my last powerpoint slide that he now wanted to talk about the working difficulties between me and the training coordinator. I said to Sam that again I found myself telling him that there were no working relationship difficulties between me and the training coordinator that I was aware of and if he could please give me dates, times, places and things that were said as well as happened that evidence this claim that there have been work relationship difficulties. Sam said that his first loyalty was to the clients, his second loyalty was to the course coordinator and that his third loyalty was to me. Sam then also said that if for some reason I ever found myself not teaching the course they would find someone else to teach it but they would be using my course content as well as my PowerPoint slides. After saying this, he suddenly panicked and pointed at the copyright sign on the slides and said frantically, "What's this Tim?, What's this Tim?", and I did not want to get into a legal tangle with him since I was supposedly already in a training coordinator tangle and therefore thought to myself "Well what the hell do you think it is? You stupid git!", but instead said, "Don't mind that, it's just part of the template design". I actually think Sam was believing this, exposing himself to be an example of something small that had been allowed to now call himself big. I then reminded Sam that all these techniques I talk about in the course will be taught to clients who come to a peer support mental health service that I wish to start, that would teach these same skills to those with mental health conditions looking for alternative ways in managing anxiety and depression on a one to one basis. Sam suddenly became very concerned and asked if I would be teaching courses as well. I replied to this question by telling him that I had never thought about it before, but now having spoken to him I now saw another opportunity. I told him that teaching courses was not a part of my original plans but now that I had spoken to him I had decided that the teaching of courses was now a part of my plans. This concluded our meeting.

Around a couple of weeks later I got an e-mail from Sam saying that he wished to meet me somewhere like a café. He gave me a date and I replied "okay". On the day of our meeting which was the 22nd June 2018 I had to attend in-house training as I was now doing some work for a support work agency. I therefore had to inform him that I could not meet with him but my friend Alistair could meet with him and he could tell Alistair what he had to tell me, and Alistair could pass it on to me. The reply to this was "No, I do not wish to explain myself to a complete stranger". I replied by saying that I could not make it and he said that he would be back in touch with a later date.

I met with my friend Alistair, one afternoon towards the end of June 2018, in a coffee shop. While Alistair was up at the counter getting served, I received a phone call. It was Sam asking me how I was doing. I told him that I was in a café with my friend, and he said, "Oh good. Just on St Vincent Street. Well I will just come down now and join you". As me and Alistair had our coffees,

Sam arrives and sits down at our table at a time when the café was bustling. Sam sat there, and for forty five minutes to an hour we got on like a house on fire and were joking, laughing, finding common ground and creating discussion out of this common ground. After around an hour of this good spirited companionship, Sam said to my friend, "Do you mind giving me and Tim some time together". My friend responded by saying that he would go sit elsewhere. Once my friend had gone Sam said that he wanted to talk about further issues between me and the course coordinator. I said, "What issues??, I've not even seen the man since we last spoke! These issues are a symptom of one's imagination! I ask again give me times, dates, places, things said etc". Sam replied to this by saying, "Tim, the course is no more". I said, "What do you mean?"; and he said, "You're fired". I looked at this man and thought "You're the guy I've been meeting for a pint with for the last fourteen years". I also thought "You're the guy who I played squash with for a few years, and now; under someone's instruction, constructively dismiss me". I thought to myself "No wonder I don't commemorate armistice day". I replied by saying to him that he ought to feel ashamed. I said that what he had done was dirty, corrupt and an abuse of my human rights as there had been no specific accusation of any event, that took place at any time, that substantiates working difficulties; and that I had not been given the opportunity to an investigation that involved the cross examination of the course coordinator's accusations and a cross examination of my defence. Sam said that since the last time he met me, I had been e-mailed by the course coordinator, and that I did not reply to him, which showed an attitude and evidence of work difficulties. I said that I had never received an e-mail and that this was a lie. I told Sam that I would shame his name by exposing what he had done to me to the Neurological Alliance, the Charity Commission, the people his charity get their funding from as well as the lottery , my Member of the Scottish Parliament, the Equality & Human Rights Commission; and that he would not walk away from this without major injuries to his name. I then told him to kindly remove himself from my sight, using a tone and body language of a man who was one increment point away from throwing him in front of a bus. Sam did just that and left. I texted him and told him to forward to me the e-mail that the course coordinator had supposedly sent me. When I got home, I had been forwarded a fabricated e-mail which had been fabricated using a word document. I knew that this had been fabricated as it is always the case that in an e-mail that has been sent to someone where correspondence copies have been sent to others, the correspondence e-mail addresses are listed beside or underneath the "original recipient" address. In this "forwarded e-mail", that had supposedly been sent to me as original recipient; and "CC'd" to Sam from the course coordinator, there was no listing of Sam's address just mine. When I responded to this finding by asking Sam to send me the original e-mail and not a fabricated e-mail, he responded by phoning my father the next day and said that he apologised as the e-mail had never been sent and what had happened was that the course coordinator had forgotten to put my e-mail address in the e-mail he sent me. I immediately knew this to be a lie, as never would an e-mail send without an original recipient address. A message would always immediately come up on the screen saying that message did not send; or the sender had forgot to put an address in the original recipient box, therefore it would be impossible for someone to think that they had sent an e-mail after failing to put in the address of the original recipient, especially when they would have been at the computer screen at the time of pressing "send". It would also be impossible for that somebody who forgot to put in an original recipient address to not be made aware of this when they would have continued to access their e-mail account between "sending" the e-mail and sacking the worker a number of days later. They would have had an e-mail sent to them almost immediately saying the e-mail didn't send if there was no immediate notification appear on screen informing the sender that the e-mail did not send. I could also conclude that this forgetting to put my address in the original recipient box was a lie as how do you explain the e-mail Sam had sent me. I also asked why if this e-mail had been sent on the 29th May, and it was the 19th June that me and Sam met in the café where I was sacked, why had the course coordinator not sent me another e-mail, or even better pick up the phone. Due to not getting any answers to my questions concerning the legitimacy of the e-mail, supposedly constructed by the course coordinator on the 29th May 2018 that Sam Whitmore "forwarded" to me on the 19th June; as well as why there were no follow up attempts made to contact me, combined with the fact that Sam had decided to talk to my father instead of me concerning private and confidential information concerning me, I decided to put in my complaint to the directors of Epilepsy Connections for both constructive dismissal and breaching of the Data Protection Act, where I was looking for dismissal of both members of staff. At the time of writing, there is currently an ongoing investigation and I am taking my local political councillor Graham Hardie with me when I am asked to come and give my evidence. My parents have put in their complaint as well as a result of the collateral damage done to their relationship that the damage done to me has caused. I have told this charity that if I don't get the result I want I will be going to third parties, and I will let them worry about what that means. The outcome to this case can be found in a later chapter as the case is ongoing, and the book will not be published until this case comes to a conclusion.

NEVER MIND ME, A LITTLE ABOUT ALISTAIR

As Alistair was mentioned in the scene where Sam Whitmore constructively fired me from my post of consultant trainer, and as I feel a loyalty towards Alistair as he has been the only true friend I have had in years, I thought I would tell you a little bit about him. Alistair was a former client of Fairway Advocacy and has learning disability, and as I advocated for him on so many issues we decided to stay in touch with one another after the closure of Fairway Advocacy. It makes sense to me that someone from the far right of the functionality continuum would be good friends with someone from the far left, it also makes sense that someone who is far removed from the ideal very light grey, as a result of having been through a lot of personalised life experience i.e. making them a very dark shade of grey, will be good friends with someone whose life path has been very unique due to an impairment in development of life skills and knowledge making them far removed from the ideal very light grey. Incompatible shades of grey exist at both ends of the functionality continuum i.e. learning disabled and high functioning. Learning disabled people and high functioning people, will be people who have life experiences and ordeals that the mainstream do not have, thus, making them both score high on individuality and undergo a lot more character development. Many of these life experiences and ordeals will be experienced by both ends of the functionality continuum, giving these two populations a lot in common, at the same time as being very different. One of these shared experiences being social exclusion and another being difficulties with boundaries. People from the learning disabled end of the continuum don't understand the boundaries due to neurodevelopmental issues, and the dark shades of grey from the high functioning end of the continuum see the boundaries as being illogical and frustrating resulting in both groups crossing these boundaries and having major fallouts with society and its foot soldiers.

Alistair is very charismatic and the most outward going guy I have known. He introduces himself to everyone, and after going for one meal in a restaurant, he will be able to go back to that restaurant on another day to say "Hi" to the manager, and the manager will love meeting him. He is a real character!! And by far a more interesting person to have the company off than most mainstream people. As Alistair has learning disability, he can't put himself in someone else's body and see the world through their eyes, and therefore, is not concerned over how others may perceive him, as he is not aware of others having a perception of him. As a result of not being concerned about how others may be perceiving him, Alistair is not self- conscious like most people are, and does not concern himself with how he compares with others. As a result of this Alistair does not experience any anxiety over what other people may think of him, which means he is confident, outspoken, opinionated, non-conformist, scores high on individuality, calls a "spade a spade", funny and is not fearful about engaging in large talk subjects; as even though his knowledge is limited on these subjects he is not worrying about what others are thinking about him because of his ignorance on the subject, and while he is in an ignorant state he is being fed new knowledge by myself, thus, erasing this ignorance. It could be said that because of their condition they have not had the skills to personally develop as much as the mainstream, therefore making them a shade of grey far removed from the ideal grey i.e. remember the shades of grey theory; thus meaning they have an experience of the world that is very unique to them brought about by their lack of life skills and therefore their character development is shaped by very personalised experiences unique to them. Remember they are not a "very light grey" like most people are, and they are not trying to be the "white" that everyone else is trying to be like as they are not aware of there being such a hypothetical pure white, as they are so removed from it, and their learning disability makes it too impractical for them to come anywhere near close to being ideal grey. I therefore, have to admit that I do from experience think that those with moderate learning disability, which is significantly more disabling than mild, are actually far more interesting people to spend your time with than the mainstream, that are all in my experience shaped by the same manipulation and insecurities due to lack of personalised life experiences, resulting in them developing into one of the many, as opposed to a one in a million e.g. they all love torn denims, they are seduced by designer clothing; despite it costing four times as much, they all want to be professionals, they don't dare have an opinion that is not the same as everyone else's, they have the same likes and dislikes as everyone else, they cut corners because everyone else cuts corners, many feel the need to be married by an age with children because everyone else is etc etc. This could go on and on with a universe of examples. I don't have any formal training in learning disability, I am instead learning all of this through my meditation practice as they say with meditation you will develop a greater mental understanding of yourself, other people and the world. The world with meditation becomes more transparent. The subjective becomes, more, and more objective i.e. you start to see more and more shades of grey in the form of what are called 'Spiritual Awakenings'.

CHAPTER 32

I have now been meditating consistently for a year, morning and night for 45 minutes, and I have found that strange things have been happening with the epilepsy. As a molecular biologist by training, I believe that there may be what is called 'neuroplastic changes' going on in my brain, where there are structural changes taking place. It is known that meditation brings on a process called 'Neurogenesis', which is the process behind the production of new grey matter. It is therefore evident that meditation brings about increases in brain volume, and as well as this, changes in brain anatomy. For example, it has been proven in studies using Magnetic Resonance Imaging (MRI) Scanners that with meditation, the part of the brain responsible for memory, known as the 'hippocampus', becomes larger in meditators. These research findings are certainly supportive of the claim that habitual meditation reduces the chances of, as well as prevent the development of conditions such as dementia as well as age related memory loss.

Over the last year I have found that there has been a lot of sudden epileptiform like activity during my meditation sessions. I have been able to articulate what this epileptiform activity is like as I have continued to consistently meditate twice per day. In those with epilepsy, the seizure threshold is low, and for those without epilepsy, the seizure threshold is high. If your susceptibility to having a seizure (seizure odds score) is rising and goes through your seizure threshold you will have a seizure.

During my meditation sessions I have felt my seizure threshold drop and my seizure odds score rise. My seizure odds score has risen while my seizure threshold has lowered to the point where my seizure odds score has gone through the seizure threshold; however, I have not had a seizure. Instead, I get a very subtle feeling of the seizure world, that just comes, and gently subsides. It's weird. It's like the seizure world is a nucleus with the real world surrounding the nucleus where I am in the real world at the same time as experiencing this small nucleus where the seizure world is found. During a seizure, this seizure world is the whole world, whereas during these meditations, the seizure world is just the nucleus with a universe of real world around it where it could be described as me having a "toe" in the seizure world, but the rest of my body in the real world, where because my toe is in the seizure world, I get a very real convincing feeling of this world being real at the same time as knowing this world not to be real since the rest of my body is in the real world. I don't experience fear or distress, and just instead a very real appreciation for how freaky and real this seizure world feels before subsiding, where my metaphorical toe is back with the rest of my body in the real world, where I am now back to being totally convinced that this seizure world is not real, and is just a very overwhelming powerful illusion brought on by a disturbance in electrical activity.

 Up until nine months ago, I was getting warnings during the day, but the climb from "1 to 6" was decelerating, as opposed to accelerating, and the deceleration was not accompanied with fear and anxiety, but instead a feeling of curiosity and a perverse feeling of escapism, where I could feel the climb from 1 to 6 being confident that the warning was going to arrest and I was not going to have a seizure. I no longer get these feelings during my meditation nor during the day and all I can say is that I am now going much longer stretches of time without seizures. All I can say is that at the time of writing I have stopped recording seizures as they have become so rare and I just tell people now it's one every ten days more out of habit than as a true reflection of my seizure frequency. The last post-ictal state i.e. amnesia, that I can remember having at the time of writing i.e. 15th October 2019 was around four weeks ago instead of just over a week ago, and my last seizure that I have taken upon getting out of bed in the morning while getting dressed is over two years ago. Meditating once daily up until September 2017 was enough to put away the first thing in the morning seizures. The irony is that, that last first thing in the morning seizure taken around two years ago happened in the midst of a meditation session. I can remember sitting there with my eyes shut and feeling my seizure odds score, and seizure threshold colliding, and suddenly I took a seizure. It was the only time that the meeting of the score and the threshold resulted in seizure during a meditation. I was meeting my Dad in the Commodore Hotel at 10.00am for a coffee that morning and arrived at 10.40am due to the post-ictal amnesia; however, it was the last first thing in the morning seizure I have had. I would have to conclude from this sitting here typing away two years later that this seizure was a one step back to be followed by a thousand steps forward seizure. You may wish to draw different conclusions.

There needs to be more research into meditation and epilepsy. Some doctors have said it makes it worse, whereas some doctors have said it makes it better.

All I can say is that I have had a very temperamental epilepsy that was very unforgiving, and now I consider myself to not be epileptic in practice even though I still am in theory, and how dare the epilepsy connections constructively dismiss someone like me who can depart and share this knowledge with those affected by epilepsy especially when I had designed a session on Meditation.

The content of the above paragraph combined with living in a risk averse society, would have many say that meditation is causing some type of epileptiform activity, and that people with epilepsy should stay clear from the practice through fear that it will exacerbate their epilepsy, however, another lot of people would think all the things mentioned and say the evidence is certainly more supportive of it being therapeutic than harmful and that maybe in life you have to take a risk in order for things to improve. It's called coming out of your "Mental Comfort Zone", which human beings are not very good at doing.

CHAPTER 33

Towards the end of July 2018, money was becoming a big issue, both as a consequence of Fairway Advocacy coming to a close in August 2017 and the unfair dismissal by Epilepsy Connections that took place in June of 2018. I had decided that I needed to look for a job as a support worker looking after those with learning disability or other disability in the community. I got a job working for an organisation called the 'Richmond Fellowship', as a community support worker, in September 2018; and towards the end of September 2018, I did their in-house training and was given a post in a team that worked from the main office. It was on the day that I started that I was asked if I could provide my new employer with a new second reference. I had given them the name of an organisation that I worked for in 2004, called Fair Deal who I left on good terms with, when offered a job as a training officer at Disability Information Greater Glasgow. My new employer told me that it was too long ago and they wanted a more recent reference. In response to this, I gave them the name of the ASA agency that I worked for when I moved back up from Slough, which was when I had the seizure related injury to my head in my bedroom which resulted in me never being invited back for another shift.

I had decided when I applied for this post with the Richmond Fellowship that I would not tell anyone about my epilepsy which was my right under the Equality Act 2010. This meant that if I had a seizure at work they would not have to put in place adaptations to my role to help me keep my job and that they could dismiss me if I had a seizure, but they could not dismiss me if it ever got out that I had epilepsy without telling them. I therefore had my anxieties about giving them ASA agency as a second reference, but the problem was the Epilepsy Society wouldn't have provided me with any greater reassurance since they set me up over my medication training; blaming my cognition for the reason behind me not being allowed to administer medications as well as used my cognition as an excuse for sending me home with instruction not to come back to work until I had been given clearance to do so by occupational health.

After providing my manager with the name of a second reference I noticed that everyone at work was constantly asking me if I was still enjoying my job as though they were anticipating a day where I would tell them I was hating it. They all had cheesy smile on their faces, and there was a tone of cynicism in their voices, whenever I was asked this question. It was constant. It made me feel that they were being deliberately very clingy. This questioning was accompanied by other bizarre behaviour and practices that I could see as having the potential to create a situation for me where the blame could gravitate onto my shoulders and see me sacked for professional negligence. It made me feel very insecure. At first, I thought that I might have been paranoid, but the evidence that was mounting certainly suggested that I was being very rational in my belief. The first example of this was when one of my managers said to me that the rota had been changed, and that instead of me working with a client in Pollok the next day at around 3.00pm, I was instead to be in the office writing up my notes. I came back to the office that next day at the time instructed, and while sitting in the office, the manageress said after having a friendly lengthy conversation with me that she was currently working on the rotas and that she had become aware that I should not be in the office writing up notes and instead be elsewhere.

I said to her, "Where?", and she told me that I should have been at a client's home in an area of Glasgow called, 'Cardonald'. I responded to this by saying to Charlene that when she had spoken to me over the phone the day before, she told me that I was originally to be working in Pollok at 3pm but this had now been changed and that I was to be in the office instead writing up my notes. Charlene responded by saying that according to the rota, me being in the office writing up my notes was not the case and that I should have been in Cardonald, round at a client's home. I told her that this was not consistent with what I had been told by her yesterday, and Charlene could only say to me, that it was my responsibility to keep an eye on the rota at all times so that if there were any changes to what I was told, I would become aware of them and not require anyone to update me about them. Charlene then said that unfortunately someone had gone without their care and that this was not to happen again. I just bit my tongue thinking to myself how other peoples' incompetence lands on the shoulders of others.

It was just a few days later and I was sitting in the office writing up my notes after seeing that morning's clients and suddenly Charlene said, "Tim, where are you supposed to be right now?" and I said, "Well according to my rota I am here right now", and again, Charlene showed me the rota that had me down for being elsewhere in another client's home in another part of Glasgow's southside. I was again told that I should always keep an eye on the rota and that this was not good enough and it was now the case that two clients had gone without care because I did not keep myself up to date with the rota.

 It was only a couple of days later that I was out in Cardonald, visiting a man with learning disability who was only allowed to work with men due to him sexually exposing himself to women. I received a phone call on my way up to this man's flat and was told over the phone by Charlene that all the shifts in my diary for next week had been rearranged and that she felt she needed to phone me because she could not have confidence that I would check the rota. Charlene communicated to me all the shifts that I had been down for, which were the ones I had in my diary and told me to score these out as she had a new set of shifts for me. I put these new shifts down in my diary and thanked her for the update thinking to myself "Bitch". I then went to this client's home where I was later picked up from by my team leader who said that because I had worked in challenging behaviour in the past they wanted to make me the keyworker of a new client, and that we were going to meet the client and his social worker round at his home. When we arrived at the house, the client opened the door and let us in, where we waited with him until the social worker arrived, but the social worker never turned up for the meeting. My team leader said that we would carry out the new client consultation in the absence of the social worker. The client was Asian, and did not speak good English. He had a diagnosis, if memory serves me correctly, of schizophrenia; and when we asked him how he kept himself safe he pulled an axe out from under his pillow and started waving it. The client motioned what he would do if someone came in the flat. The client went through the motions of grabbing a person's hair, yanking their head forward followed by beheading them. My team leader said nothing. I didn't look shocked, and told the client that I would be his keyworker, and would be responsible for creating his care plan, and ensuring he got good quality care from myself, as well as others who cared for him, and that I would be the bridge of communication between the client and the wider team composed of people such as social work and other allied professionals. When we left, I was asked if I was okay with this client, and I said, "No way". I told my team leader that this breached all protocol, and that this man in my opinion did not have the cognitive capacity to be in the possession of an axe in the house, there was no need for him to have an axe in the house, there had been no risk assessment carried out, meaning that if someone got attacked and experienced trauma or severe loss they would have a right to claim compensation on the grounds of professional negligence, and the first thing a lawyer would want to see would be a risk assessment, and that I as the keyworker would be blamed for not bringing it to everyone's attention that no risk assessment had been done, and that I would end up being sacked and made unemployable. With all the denial coming from the Richmond Fellowship over providing me with misleading rotas despite this misleading information being provided to me in person as well as over the phone, I believed that the team leader I was with would deny ever seeing the axe at the consultation and that that was probably the reason as to why the social worker did not show up, as if there was going to be a stitch up orchestrated by the Richmond Fellowship, then the Glasgow City Council social work department would most likely want to have nothing to do with it. This would especially be the case if there was anyone from Glasgow City Council social work department who remembered me from back in 2008 where they had been involved in setting me up over my epilepsy. I therefore said that until a risk assessment was put in place, I was going to exercise my right as well as abide with the law, which was to not go anywhere near this man's house without a risk assessment being carried out to determine the right level of support. The team leader told me that a risk assessment would be arranged and that no one would be expected to work with this man until one had been carried out. I thought to myself that there was so much not adding up, and that I had to keep my eyes open like a hawk because either these peoples' moralities or competencies could not be trusted.

It was only a couple of days later that I was sitting in the office and my colleague asked me what I was doing with my weekend as he was coming off shift, and I said, "I'm going to go to the gym. All these 5am rises in Helensburgh have caused me to go three weeks without the gym as my body adjusts to this new way of life". My colleague said, "Good luck with that, and I will see you in a few days". I said, "Cheers", and thought to myself, "that guys a decent guy, there are some decent people". This statement was to be followed by a voice from the back of the office saying, "Tim". No prizes for guessing who this was! "Tim, why are you here?" and I replied, "because Charlene, I was told to be here at this time, on this day, when you phoned me up the other day telling me that all of the shifts in my diary were to be replaced with new shifts, that had me down for being in different places as originally planned and the new shifts have me down as being in this office at this time". Charlene replied, "Let me see your diary", which I showed her and she denied ever giving me any of these new shifts. Charlene also denied ever giving me the phone call that I had received. I said that I could evidence her call from my call log, but she just replied by saying, "That's an office number and does not prove that it was I who had phoned". I told her that I had a clear memory of speaking to her, and asked her to explain why I had one set of shifts scored out in my diary, which were the shifts she was now telling me that I should be doing, and the listing of a new lot of shifts in my diary, which she was denying ever giving me. Charlene replied, "That's a question only you can answer", and I said, "I think I must be needing a neuropsychology assessment, as I seem to be having many false beliefs, and acting out on false memories". I further went on to say, "Charlene, I'm worried that I must have some sort of early onset dementia". Charlene responded, "What an attitude problem you have!". Charlene pointed at a room across from her desk and said, "Get into that room now!". I went into the room with her and she said to me, "Tim, I know you are new and only have been here a few weeks but you have been making a really bad impression of yourself." Charlene continued, "I know you are new but that is not an excuse for being unreliable, being late and not being where you are supposed to be. There have been two previous occasions where clients have missed their care, and this has now happened to a number of clients today, as you not only should not be in this office at this time, but you should also not be doing the shift that you are currently doing". I responded by saying, "Come clean! You set me up by fabricating evidence against me! You set me up the first two times and this is an incredibly desperate attempt at setting me up for the third time". Charlene responded by shaking her head and saying, "Oh no you don't! How dare you accuse me of setting you up by fabricating evidence". Charlene continued, "Tomorrow you, me and your Team Leader are going to have a meeting about you, your unreliability, the need for immense improvement and what consequences you face if you don't improve". I thought inside to myself "Charlene, there will be no such meeting!". I said, "I am going home now as my time for going home has come according to the shifts you gave me and the shifts that I wrote in my diary. I will see you at tomorrow's meeting and look forward to discussing this "misunderstanding". I had decided that I was resigning, but I did not want to tell her that. I said to her, "Charlene, do you know what the term 'collateral damage' means?". All Charlene could say in response to this was, "Don't patronise me". I asked her this question because what angered me was that all this woman could see the outcome of constructively dismissing me as being, was me not working there anymore and having to look for another job. I knew for a fact that it would have never crossed her mind what impact me losing my job might have had on the possibility of being able to meet a future partner or the long- term success of any current partnered relationship I was in. This woman would have not considered what the effects, caused by the constructive dismissal, would have been on any dependents; such as wife and children, and what effects it could have had on their education, future employment and social connections; if finding new employment meant moving elsewhere. This woman, who had been promoted to a position way beyond her abilities, would have no knowledge or awareness of the effects her treatment of me could have had on the mental health of any children of mine, living in a home where the financial hardship caused by the constructive dismissal could create so much domestic pressure; resulting in the break-up of Mum and Dad because of an emotionally unstable environment, resulting in poor school performance, delinquent behaviour and brushes with the law etc. It's like I said to my local liberal democrat councillor, one thing I've learned in life in recent years, especially through my meditation practice, is how frighteningly little you need to know to get a role in society that grants you powers and responsibilities that requires you to know so much to adequately exercise. It's why our society is so dysfunctional and stands on its head. It's why I describe our society as like a "Bull in a china shop, with a blind-fold on", and we allow that "Bull" to have so much control over our lives, by the granting it of so many powers it is too life uneducated, life un-skilled, too ignorant and/or too low IQ combined with too little ability to apply intellect to practice (AAIP) to exercise responsibly. Most people that I have come across who give orders, but also those that take orders, are too lacking in initiative, intuition and insight to truly know what they are doing. The powers to give orders as well as make autonomous decisions in the wrong hands creates for the rest of us a very dangerous society; resulting in recessions, austerity, mental health epidemics, drug and alcohol addiction, compromised physical health of self and others; poor housing, poor educational amenities, privatisation of essential services, industries under the control of the underworld, overcrowded prisons etc. Psychiatrists would say that this analysis of the world is symptomatic of depression when in fact it is evidenced as the truth from my life experience and education, and this term depression is just a big brush to sweep the real issues under the big rug.

The next day, I woke up at 5am, and wrote my letter of resignation, made my way to work, and walked in the front door, into the main office, full of people who had been asking me with grins if I was still enjoying my job. I said, "Don't ask", before they could ask, and I said, "Inside this envelope is my letter of resignation. I don't have a job anymore for you to ask me about, as I no longer wish to work for you. I have been treated dishonourably, by dishonourable people; therefore, this is no place for an honourable person like me. The letter explains it all. Good Bye", and I left.

All I knew at this workplace was that I had never offended anyone, or stood on anyone's toes while I worked in this place for the very short time that I did. I am a very conscientious person, and speak to as well as treat others exactly the same way I wish others to speak and treat me. I did my job and never gave anyone any grounds to have an issue or complaint about me. All I can say is that they wanted me out only three weeks after starting. You can't say job performance was their reason for wanting me gone as there is a probationary period which is six months, therefore, unless you do something really bad there was no legitimate grounds for pushing me out the door so soon in a "jump before pushed" fashion, therefore, there must have been a real concern that suddenly emerged in the three weeks between offering me the job, and me handing in my resignation. All I can say is that during that three week period there was a request for another reference from an employer who would have known about my epilepsy, and I wonder what had been shared. I do recognise that people like me apply for jobs that we would have not applied for thirty years before our time. A graduate in molecular biology from Glasgow University would never have applied for a support worker post in the 1980's. It was the Blair Government of the late nineties that discredited the university degree by inventing so many university degree specialties, having people go to university to study degrees in subjects like television studies. It's a good example of how most people don't question logic and just choose to conform by believing that this must be a good idea as the person in authority thinks it's a good idea and it is therefore, just taken for granted as being a good idea. That "good idea" being the invention of degree subjects, that can only be described with one word, and that is "non-sensical". As the rest of the world can't appreciate the difference between a degree in a subject related to finding cures to cancer and a degree that is in a subject that is related to painting nails, people like me have had to apply for jobs that are well beneath our level of education and skill set meaning that we have had to work in jobs where people of our level of education inevitably make others feel less educated, giving them chips on their shoulders that result in the rejection of people like us, causing us to get bullied/tormented out of these jobs. I therefore, see this as being a potential reason for why I had to jump before be pushed. It was a job where my last job was working for myself running an advocacy charity and as well as that it was a job where my team leader became aggressive towards me when I shared with her that I had a molecular biology degree. The Richmond Fellowship experience could possibly have been a repeat of Epilepsy Connections in as much as it could have been an experience encountered as a result of someone above me feeling an insecurity as a result of me having an experience of something from more than one perspective, unlike they who had only had experience from one perspective. With Epilepsy Connections I had professional as well as personal experience of the condition, and with the Richmond Fellowship I had advocacy, educational as well as support work experience of working with vulnerable adults, and I have also in both cases been more educated than the authority above me. My meditation practice has made me aware of how much insecurity and self-loathing people are guilty off and therefore cannot rule this out as being a reason behind the Richmond Fellowship experience. If your reaction to me saying that I am too educated for the role of support worker as well as saying that in the 1980's never would someone with a science degree apply for a job as a support worker, is for you to say that I am being arrogant and obnoxious, then I am afraid to tell you what you already know, and that is you are in denial probably because of the very insecurity that I say exists in others. I ask you this, "Do you honestly believe that if you told someone who had just graduated with a molecular biology degree that they would be a support worker in twenty one years time, they would feel that their four years at university had been well spent?". I also ask you to be honest with yourself, and consider what words would go through your mind after asking someone what they were studying at university and their reply was, "I am studying a degree in the history of aircraft carrier ships". Precisely! I've made my point.

It was after this letter of resignation that I decided that I was no longer going to apply for jobs and that I would actually rather go to prison than work for someone. My life had got to the point where I saw prison as just being another department in the "University of Life", that if I ever found myself in, I would just stop my meditation practice, as I would be in an environment where rage would be an asset. I also saw time spent in prison as being a place where I would learn new knowledge and skills that would be transferable to a world that was full of people like me who had been socially excluded, and through their social exclusion had developed an "every man for himself" ethos. Remember what I said about "High sense of self". I had a very high level of fitness. My resting pulse rate was forty seven, and has been as low as forty four. An Olympian athlete's heart rate can be as low as 38 according to a heart rate monitor book that I had bought, which made me realise that I must have been fit enough to be in the army, even in the higher more physically demanding regiments, and saw this as being a potential vocational asset, especially when combined with rage; therefore, being given a name of someone that would give you the opportunity to maybe "rough someone up" for a living was what I saw myself doing if I ever gravitated towards criminality. I'm sure that someone in prison would know someone on the outside looking for someone to play such a role at the time of my release. It just shows you that society criminalises people, and feeling like I was on my last law abiding legs evidences this. That's why I look at the police and think "God, you are such simplistic beings who have no idea how complex this world is, and for some, law abiding behaviour is impractical, and it's your own very society that the judicial system protects that makes law abiding behaviour impractical for those you end up imprisoning". My last word I then think to myself when I see a police officer is "Mug!"

As I had not given up on living a law abiding life, I had decided that I was sticking with my plan, which was to start a peer support service, treating others with mental health problems by teaching them the self- help strategies that I have taught myself, and have been able to use successfully to self-manage my depression and anxiety. One thing I can say throughout all these experiences that you have read about is that I have developed a vocational skill from them, and that vocational skill is the skill of "self-help". If it were not for meditation, aerobic exercise, distraction, thought blocking, positive thinking, slow breathing; I would have taken my life back in 2013, which was when I nearly met my life intolerance threshold before taking up meditation. Up until 2013, if it were not for age and aerobic fitness, I would probably have suffered from heart attack or stroke as well as having had a few angry spells in prison, where goodness knows what vocational skills and influential people I might have met in there. I therefore, see myself as seeing the option of social exclusion as being the best option for me, creating my own opportunities; which would not be possible for me to endure without my meditation and aerobic exercise. I can go up to three weeks without a conversation because of social exclusion.

Despite coping, I feel society still owes me compensation, as society has provided many with so much, and has provided me with nothing, and therefore, see universal credit and personal independent payment (PIP) as being a means of being compensated for, living in a society that disables me, as opposed to my epilepsy, depression and anxiety. I am still alive today, and kept myself out of prison because I managed to survive a "beating-up" by society through the use of meditation and exercise; however, no one should ever find themselves being alive and enjoying whatever liberty they have because they found a way in surviving a "beating" by society, and this finding a way does not let society of the hook with what it has done, thus, does not make you less deserving of some form of compensation. I therefore, apply for universal credit and PIP with the aim of getting both compensation and a financial helping hand in enabling me towards moving away from relying on a society that shows nothing but intolerance towards me, and instead, moving towards becoming a self- sufficient independent social recluse who enjoys having no relationship with mainstream society other than the clients who use my mental health service, who will share a lot of my sentiment.

As I have already said I do believe that I would have done a number of spells in prison without the meditation. In fact, it might be a lengthy stay for something like murder. Remember the incident with my father in 2016! I have also said that I would rather a spell in prison than work for someone else, and therefore I have told the universal credit medical examiner that if I ever got another job and someone ever pulled a stunt like the others have done in the past I would do the judo throw on them that I did on my father and I would ensure that I gave them a lasting injury to remember me by. I have said, I would throw someone and damage their head and put them in a wheel chair and can't promise that anything that involves a blow to the head will not result in death. What I can tell you is this is the truth as the only justice that appears to work and put closure on things for people like me is "Rough Justice". I will leave it to you to decide if my decision to do this to someone comes under 'Mental Health', 'Pragmatism' or 'Social Justice'; or you could be really unfair and despicable and call it "Criminality". I put this word "criminality" in quotation marks as it is a word that requires redefining. It is a word that assumes the authority is always the good guy and the powerless the bad guy. As a biologist I would say, "If the rules don't work for you, then break them!". It's called "SURVIVAL". Rules create unlevel playing fields. When the rules advantage one party, the breaking of rules by the disadvantaged party should be allowed, until the playing field is levelled for both parties !!!!!! Therefore, breaking rules is very often "Justice", and not always "Criminality". The two words get confused and wrongly used. They are very different, but both share a common trait, and that is: They both involve breaking rules!

CHAPTER 34

It is now Monday 3rd December 2018, and I am two days after being interviewed by Epilepsy Connections over my complaint regarding Sam Whitmore's and Peter Dale's unfair and dishonest dismissal of myself, as a trainer on the 'Epilepsy Futures Course'. I attended this meeting with my local Liberal Democrat Councillor, Graham Hardie, who I decided to approach for help with representation as he was the only male councillor in Helensburgh, and had also been at the same school as me. Graham had also gone to St Andrews University, where he transferred to Glasgow University, just like I had. I've been meeting him for coffees over the last few years as we both tried to start a social isolation group, where we sat there and had a good, male version of the word, "bitching" session about our former teachers. Upon our arrival we had the Executive Director of Epilepsy Connections whose name was Shirley Maxwell, an employment lawyer and a director, whose name I cannot remember as she said nothing throughout the hour-long meeting. This was a meeting where no minutes were taken and, therefore, I had to ask my councillor to take notes. When I asked my local councillor, Graham Hardie, to take notes all I got from the Epilepsy Connections side of the room was 'tuts and exhalations' of objection, as they obviously, somehow saw this as evidence of me being really forward. They knew I was a former disability advocate which is probably why they immediately appeared to be on the defensive. In my opinion they should have had a secretary in the room take the minutes, but obviously they wanted no record of this meeting. The meeting started with a really patronising, "Welcome Tim, we received your complaint and we have come to a conclusion regarding the outcome of your complaint.". "I would like to start off by saying that you must have had a terribly difficult life, and that you have lived with the enormous burden of very disturbing seizures that have seriously reduced your employment prospects". I thought to myself. "No, I do not. It is not my seizures that affect my employment prospects it is in fact the attitude of others towards my seizures". This evidenced an immediate failure of hers to recognise the number one enemy of living with epilepsy, and that is public attitude. This immediately evidenced them as a charity not being fit for purpose, in terms of anything they say about being a charity that shows concern for the human rights of those with epilepsy.

I was told that the meeting would start with the conclusion of the outcome and that I would be told the rationales for why they had come to these conclusions. The lawyer said to me with a smirk, "Mr Bone, you raise in your complaint 'subsection 3, of the Human Rights Act', which refers to you having a right to be treated in a way that is free from torture or inhumane treatment, as well as your right to be treated with respect and dignity. I have to inform you that this right does not apply in this case as the Human Rights Act does not apply to employment law.". I responded to this and said, "First of all, could someone start taking some notes as minutes are not being taken.". I asked my councillor to take notes which they showed objection to but did not prevent us from doing. I responded to this news about the Human Rights Act and said, "That is wrong. I Know from my research that the Human Rights Act was enshrined into Employment Law and now this Act applies in all work settings." The lawyer said, "It only applies to public bodies, which Epilepsy Connections is not". I know that Epilepsy Connections is, as it provides public services to the public, and therefore qualifies as a public body. I made the lawyer aware of this, and he said, "Please Mr Bone. I do this for a   living". I replied, "Regardless, the human rights, subsection 3 applies, and with the suffering I have experienced, Mr Whitmore and Mr Dale have both broken this Act". I then said, "If you are going to tell me that the Human Rights Act does not apply then myself and my councillor here will have to go away and get a second opinion on that". "The beauty of the internet", I thought to myself. This information could actually have been checked there and then on the mobile, but I decided not to do it that way and let them worry instead. The three of them all looked at one another with, "This isn't working" expressions on their faces, and looked very worried. The lawyer then went on to say, "You claim that Mr Whitmore breached the Data Protection Act. I must say that the Data Protection Act does not apply here". The lawyer said that, "As Mr Whitmore had evidence in the form of an e-mail from your father that you had informed him of what had happened it was right that Mr Whitmore believe that you had no objections to Mr Whitmore sharing information with your Dad about you without a signed mandate". I told him that Mr Whitmore had shared information without a signed mandate, and that that was in breach with Data Protection. My councillor said that if he had a constituent come to him over any matter, he could not share any information concerning that matter with anyone without his constituent signing a signed mandate. I then said that for all Sam knew, my father might be a very nosy man who had read a diary that I keep causing my Dad to contact him over this matter without my knowledge. The lawyer looked at me with a, "I can't answer that" expression, and shut up. Again, all three looked at one another with helpless facial expressions realising that this meeting was not going to be the walk over that they believed it was going to be. I then said to the lawyer that this talk was farcical. I reminded the lawyer that we were here today because I had a fabricated e-mail in front of me that can be evidenced as being a word document, and not an original e-mail. Peter Dale never sent me this e-mail dated the 29th May 2018, that Mr Whitmore sent me. It can be seen in the fabricated e-mail; supposedly sent from Peter Dale, to me, on the 29th May 2018; that Sam Whitmore's address does not appear in it as either a correspondent recipient, therefore how could he have received a copy of this from Peter Dale, to forward to me. I also said that the header of Sam Whitmore's e-mail had a link to his e-mail address, whereas the header of the fabricated Peter Dale e-mail, does not provide a link to his e-mail address. I said that regardless of the Human Rights Act, as well as the Data Protection Act, I had in front of me an e-mail that could be proven to not be an original e-mail, and instead a word document that had been fabricated to look like an e-mail to legitimise dismissing someone. I then asked the lawyer if that was legal. Again, the lawyer looked at the other two with the helpless expression.

Shirley Maxwell said to me that their complaint procedure is for service users and that I am not a service user. Shirley said that they had to tailor a complaint process for me where my understanding was that she was trying to suggest that they did not need to investigate my complaint simply because their complaint procedure was only open to people who were clients and that this investigation was not an obligatory one, and done purely out of good will, and therefore I had no right for this complaint to be investigated nor come to a justifiable outcome. I knew that this was rubbish, as according to this theory, if Mr Whitmore spat in the face of an old lady while out with his clients then this old lady would have no right to complain as she is not a client. My councillor said that if I had done fourteen years of service for Epilepsy Connections in the form of befriending, delivering courses and delivering public talks on living with epilepsy, then he did not think that Shirley Maxwell, the lawyer and director could sit there and say that no complaint process investigating a complaint of mine and coming to a justifiable outcome was obligatory. I said to them "What was the actual outcome then? Have these two shameful characters been allowed to keep their jobs?". Shirley Maxwell said that

Epilepsy Connections had a duty to protect the confidentiality of Sam Whitmore and Peter Dale and therefore were not allowed to share the outcome of the investigation in terms of what happened to Sam Whitmore and Peter Dale. I responded to this by summarising my interpretation of what they were saying and that was that I make a complaint and that due to confidentiality I am not allowed to know the outcome of that complaint. Shirley and the lawyer both said, "Yes". I said, "So, does this mean you could therefore keep them on your books without me knowing?". The lawyer said, "It is a private investigation, being carried out by a private organisation, which by law is not obliged to share any information about with the public". I said "How can you have an investigation where you interviewed the accused, but did not interview the one making the accusations?". The lawyer said, "We have your complaint in paper. We don't need to interview you". I said, "Yes you do, as they could have countered what I had put in my complaint with made up lies. This whole investigation is about their dishonesty for heaven's sake". I said that being a part of that investigation I should have been interviewed, and being the one making the complaint, I am not a member of the public, therefore, I am entitled to know the outcome of the case. The lawyer looked at me with a sarcastic smile and said that it was a private investigation, carried out by a private organisation and therefore for reasons of confidentiality they could not share with me the outcome of the case. I replied, "Yes you can, and you should, as I am not a member of the public being a former consultant trainer of your private organisation who was the one that kick started this complaint". I said that we would just agree to disagree and that I hated to inform them that this meeting had not brought this case to an end and that it was in fact day one of a battle where I would be using media to expose a big name in the voluntary sector as being corrupt, dishonest and be prepared to constructively dismiss a person with the very condition that they say they are there to protect the interests of those living with. My councillor said, that I had put in fourteen years of commitment into their charity and that they had demonstrated themselves to be the opposite of what they claim to be, which is a charity that helps enhance the lives of people with epilepsy by skilling them and opening up opportunities for them, as well as provide facilities and services that promote their mental wellbeing.

Shirley Maxwell looked at me and asked me what I would like to see as an outcome to this case. I replied, "The dismissing of these two individuals". I looked at the lawyer, and said to him, "I have written a book called 'A Fitful

Life' which I gave to Mr Whitmore in May 2018 to read the first draft of, and in that book I share with the reader all the discrimination and prejudice that I have experienced all my life. I told him that I was on a social work course and got discriminated against, been discriminated against at St Andrews University because of visual memory difficulties related to my epilepsy, had been discriminated against by an agency that I worked for; after I had cut my head of a mirror during a seizure and bled badly, and that there was a huge list of other incidents that I was not going to go into. I told him that Mr Whitmore read my book and knew about all the injustices I had, had to live without closure on; and how these injustices had pushed me to having panic attacks, and suicidal ideation, with me belonging to a suicide risk group that has a one in seven attempted suicide rate, according to a University of Western Ontario Study, carried out by a psychiatrist called Garcia. I said that despite Sam Whitmore knowing about this he still went ahead and decided to participate in the constructive dismissal of me in June 2018, just a month after reading my book. I told the lawyer that I was a meditator who had been meditating since September 2013, and that without this meditation, I would be dead, as if I miss as much as two sessions, I am wakening up in the middle of the night overwhelmed by feelings of isolation and being trapped in a hell, where I see only one purpose in being alive, and that is to die. I looked at all three of them and said that because of this, Mr Whitmore is in no fit position to be working with anyone with epilepsy, whether that be a colleague or a client, and that I would do everything, and never rest, until I have named and shamed him, as well as their charity. I said, "We have all the winning cards. The fabricated e-mail, the Human Rights Act subsection 3, the Data Protection Act; and as well as this, a community mental health referral on the 11th December 2018, where I will be telling the community mental health team everything that Epilepsy Connections has done to me in terms of me not being able to work for anyone anymore, as the trustworthiness and true intentions of people; both colleagues and employers/educators, have become so discredited by so many years of being exposed to people in positions of trust behaving dishonourably towards me". It is now my intention to apply for Employment Support Allowance, as I no longer wish to ever work for anyone. I would rather go to prison than work for a person, and I am glad to say that my parents have wealth, as they can support me financially, as I try to start up my own peer support service. I said that I don't feel guilty nor embarrassed admitting my family have wealth that I can live off, as I am only doing what every other bitter person, who complains about people with wealth being allowed undeserved luxury, would do if they had the same access to it, and that I wouldn't call money for food, utilities, clothes, transport etc as luxury. You just need to look at the House of Lords. How many politicians spend their entire careers damning the house of lords and then accept peerage like it's in fashion the moment they are offered it. Examples of such politicians are John Prescott, Neil Kinnock and Peter Haine.

I will aim to get justice over my experience with Epilepsy Connections, as like I said, I have the winning cards, but I will not allow what happened between me and Epilepsy Connections, to distract me from working on my peer support service, as this is the future. Me alone, working towards future success, leaving behind the filthy experience of human beings that I have encountered all my life. Yes, I have become misanthropic.

I will be forty four years of age in a couple of months' time, and I am glad to say that despite all the hardship and abuse that I have received from the human race for having epilepsy, social anxiety disorder and depression; where the latter two were caused in themselves by abuse that goes back to my school days and further reinforced by all the grief I have experienced since then; I have learned a large number of self- help techniques. I have lived through this more than a storm without ever taking a single anti-depressant or tranquiliser; and I have instead used cognitive techniques in the form of meditation, aerobic exercise, distraction, visualisation, positive thinking, thought blocking and slow breathing, to control mental health symptoms. I have also developed a lot of vocational skills such as the training skills acquired from teaching the 'Chronic Disease Self-Management Course' in both Glasgow and Slough as well as the self-management course I had designed myself when working at Disability Information Greater Glasgow. I have also managed to experience four very successful years of providing advocacy for people with neurological disability if you include the months I did advocacy on a voluntary basis for, that has tremendously boosted my confidence, moral and self-esteem as well as shape me into a positive thinker that has now left me with the skills to make a success of any aim or goal I wish to work towards achieving, in the form of 'Positive Affirmations', 'Negative Thought Blocking' and 'Visualisation', while working towards these goals. I therefore, feel that I have a lot to offer other people who are struggling with their mental health problems as well as confidence; therefore, in my building of my mental health peer support service, I am designing day courses as well as one to one sessions teaching people about meditation as well as teaching them the cognitive skills and techniques one can use for confidence building, depression, anxiety, anger/rage and phobia management.

Fairway Advocacy taught me that when I am left to my own devices, where I do not have to work with others, or for others; I excel and succeed. It's just a pity that there was not enough funding to continue Fairway Advocacy; however, with the peer support service, what I earn will be proportionate with what I achieve, therefore, I have faith; being in the knowledge of what I can achieve when I am left alone, in being able to offer a self -help service that teaches people to conquer mental health problems by simply using the knowledge and skills that I have acquired through my own life experience. No one can take this knowledge, skills and experience away from me through discrimination nor as a result of their insecurities. I am a great believer in turning negatives into positives, and therefore with the using of positive affirmations, visualisation and negative thought blocking I should be able to go on and make a success of my peer support mental health service. How long will it take? Well time will be the verdict of that!

I am watching my diet, exercising and meditating to look after my mind and body so that I can reclaim lost years and be an eighty five year old hill walker and not an eighty five year old getting his pad changed in a nursing home; or being hoisted from his bedroom into a bath, having his right to be treated with respect and dignity, under the Human Rights Act, being violated by care staff, medical staff and/or social work staff. This might sound cynical but I have seen it as a person affected by disability, as a student training to work in health and social care as well as an employee; in the form of support worker, trainer and disability advocate; and therefore, have to contemplate such treatment as a possibility if I ever find myself relying on these people to help me meet my activities of daily living in old age, as a result of having a stroke, or developing an age related deteriorative condition such as dementia. My future health is especially concerning for someone like myself, as living in a world without family and friends would only expose me to such abuse and violations of my human rights without any need for cover up as who would hold these people to account on my behalf? I don't feel though that people with family and friends have that much of an advantage though, as judging by other peoples' life skills I doubt family and friends in the majority of cases would have the assertiveness and self-belief to advocate for a family member or friend if that person was being mistreated in a nursing home. You just have to look at how impossible most people find going down stairs and telling a neighbour not to drill a hole in an apartment wall unannounced when it is causing very loud, vibrating intrusive noise in that person's home. Why am I the only person knocking on an antisocial neighbour's door demanding that they ask if now is a good time for them to start loud DIY work before commencing any loud home improvement or give prior notice of loud construction work so that the rest of us who live lives can get on with our lives without sudden noise from another's home hijacking our day. If people don't have the skills to demand this respect be shown to them by a neighbour then what chance do they have of demanding a nursing home treats a relative of theirs with respect, or that a social work decision that violates the human rights of a relative be reversed and a more humane one made. This is why all people should protect their heads and other body functions, as the minute they become dependent on others to compensate for things going wrong with these functions, they open themselves up to all forms of abuse and exploitation. If you were to get every reckless driver to do national service in the form of providing support work for such vulnerable people e.g. head injury for a period of a year, these reckless drivers would start doing their observations, indicating, sticking to speed limits, wear their seatbelts; and people who make the most unhealthy lifestyle choices would stop overindulging on sugar, salt, simple carbohydrate, alcohol, excess saturated fat etc if they were made to do the same national service. Disability advocates could give them presentations on the injustices experienced and human rights lost by people who have had head injury, spinal injury etc from car accidents and other reckless behaviour.

CHAPTER 35

I have since February of 2018 become closer with my Mother. My mother has been back on the scene more, and I believe that back in 2003 when the westies became an obsession, it was her way in withdrawing from society as it had all become too much. As I am now meditating, and do not get anywhere near as distressed as I used to, it has become easier for my mother to see her son again as it was distressing her seeing me in such a state that other people had put him in. This is especially the case when these people are in positions that require care and trust.

My brother in law who is married to my younger sister wants to meet for a meal this week beginning 3rd December 2018 and I have had my father explain to me that my younger sister has had her mental health problems as she has two young sons where one is very hyperactive and never calms down nor sleeps. My nephew is going to speech and language therapy as he has delayed speech, and therefore my father asks that I understand the reasons behind why my sister might not have been in touch.

My older sister, everyone would agree, is an unpleasant person who has no empathy for anyone who struggles. My older sister has shown no empathy towards me nor has she shown any empathy towards my younger sister's troubles, and therefore, my older sister is the unpopular one in the family who doesn't spend nearly enough time with her son, who now reports to his grandparents that he is depressed, and according to my father, he was caught looking up a document on the internet about suicide a few days before my universal credit assessment.

Despite this bad news about my two nephews, it does look like family is coming together again. I won't be going home for Christmas this year as that would be too big a jump, but with smaller steps, it could be the case next year.

AFTERMATH OF CHRISTMAS & NEW YEAR

Christmas of 2018 has been and gone, at the time of writing, to the majority of the population; which is now 2pm on the afternoon of the 2nd January 2019. To Christians, this is the 8th day of Christmas whereas to the vast majority, Christmas has now been and gone. To the retail world, Christmas has been and gone by boxing day, and by the deals in the shop windows, it is evident that they are now wanting clear of their Christmas stocks for another year. I must confess that I did take advantage of this by buying three pairs of Primark denims in the sales, but these I did genuinely need, unlike others; whose strings are pulled like puppets into going into shops to take things of shelves, taking money out of wallet, and walk out of the shop, immediately into the shop next door to make the next purchase. I do live in a world, where I find myself thinking "Puppets", as I walk around its streets. Is this judgemental? Well who cares! The world has been judgemental towards me, so expect me to be judgemental towards it, but I must emphasise that my findings and conclusions that form my opinions are all evidenced by the observations that I make daily. There's no conclusion that I draw where the only evidence I have is urban myth and what I hear others saying. As a person who questions logic, I always look for hard evidence that come from observations, studies, experiences, behaviours etc. A good example of this is Christmas where it would be true to say from such hard evidence that it is a festival that is celebrated largely by unchristian people, for unchristian reasons. I know that this is not true of all people, but those who celebrate Christmas, who are of the unchristian fabric of our society, are either celebrating it because of conformity or because of a naivety. Christmas does not actually celebrate the birth of Christ, and if you research Christmas, it is a pagan festival that celebrates the winter solstice. It's a hook with a bit of bait for people to bite, which unfortunately most people do, causing them to spend money that they do not have. It is for this reason that I did not celebrate Christmas. It is also why I didn't have a single Christmas decoration up in my own home. I felt proud being the only one in my tenement close who had no Christmas tree. I thought to myself that I am of a Christian ethos, have an IQ of 120, hold an Honours degree in Molecular Biology, been a meditator since 2013; where the world has become increasingly transparent, and therefore, I should be wise enough and know better enough than to celebrate such a festival which is about "Spend! Spend! Spend!" and not what it is branded as being about, which is "Be thankful! Be thankful! Be thankful!". Christmas, which is really a pagan festival, is about "Get! Get! Get!" and is certainly not about "Give! Give! Give!". Even if Christmas were a festival where the people celebrating it were of a Christian ethos, I probably still wouldn't celebrate it since those Christians are of a faith that would have had a guy like me with epilepsy burned alive many generations ago. The bible is full of people with epilepsy being "Cured". I joined a church to try and form relationships since people are painfully awkward at forming relationships outside an already shared experience e.g. mother & baby groups, and the Institution e.g. the workplace, the sports club, the college etc. I have not shared with anyone at the church that I have epilepsy, and I would dread to think how they would react if they found out. I have therefore decided to keep my mouth shut, as people still believe to this day that epilepsy is a demonic condition. This belief is especially re-enforced considering the psycho-hallucinatory symptoms that comes with my type of epilepsy.

Throughout Christmas of 2018, I spent Christmas eve on my own. I also spent Christmas Day on my own, but for a three hour lunch with my local liberal democrat councillor, Mr Graham Hardie, at the local Indian Restaurant. I then did some card tricks with Mr Hardie and the waiter, where the waiter was the manager of the Dumbarton Indian restaurant, and said he would like to think about how he could use me, as he saw a business opportunity in me. It is definitely the case, that when I am left to my own devices, to do my own thing, without anyone else having any autonomy over my personal development, I do very well. It's when other people are put in charge of my progress, that things go pear shaped. I am definitely cut out for being my own boss and not having others being my boss.

As has already been mentioned, the remainder of Christmas Day was spent alone, and but for a coffee that I had with my father on two occasions; where my mother attended on one of these occasions, I saw no one before New Year's Eve, which I spent entirely on my own. I then spent New Year's Day on my own, where I slept throughout the majority of the day. On New Year's Eve, I thought to myself, how much on my own in this world I was, and why was I on my own. I thought of how painfully awkward people are in terms of them being open enough, to make new friends, therefore my life was at best going to be living in a clique world, where I would just be working; and sharing contact details with people, that tell you they will contact you, but then never do. I also thought that I was on my own because I could not accept my parents invite to the party they were having, and thought about the reasons for not being there. It came to me that I was without a single relationship and would never be able to have relationships with my family members as they still sat back and nearly watched a son and a brother take his life, living in a world where 1 in 7 people with his condition will make an attempt on their life. I felt that I was destined to a life of just me on my own and that I better look after my health and make a success of my peer support mental health service, as there will be no one to fend for me in the future. What I noticed was that this wasn't making me feel depressed, nor angry, and instead just had me feel impartial, making me realise that my meditation was working tremendously and stopping me from going down a "mental downward spiral". My meditation was also stopping me from "circulating" the mouth of a downward spiral.

After realising this huge improvement in me, I decided to just go to bed and turned the light off, where I then had a seizure. To hell with the seizure; living with 24/7 anger that is a few increments below your rage threshold, as well as; depression and anxiety combined, is a far more frightening thing to even imagine having to live with. Having a seizure in a shopping centre frightens me, in terms of consequences, but so does going into a shopping centre and gunning down a huge number of people. The consequences of a seizure in a shopping centre could be six months in prison, but the consequences of a rage pushing you towards gunning down a huge number of people in a shopping centre, would have you never see the light of day again.

I slept on the couch for the majority of New Year's Day and lay there thinking that I still hadn't received a phone call from either of the parents to check on how I was keeping as they have little awareness of how well my meditation was working, and I still by the evening of New Year's Day received no Happy New Year from my mother. I had received a text message from my Dad, Bill and my older sister which was so quickly put together she couldn't even find the time to personalise the text by greeting me by my name. I received nothing from my younger sister, who never looked me in the eye and spoke to me when I went to visit her a couple of weeks before; and who, my father had said in a previous conversation, has never been able to forgive me for throwing him and giving him a near head injury back in July 2016. I saw this lack of correspondence as evidence of my younger sister still not being able to forgive me. I also thought my mother will be dancing and drinking, and not giving a toss that her son has spent all of New Year's Eve and New Year's Day alone which was not easy for me to do. I thought of the reasons behind this and felt that I could never repatriate with family. It is the case that if "1" is on route to suicide and "10" is suicide, my family had me at "13", and I remain to be at "13". What does this mean? It means that I should be dead; but because of the meditation, I neither feel the pain of being "13" and continue to remain alive with hope as well as a whole load of aims and objectives ahead of me for the year 2019. I do therefore see my family as being people who have what I would call "Invisible Blood" on their hands, as they are responsible for the "Suicide that never happened", and this is something that I could never forgive them for, especially when they show no signs of recognising their sins nor seeking forgiveness. I heard in my mind what Graham Hardie would have been saying to others if I had killed myself, and that was, "His family had just ignored him". As a result of this, when my father came to my home with my television on the 2nd January 2019, I turned him away from the door by telling him that he in theory had a television with him but in practice it was a" broom and rug" that he was just using to sweep issues under the carpet with. I told him that I now only wanted him for two things in my life. One of these was money, and the other was as a "second brain" to help me with any task I had difficulties with. I told him that my relationship with family was a bit like BREXIT. I needed a severance deal that helped me become 100% independent of anyone, allowing me to live in a world where there would be no one to ask these questions or get such help from after he had gone. My Dad started behaving in an incredibly wet way by covering his face and crying. My father then walked back to his car. I felt positive and optimistic as I now see my life being the running of a peer support mental health service, Card Tricks, Writing and possibly Comedy; as meditation has made the world so transparent to me that I see all the irrationalities and non-sensical nature of everything going on around me that helps me take things with a pinch of salt and also has had me laughing at the world instead of being angered by it, giving me lots of material to make jokes out of. What was my "inner critic" and "inner cynic" has increasingly become an inner comedian. There's a live entertainer in my mind now that can make me laugh. None of that involves family. I will now be heading back up the stairs to my flat where every step is a step closer to achieving my long term goals which will either be a destination reached in the year 2019 or a destination that the year 2019 will take me closer towards reaching. I think "upstairs for positive affirmations and visualisations" and get a real feeling of the neurotransmitter Dopamine being released.

I must say that there is a lot to be said about the saying: "IT WILL EITHER MAKE YOU OR BREAK YOU!" and I go about making sure living with Epilepsy, Depression and Anxiety MAKE ME!, using Meditation, Visualisation, Positive Affirmations and Aerobic exercise in both a therapeutic capacity as well as in the form of a vocational skill that I can make a living from by teaching mental health symptom self- management. It is a sad truth about the relationship that I have had with the human race, that it could be said that I have had a healthier relationship with epilepsy, depression and anxiety; as living with these three conditions has taught me knowledge, skills and given me personality attributes that have greatly increased opportunities for me in the self- employed world by making me independent minded with an ability to cope without peers; walking a path in isolation, where every day I have survived some form of attack and have been left to my own devices to develop coping skills, knowledge and experience as well as grow a thick skin. Unfortunately, the human race has done nothing but cause damage to me, as well as create chaos, that has held back any formal education I have been in receipt of by others, as well as personal development opportunities that other people have been responsible for the managing off. Time has consistently taught me that I excel on my own when others just keep out and I refuse to give any human being other than myself the responsibility of educating me or being in charge of my personal development. The scientist in me has drawn evidence based conclusions on others' ability to be put in charge of my education and personal development from years of observations. These observations have allowed me to conclude that the people in my life who have been allowed such responsibility have only being capable of causing destruction and have not had the skills nor attitude to grow me as a person with knowledge and skills. People have consistently proven themselves to be ignorant, prejudicial, naïve, lacking in intuition and insight, intolerant, sadistic, plagued by insecurity, non-independent minded, lacking in leadership etc thus having me conclude that they are not fit enough to be allowed to be given roles and responsibilities that involve shaping my future and determining my long-term wellbeing. As I have watched myself grow and develop when I have been the only person in charge of my education and personal development, I have been able to make decisions regarding my future relationship with the human race that enhance quality of life and maximise opportunities for the full fruition of my potential. One of these decisions has been to effectively "sack" the human race, and give it its "P45" for incompetence and unprofessional practice in the fields of future education and personal development. Life is truly what you make of it, and decisions such as mine; to fire the human race, evidence such a claim. Many people reading will relate with this relationship with the human race, and I would hope that this would have an empowering effect on them to take on more responsibility for their own personal development. Most celebrities would tell you that they struggled in a society that offered them no opportunities other than hardship and it was only once they became aware of a talent that they either were born with or developed through self-investment that opportunities arose for them to rise to fame. I go to make sure such people who are "self-made" inspire me as opposed to people who blend with the rest dishearten and destroy me.

I do recognise that you do need to network and form relationships with others to even make your own self-made attempts work in your favour, therefore, in this world; people like me have to pick their companions very, very, very,………… carefully. It does make you think "Are people like me Saints born in hell?". I have become very religiously open minded.

FINALLY SOME CLOSURE AND EVIDENCE OF MOVING ON

It is now the 17th January 2019, and I have had a phone call from my father, who put in his own complaint in relation to the treatment that I received from Sam Whitmore and Peter Dale at the Epilepsy Connections charity back in June 2018. My father's complaint was that the injustice that Sam Whitmore subjected me to had caused me to react in a way that created a lot of stress for my mother and father. When my Dad instructed me by text to phone him, so he could update me on a development that he wished to make me aware of, I did exactly that, and learned from my father that Sam Whitmore had been sacked from Epilepsy Connections; and the director, who had said nothing during the meeting on the 30th November, had resigned.

This is the closest experience of justice I have ever had in my life in relation to disability discrimination. I do however ask if the right head rolled at Epilepsy Connections for the way I was treated. I wonder if the injustice had been passed onto someone else's shoulders. I do find it very inconsistent that someone who was your friend for fourteen years fires you by becoming a part of a setup. I have also wondered if Peter's awkward blushing face with a look of despair every time he saw me with a refusal to show a desire to form any kind of bond between us might have been a symptom of being in the knowledge of some dirty pre-determined decision to do something unlawful that he would be playing a proactive role in under someone else's instruction. There is a lot of chauvinism towards men in the voluntary sector and if you look at the many charities staff lists there is an under-representation of male staff. There is therefore nothing a female chauvinist hates more than a man who she feels knows more than her and who she sees as probably being more qualified to do her job. Remember, Sam Whitmore did say in 2004 that I should have had his job. Sam probably shared this with Shirley. There was always an aversion like response shown in body language and tone of voice by Shirley when she said hello to me every time I showed my face at Epilepsy Connections. There was certainly a noticeable difference between Shirley's response and the other member of staffs' responses. I know that it would be consistent of the voluntary sector culture for the female head of an epilepsy charity to not like a man giving talks to social workers, nurses, teachers and other people who come into contact with people with epilepsy on 'Living and growing up with Epilepsy'. This is especially the case if the male is also an epilepsy rescue medication trainer for a rival epilepsy charity, as well as a symptom self-management course trainer that was run by another charity. It has already been mentioned in a previous chapter that the head of the unit that I worked in at the Epilepsy Society, which is also a part of the voluntary sector, refused to drug train the men; and then played the dirty stunt with me over my medication training, thus, denying me my role as an epilepsy rescue medication trainer; and then tried to get rid of me by making accusations about me being cognitively impaired, which I knew was the beginning of her bringing my epilepsy into the equation, when she decided to get occupational health involved, with the aim of making me look too unfit to practice as a support worker.

CHAPTER 36

In October 2018, I had decided that I wanted the mental health conditions that have plagued my life, as a result of how people have treated me in both education and employment settings, to be officially diagnosed for the purpose of claiming universal credit; as I had no income, wished to never work for anyone again, and decided that I wished my full-time job to be growing and developing my peer support service. I knew that for the claim that I was making to appear genuine, which was that I could not work because of anxiety and depression; I would have to have demonstrated to the Department of Work & Pensions that I had tried to seek treatment.

I was invited to the Jeanie Deans in Helensburgh, for a psychiatric referral on the 8th January 2019, and at this appointment, combined with a follow up appointment on the 5th February 2019, I gave the psychiatrist a three hour history of my upbringing, my experiences of education and employment, as well as my experience on the sports field as a child that had scarring effects. I told him that this had resulted in social isolation, as well as the developing of anger and rage issues when dealing with criticism and working with awkward people. I told him that having had an overly critical upbringing had also resulted in the development of anxiety in performance settings, causing avoidance; which is a classic symptom of the anxiety disorder called 'Performance Anxiety', which is a subtype of 'Social Anxiety Disorder'.

After providing my psychiatrist of a complete history of my background and my experiences with people in positions of authority, as well as the odd bad experience with peers; I was told at the end of the appointment, on the 5th February 2019, that I was the way that I was and experienced the issues that I had because I had a 'Personality Disorder'. I asked the psychiatrist what the cause of personality disorder was, and he said, "Genetics combined with environment". This diagnosis of personality disorder is a way in saying that it is me that is the problem and not the way people have treated me. I was told that my reactions to my traumatic experiences and the depth of my scars were disproportionate, and that the average person would not have been as affected by the same experiences I have had; and therefore, my levels of anger, rage, anxiety, depression etc were all down to a dysfunction in me. I woke up that night thinking a guy like me is not allowed to have depression, nor am I allowed to have anxiety, anger or rage. I thought no matter how proportionate my anger and rage is, it will always be labelled "disproportionate" and a symptom of me having personality disorder. When I say, "A guy like me", I mean "A guy with complex partial epilepsy" or any other hidden disability that will create for someone vocational and educational difficulties causing them to face social exclusion. I felt that this diagnosis of personality disorder was a way in sweeping the real issues under the carpet and possibly originally invented in the 1950's, protecting those responsible for the scars from having any legal action taken against them. It is very convenient for the scarred to be labelled "disordered", especially when many of the people who are responsible for other peoples' scars are public sector workers; like the psychiatrist, and I felt it was a bit convenient that I was diagnosed as having "paranoid personality disorder", meaning any claim made by me against them plotting against or picking on me, would be attributed to my "organic paranoia". There's this taken for granted assumption amongst our general populace that paranoia is a fear stemming from an irrational interpretation of ones' mind, but I ask this; would "paranoid" be the wrong word to describe someone dangling above a tank full of piranha?

It certainly supports my theory mentioned earlier on in this book that personality disorder is just a way in discrediting someone's claims, views, beliefs, suggestions, advice etc; protecting those in power from rebellions that are led by those more outspoken and principled than the rest. In fact, while doing an internet search for stories regarding organisations that are "anti-psychiatry" in the western world; to defuse a feeling of rage towards psychiatry, I discovered a page titled *"30 years after Prozac arrived, we still buy the lie that chemical imbalances cause depression"*, that was written back in December 2017, by a lady called Olivia Goldhill, who is a philosopher that mentioned that President Nixon who was president of the USA between 1969-1974 had told psychiatry that putting peoples' depressive symptoms down to personality disorder was more politically palatable than putting the depression of others down to the real issues that were poor housing, lack of meaningful employment, isolation/loss of community, poor nutrition and many other politically sensitive issues. According to the same reference this instruction from President Nixon suited psychiatry perfectly at a time when psychiatry was trying to justify itself as a medical discipline to the other medical disciplines. The theory of personality disorder created the illusion that there was science behind psychiatry, when in truth, psychiatry was a way in political coverup. Psychiatrists would say organic dysfunctions in the blood brain barrier causes depression and stress related anxiety, when in fact it is the politics of society wearing down the blood brain barrier that causes these two conditions. It is like what the famous Scottish psychiatrist Ronald David Laing said about those experiencing depression, anxiety disorders and personality disorder; which was, "There's nothing insane, about being sane, in an insane world", meaning that mental health conditions are just sane peoples' emotions, brought on by evidence based outlooks on the world. RD Laing's quote is consistent with what I say which is, "I'm an upright guy in an upside-down world". It is also consistent with my arguments about so much psychiatric theory being flawed as a result of psychiatry doing no studies on normality, which if they did, they would realise how insane normality is and how sane their patient is!!

Psychiatric theory gets its credibility from engrained beliefs from childhood. This engrained belief is: "I'm beneath everyone else, therefore I'm going to be less like me and more like everyone else". As a result of this everyone grows up believing the majority way is the correct way and the minority way is broken, defunct, impaired, mutated etc. As a result of this, it is just taken for granted that if your behaviour, reactions, thoughts, views and beliefs are inconsistent with the majority, then you are defunct, broken, impaired, mutated etc. It is this taken for granted belief that you are defunct, broken or impaired, if you do things the minority way, that legitimises in the eyes of psychiatry the name-calling of people who do things the minority way. The name psychiatry chooses to call those who do things the minority way is 'Personality Disordered'. The irony is this label comes from not being affected by the deep rooted insecurity to break ranks with the majority, that most people are affected by, when they disagree with the majority. How many people, per hundred, if put in a room of fifteen would dare put their hand up to say they are 'against' when the other fourteen have said they are 'for'? This fear of others to put their hand up when they are 'for' and everyone else is 'against', is the reason for those who do have the courage to put their hand up, when they are for and everyone is against, being labelled Personality Disordered. Personality Disorder is basically a term used to describe people who have a confidence others don't have, and therefore are seen as the trouble makers; however, imagine we lived in a world where most people did not have a fear to put their hand up when others are keeping their hand down. There would be far more many people who would vote 'against' when everyone else appears to be 'for', and therefore, the trouble makers would be in greater numbers; meaning the exploiters in our society would be up against a greater force and as a result of this, the street civilian would enjoy far more many rights as well as distribution of wealth. People with paranoid personality disorder are people who recognise, and are prepared to shine light on, people who do not have the best intentions as well as put on fronts that fool other people into trusting them, resulting in abuse and exploitation, which are the two tools that the world's economy uses that are responsible for inequality of wealth and lack of human rights. Those that point it out and then confront it are labelled 'personality disordered', as they are behaving in a minority way i.e. retaliation and are referred to as 'paranoid' to discredit the claims they make about people in charge exploiting and abusing workers and civilians. We need more people with paranoid personality disorder. Psychiatry is politics and not medicine.

Originally personality disorder was a medical condition of mind, that was probably created for the purpose of avoiding politically sensitive subjects that politicians did not wish to discuss nor be held accountable for; but I believe the survival of this theory has continued amongst modern psychiatry as a result of the need for approval that the vast majority of our population are forever seeking. The average person will go as far as walk into a shop, buy a pair of denims with a gaping hole in them large enough to put your fist through; and pay the same price as a week's worth of food, in order for them to get the approval of others and fit in with their friends. This need for approval has people behave in an insane way that lacks logic or any kind of rationale, other than the need to be like everyone else, to guarantee getting approval by everyone else. These people who wear such clothing for these reasons, and commit a huge list of other seriously daft behaviours for the purpose of getting others' approval, such as covering their bodies in an inch thick of fake tan that makes them look more like a frankfurter than someone from the Mediterranean, or become a psychiatrist so that they can say they are a doctor at a party; have been allowed to hold positions where they are forming judgements and coming to conclusions about others, simply by observing their behaviours. I am confident in saying that anyone who is in such need of approval will have a very impaired ability to make accurate judgements of others, as a result of being so intoxicated by human insecurity; and it is this human insecurity that has convinced people into believing that the human body has a heart for circulation, lungs for breathing, liver for detoxification, brain for regulation of all body functions, kidneys for correct blood water/ion concentration and the **"Personality for approval by others"**. I put "personality for approval by others" in bold as this belief in what personality is for is wrong. Personality is not an organ, nor does personality have a function. It is believed in psychiatry, yet psychiatry would never admit to this; and amongst mainstream society, that the personality exists to win the approval of others, and if your personality does not win the approval of others then your personality is somehow defunct, and you therefore have what is called a 'Personality Disorder'. It is this false logic that stunts individuality, fuels conformity, destroys potential, causes history to repeat itself and allows for a status quo to remain that is about the exploited continuing to be exploited by the exploiters; and anyone who dares goes against the grain ends up in prison or face down with bullet holes all over them, either put in them by criminal or politician. This description of what the false logic behind personality results in, sounds very cynical; and if I am correct, 'cynicism' is labelled as being a symptom of depression by many psychiatrists. It can therefore be said that anyone who goes against the unhealthy grain, or starts to draw attention to the unhealthy grain, gets labelled "mentally ill" simply as a way of discrediting them as well as stigmatising "going against the grain behaviour" so that others don't follow suit.

In my opinion, modern day psychiatry has got it all wrong about personality. Modern day psychiatry sees the personality as the "6th organ" of the human being that serves to win the approval of others, which is where the labelling of people as "Misfits" comes from, but personality is in fact a "destination" and not an organ that serves no purpose. Life is a journey, and each journey takes you to a destination, and the destination of life is not death, the destination of life is the "Here and Now". No two journeys on this planet are identical, and therefore no two personalities should be identical. A person's personality is their "here and now" character that has been shaped by a journey that has been made up of events, encounters and experiences; where things have been learned, outcomes have been achieved, there have been losses but also gains, evidence based views/beliefs/principles have developed, life skills such as self-advocacy/problem solving/socialising etc have developed; and characteristics such as introversion/extroversion/openness to new experience/outspokenness/funny/angry etc have developed. Every personality has these features, which could be scored on a "1 to 10" where future events, encounters and experiences will cause these scores to go up and down. Just like geographical destinations change in population, surface area, annual festivals, climate, language mix, currency, price of housing etc; with time, so do our personalities, due to the continuing of new experiences, encounters and events affecting the scores of all the mentioned features of personality. Therefore, just like there is no such thing as a "right" or a "wrong destination"; or a place that has less of a right to call itself a destination than any other place; there is no such thing as a "wrong" or "right" personality, or a "lesser personality" than any other personality; therefore the psychodynamics of both personality and personality development expose the theory of personality disorder as being deeply flawed, where the only difference between what psychiatry would call an "unhealthy personality" and a "healthy personality" is that one personality gets more approval by others than the other personality gets. Remember though, personality is not an organ, and was never formed for the purpose of approval by others. Psychiatry in my opinion is an area of medicine where they are operating on the wrong thing. The thing psychiatry should be "operating" on is the roots that give rise to the events, experiences and encounters that lead to the development of a personality with feature scores that create incompatibilities with society; but that would involve political campaigning more than it would seeing patients in outpatient clinics. Now I'm starting to sound like President Nixon's opposition!

As a result of this psychiatry appointment, the only help that can be offered; I am told, is strong anti-depressant and tranquiliser medication that will reduce my seizure threshold, possibly bringing back daytime seizures. What an answer; which raises far more many questions than it provides answers to. I just thought to myself "Thank God I meditate. Thank God I am only here to make my universal credit claim look genuine, and I never came here wishing for their help. These people are useless!". I felt like visiting the Buddhist temple on my way home thanking the Buddhist Priests for their discovery, and how it has saved me from the toxicity of psychiatry.

This psychiatry appointment confirmed in me the need for alternative therapy services for those with both depressive and anxiety disorders as well as my future role and purpose, which is that of a 'Peer Support Mentor' who can teach others the self- management techniques used to treat depressive and anxiety disorders, protecting those not just from the potentially life wrecking effects of these disorders but also protecting them from being exploited by the pharmaceutical industry and the bad decisions made by psychiatrists borne from an ignorance of the real issues that cause these disorders i.e. societal and/or neurological. I therefore, hope that this book is read by mental health professionals, those affected by mental health conditions, educators, employers, social care workers, neurologists, parents and other relatives etc so that these conditions become more transparent; and that those reading will have a greater understanding of the issues, conditions and alternative treatments that can only improve the lives of those affected by such conditions, as well as make the services that those affected by these conditions are in receipt of more holistic. I would also hope that this book would be an eye opener to politicians who do not give disability high enough priority. I can follow an entire election campaign on the news, television debates, BBC Question Time, newspapers etc and not hear a single politician make any reference towards what their party has to offer those facing social exclusion because of their disability. This is especially the case with hidden disability. It is believed that if the disability cannot be seen then it does not exist. A person with epilepsy who sits on a disabled seat on a train where there is lots of floor space around the seat gets rude stares when the person with a zimmer comes on the train; however, what people don't realise or even consider is that this person has epilepsy and is at risk of a daytime tonic-clonic seizure at any time, and therefore, needs a seat where there is the space for him to fall to the floor, where there is enough floor space for violent contractions of arms and legs, and then enough floor space for being put in the recovery position. It is also important for the person with epilepsy to be sitting in this seat, as falling to the ground from a seat is far less likely of causing injury than falling to the ground from standing. This is an excellent example of how the public believe if the disability is not obvious to the naked eye, then the disability does not exist; and it is this naivety that causes our politicians to never be heard speaking about or being questioned on hidden disability, in any context by the media.

CHAPTER 37

As I finish this book, I am just about to text my friend Alistair, who has moderate learning disability; as well as had frontal lobe epilepsy, which he grew out of when he was a child. I am due to visit him as he has been admitted to a mental health ward in the north of Glasgow after trying to take his life just 72hrs ago. The frightening thing is, it was only four days ago I was sitting with him in Helensburgh, after the crisis team sent him to me; as he had just been discharged from hospital, after taking an overdose.

When I visited Alistair in his mental health ward, he had knife wounds to his abdomen. Alistair had tried to stab himself and was now being kept in the mental health ward for an indefinite period of time. Alistair kept complaining about being thirsty and how no one was giving him anything to drink. Alistair claimed to be suffering from dehydration, and when he reported this to the nurse all the nurse could do was say, "No you're not, Look"; and then pinched and pulled his skin on his forearm and said, "See how your skin just springs back to its original shape instantly. That means you are not dehydrated". I thought to myself "Yes, it means you have not yet reached a certain severity of dehydration, but dehydration begins long before the elasticity of your skin starts to show symptoms". In fact, dehydration begins before you even start to feel thirsty, which is why the majority of the public fit the biological definition of dehydrated even though they would not report feeling thirsty. We spend most our lives in a dehydrated state. Thirst is in fact a very poor indicator of hydration levels. The sensation of thirst comes from a part of our brain that has not evolved well, which is why you should aim for 2.5 litres of water a day, whether you feel thirsty or not. I therefore asked the ward staff if Alistair was getting his 2.5 Litres of fluids per day and the answer was of course a "Yes". With the severity of Alistair's learning disability, I would be surprised if Alistair knew what 2.5 Litres looked like. I said good-bye to Alistair after telling him that I would see him soon. I have, since visiting him, tried phoning the ward to ask how he is doing, but the Data Protection Act stops the ward staff from sharing information with me. There is a need for Data Protection but like all things, this need for Data Protection is never practiced in moderation and is always done to extreme, thus, causing lots of red tape that disallows anyone advocating for a vulnerable person to make enquiries without signed mandates. This creates a boundary to information that too often favours the exploiter, especially if the exploiter does not make the vulnerable adult aware of the need for a signed mandate. You could probably write a book on the failings of this act alone.

Three months has now passed since I saw Alistair, and I have been informed by one of Alistair's contacts that he is still in hospital with no plans for discharge, where he is "up to the eyeballs" on medication, does not recognise anyone he knows as well as becomes very distressed when anyone visits; and the medical staff see Alistair being there for the long term. I know that a number of people from different disciplines will be involved in making decisions about Alistair's future, as well as the long- term plan for Alistair in terms of living and care arrangements; and these disciplines will be psychiatry, mental health nursing, social work, support work, housing and General Practice medicine. I also know from my previous experience of advocacy work and other health and social care roles I have had, that there is the potential for decisions made; not to be made in the interests of Alistair and more in the interests of community resources and savings, especially with Alistair being someone who does not have anyone fending for him, as he has no friends capable of fending for him and his relationship with family could not be described as close, who have accused him of being child- like. An example of Alistair being accused of being child -like is his brother in law accusing him of being a child because he chooses Ribena over lager at family get togethers. Alistair informed me of this and found what had been said to be very upsetting.

Alistair will also have told everyone involved in his care that I was his advocate as he did have a tendency to describe me to others as his advocate even though I stopped advocating for him as long as two years ago, therefore, there is a chance that all people involved in Alistair's care will think I am his present day advocate, which might explain why there has been a reluctance to share any information with me as to his whereabouts and their plans for him. I, therefore, do worry as a result of my personal as well as professional experience that Alistair being kept in hospital for an indefinite period, where he finds himself on high doses of medication, might not be a psychiatric decision and possibly a joint social work/housing association decision. I do worry that the housing association would rather give Alistair's two bedroom home to a family of three, than have a person with learning disability living in it on their own; and that one way in achieving this would be to put a case together that would legitimise keeping Alistair in residential care for the rest of his days. With demand for housing outstripping supply, this is a stunt I would not put beyond social work and housing. I have had clients with depression on 'Employment Support Allowance' when I was an advocate, come to me with threats of eviction from their housing association, after housing officers had made surprise visits accusing them of not keeping their flats clean, as a result of finding lots of clutter in their home. I visited these homes, and yes, there was clutter; but it wasn't clutter that made the place unhygienic, it was just newspapers and magazines from last week lying on sofas and on the floor. These were homes, that I believe, the housing association would rather a family of three lived in, who were economically active, than a person on benefits who is economically inactive. These stories about Alistair and my clients with depression being threatened by their housing associations are examples that are consistent with the life experiences I have had living with epilepsy, that demonstrate and evidence the dangers of living with a hidden disability/condition in British society. I am afraid to say it but Britain, regardless of whether it is a Tory, Labour or Lib- dem Westminster Government; Labour, SNP, Lib-Dem Scottish parliament or Plaid Cymru Welsh Assembly etc; is an incredibly right wing country to live in for a person with a hidden disability that has a lot of stigma attached to it, combined with a lack of public understanding. The only left- wing discussion that goes on in this country, is discussion in the context of inequality of wealth and gender rights. Many of the arguments over better gender rights can sound frighteningly right wing. There is no discussion over inequality in human rights between disabled people and non-disabled people, and as a result of this, there is a treatment of those of us with hidden disability that is worthy of imprisonment; yet as this is not recognised, too often it is the person with a hidden disability that ends up being imprisoned. When you look at the damage, as well as collateral damage that discrimination causes to peoples' lives; I believe that discrimination should be recognised as a crime, and that criminal law should cover discrimination cases where the perpetrator of the discrimination, as well as accomplices, could face a prison sentence. If their actions have the potential, in some cases, to be the tipping force that causes someone to go home and take their life, then that is criminal law in my opinion, and not civil law. These people quite literally cause mental torture for those living without closure, especially those living without closure on a number of previous incidents. These discriminators also cause physical torture if the mental torture is exacerbating symptoms such as seizures, when the person has a disability such as epilepsy, where the disability's symptoms are exacerbated by mental stress, which then creates a second source of mental torture along with the continued first source i.e. lack of closure. This also causes mental torture for those closely related to the discriminated against person, causing physical symptoms in them such as compromised immunity, heart health problems, malnutrition, addiction, sleep deprivation, affected judgement; resulting in increased risk of accidents etc. You effectively become a victim of the same trauma as prisoners of war do i.e. mental and physical torture. If torturers in prisoner of war camps have been convicted for war crimes due to the physical and mental torment they caused in others, then discriminators should be convicted for crimes related to inequality that has involved human right violations. 'Human rights' is where these two areas i.e. war and inequality, cross paths.

How Scotland can describe its political orientation as "centre-left"? What a joke!! If this country is centre-left then what the hell is the right? Let's just say, I would rather not find out.

CHAPTER 38

In a previous chapter It was mentioned that my family was a family where members only met up for novelty events like Christmas, New Year, landmark birthdays e.g. 50th , Weddings & Funerals; and I said that if you were to tell me on any given day that over the next few weeks I will find myself under the same roof as all my family members when it will not be a 50th, someone's wedding, Christmas day or New Year; then my reaction would be to say, "Who died?". Well, my claims about family have been evidenced to be true, as since writing that chapter up to the present moment I have not seen any of my family members, other than my father, and only very recently my mother when she is dragged along by him. It is also the case that I have just been informed that my Uncle Ralph has died and his funeral is in a couple of weeks' time. I have decided that I will not attend, and I am telling my cousins that I will not be able to attend, as to attend would involve crossing paths with my sisters and brother in laws, alongside my mother; whose presence, when my father brings her along to meetings, I find to be an endurance test which one could not afford to go wrong at a funeral.

 I will write to my cousins, explaining the difficulties that I will have attending; making them aware that I was abandoned and neglected, and that this caused me to have a very strained relationship with my father, and therefore, even though I had his support in theory, I did not have his support in practice due to it being a relationship that was very strained by the absence of the others. I will say that without my meditation sessions I would be dead, and the last time everyone in the family would have been together would have been my funeral, which would probably have been as far back as 2013.

I also don't want to go to the funeral as there will be a lot of people at the funeral, as my uncle was a very highly thought of man being a former teacher and Dean of Education at Leeds University who had many social connections; and the number of people at his funeral would only act as a reminder of what a socially excluded guy I am and how I have no social connections, which would anger me as its been such an injustice. I need to instead move on and come to terms with the fact that I was born with no supportive family, don't attract friends, live in a society which for a man with a disability is like being of a different ethnicity in a racist culture; and get on with my projects, as I have now decided to add Chemistry & Biology tuition as another service that I will provide, as well as, running my peer support service; and give myself the life I truly deserve, where I cannot be touched by the insecurities; ignorance; intolerantly rigid attitudes; the dangers of others conformity to unethical and immoral behaviours as well as the low intellect of some, and/or lack of intuition of others. I'm a "SURVIVOR" and a good person, and have increasingly believed myself to be a saint in hell where I have clung onto two rocks with one arm on each rock, that have been both my meditation and exercise; preventing me from being swept away and drowned in very deep, turbulent, freezing cold water. They used to say that "people with epilepsy are possessed by the devil", I would say that people with epilepsy are picked on by the devil; but like is the case with personality disorder, the attack comes from the outside, and not the inside. In other words, society is the devil. It's what that colleague, who I phoned up to apologise for being late at work during the amnesia phase of a seizure, that you read about in chapter 2, said to me when I first started at Thelmer Turner Homes in Nottingham back in 2003, and that was: "When you die you're not going to hell". Martin then pointed up at the sky and said, "That is Heaven" and then pointing at everything around him, he continued by saying, "This place is Hell!".

After doing a few years of meditation practice I have become much more spiritual, and had many spiritual awakenings where you experience; for a few days in a row, the world becoming more transparent to you. This has made me become very spiritual, and has made me increasingly believe that the world we live in is hell, as it preaches morality, but practices: jealousy, dishonesty, judgementalism, greed, possessiveness, adultery, hatred etc. I do increasingly think of myself as a "Saint" living amongst demons, and that there are other saints like me, who are suffering due to an incompatibility between themselves and the demons. I don't think you can get this far through the book and say that my views are not evidenced, and say that they are the conclusions of an evaluation carried out by a bitter and angry guy who just looks for anything to criticise society for. That is what psychiatry would describe me as being. It's that old 'saying' said by a French philosopher called 'Jean-Paul Sartre', and that is:

"HELL IS NOT A PLACE, HELL IS OTHER PEOPLE!"

After deciding to not go to the funeral, I chose to write my letter to my Aunt Jean and two cousins, Rachael and Tom; explaining to them the nature of the relationships between me and my family, the events that had led to the breakdown in family relations as well as the abuse and neglect that I have been on the receiving end of for many years; and that to go to the funeral would require me to cross paths with family members that I would find traumatic and could lead to conflict on a day that should be without conflict. I told my father I would be writing this letter the day before he and my mother went off for a two week holiday in Georgia. My Dad gave me my Aunt Jean's address, and left, having told me that there was no news on the date of the funeral. Over the next two weeks I only had two conversations with someone else due to the social isolation. I had only had a conversation with a guy in a bar and a police officer, who had come into my home to ask me if I had witnessed anything on a day that the person across the landing from me had had his flat broken into and had everything robbed. My neighbour had no home insurance and only had a yale lock, making it easy for the door to be picked by the thieves. Other than these two conversations, there was no other face to face dialogue with anyone, over a two week period. This did cause me to waken up in the middle of the night feeling agitated, however, my meditation practice kept me sane; and after two visits to the gym, on top of my meditation practice, I had completely ridded myself of all night time agitation brought on by social isolation.

As I am, at least in theory, seeing a psychiatrist, I thought to ask him for a supporting letter to go with my own letter, explaining that I would find the funeral too traumatic and if my absence could be excused. I was provided with this supporting letter, the day before my father returned from Georgia, where I was phoned by him the next day, to be told that tomorrow he would be going down to Leeds, which I thought he was doing to give his sister emotional support, as there was no mention of a funeral, and he had; prior to going on holiday, visited his sister in Leeds, purely just for the purpose of providing her with psycho-emotional support. It therefore, came as a real surprise to me, when I met my Dad a few days later in a coffee shop, to be told during conversation about Aunt Jean and how she was coping, that the welsh national anthem was sung at the funeral. I said, "Hold on. When's the funeral?" and he replied, "Yesterday". I told him that he had not told me when the funeral was, and if I had known, I would have got my letter off in the post much sooner. My Dad replied in a patronizing tone, "Come on Tim, it is three weeks since your uncle died" but I replied, "I would still expect a father to tell his son when his uncle's funeral is". I never pressed my Dad for the date of the funeral, as I did not know how long it would take for funeral arrangements to be made in the case of someone like my uncle whose death would be followed by a post-mortem due to the original findings being "death from unknown cause". My uncle, I was originally told, died as a result of being sent home from hospital, after being admitted to hospital with what I believe I was told was a gastro-intestinal problem. My uncle was examined at the hospital, and sent back home where he was found lifeless, lying in his bed beside my aunt in the morning. I was told that because of the nature of his death there would be a post mortem. I had thought the post mortem might have been the reason as to why three weeks had passed without anyone giving me a date. I said to my father in response to him telling me it was three weeks ago since my uncle's death that he had denied me the opportunity to send my letter to my aunt and cousins by not telling me that his visit to Leeds the day after his return from holiday was to attend the funeral". I said, "You have denied me the opportunity to explain myself purely to save your own image and the image of the rest of your family, thus, compromising my image instead". I stood up and said, "You're cheap scum!" and just walked away. At the time of writing he's been trying to contact me but I have blacklisted him on my phone and disconnected my landline. Nine days have now passed since my learning of this betrayal and still do not feel tempted to meet with him or speak with him despite my last conversation being that conversation in that coffee shop nine days ago.

I am disappointed that my cousin never phoned me to ask me how I was keeping, as according to my father he had been telling my cousin what life had been like for me. I am also surprised my Aunt didn't contact me, as I would have expected her to have shown concern and thought to herself "Not showing like this is out of character of Tim. I better phone him or visit him when I'm up in Helensburgh to find out from him why he didn't attend his uncle's funeral, and if there's anything he wishes to share and talk about". Instead there has been no response which just further confirms that we are a family that show no concern for one another and meet up more for the sake of fulfilling a societal obligation. It's "Now that that family obligation has been ticked it is now back to life as usual". Well I'm a genuine person and I don't say, "I am" when "I am not"; therefore, I won't say, "I'm family" when we are not. Family is just a lie that many of us are taught from a young age to result in disappointed heartbroken people in later life. Why do you think if a person is murdered, that persons' relatives are first on the suspect list. The next most likely people, after relatives, to kill you are friends. That would be consistent with how Sam Whitmore treated me. I could have killed him.

I see the lack of response to my absence as well as not telling me when the funeral was, as evidence of there being a real attitude problem towards me in the family which is not good for my confidence, therefore, since my life is the kind of life where it is crucial to be feeling confident about yourself, since there is no one to advocate or fend for you; I wish no involvement with my family since they show an attitude towards me that is demeaning and demoralising. I do believe that my Dad being a former neurologist, and my mother; a former learning disability teacher, has made them very judgemental towards me.

I have also learned to identify with being this really depressed guy when I am in the company of my parents which means I just dip into a depressive dive when I see them which means they have a toxic effect on me especially if I am having a good day before they arrive. They just re-open healing wounds.

 My family were always judgemental towards a great aunt of mine, who we called Katie Anne. Katie Anne suffered from depression which made her very vulnerable due to low confidence, and all my family could ever do was be rude about her, including my psychiatrist uncle. They just cracked jokes about her behind her back, and used to crack jokes about her being dirty, as she didn't wash. Having experienced depression, I now know why Katie-Anne didn't wash, as this is one of depression's major symptoms; and just like my psychiatrist uncle couldn't recognise my social withdrawal, which is a major symptom, he couldn't recognise Katie Anne's lack of personal hygiene; or maybe he was just very judgemental of people with mental health problems. Katie Anne, could also become grumpy at the family get togethers, but that was because unlike myself, who could socially withdraw to my bedroom, Katie Anne couldn't socially withdraw; meaning she had to endure a whole day of companionship, coping with a condition that makes being a member of large groups difficult. Again, my psychiatrist uncle could not combine her grumpiness, with lack of personal hygiene, to identify my great aunt as being depressed. Those affected by depression become drained; especially if they sit amongst people who they share a relationship with, where a lot of baggage can be found. My family were very judgemental towards Katie Anne, as my older sister used to say to me, "Katie Anne used to make Great Uncle Willie's life hell". My older sister continued, "Katie Anne's behaviour was always challenging, and she had to be hospitalised on a number of occasions. Poor Uncle Willie!" This would explain why my sisters can't forgive me, for the effects the strained relationship between me and my father has had on my father. It will be something like this, that the nephews I barely know, will be saying about me in the future: "Uncle Tim made Grandad's life a living hell!" followed by, "You know, he attempted to kill your grandfather by throwing him over his shoulder, cracking his head causing Grandad to require emergency hospital treatment!".

CHAPTER 39 ACHIEVEMENT VERSUS SUCCESS

https://smallbusiness.chron.com/set-up-website-sell-things-48826.html

I'm going to finish off by saying that after having written this book I am proud of what I have managed to live and cope with. When I look at the difficulties that epilepsy, depression and anxiety have created for me living in a very intolerant society, all I can say is that living with each of these conditions is a real test of character, and anyone who has lived with these disabilities; and is still fully functioning i.e. they have aims and goals, ambitions etc, is to be praised and recognised as being a coper with a high emotional pain threshold. I don't see epilepsy, depression or anxiety as being disabilities. I in fact see them as mountains, which those who cope with can boast to have got to the top of; and therefore, have turned the epilepsy, depression and anxiety from being a disability into a medal that can be worn around one's neck.

I have developed an outlook on life that I would never have developed without having the view of the world as well as life that I have had as a result of living with these conditions. In other words, living with these conditions has made me a smarter, as well as much more experienced person.

One thing that living with these conditions has taught me, combined with the meditation practice making the world and life more transparent, is that there is a difference between ACHIEVEMENT and SUCCESS. 'Success' is an outcome, whereas 'achievement' is the surviving of a journey, and there is no relationship between size of achievement, and size of success. The Lottery is a good example of this, where the person who wins it will have an expensive house, expensive car, expensive clothes, etc, thus, making him very successful; however, the size of the achievement behind the huge success has been no greater than going into a shop and buying a lottery ticket, therefore, winning the lottery would be a good example of experiencing huge success without any achievement.

There are then examples of where success is not great, but the achievement behind the success has been huge. An example of this would be where the experiencing of modest success requires one to face a phobia that has plagued their life for years, where they manage to face as well as overcome their phobia, so that they can experience modest success. In such an example, despite the success being small; the achievement is huge as it has involved overcoming a lifelong phobia stemming from a very deep mental scar. Another example would be having a good attendance at your lectures at university, which one would not describe as being a huge success; but for the person who can't get to lectures because they have a fear of seizures in a lecture theatre, or they have depression and are too drained; or have social anxiety disorder and are terrified of public places; becoming a regular attendee at lectures would be a huge achievement, therefore, living with epilepsy, depression and anxiety has taught me that there is no relationship between achievement and success. A person can have experienced a huge amount of achievement in their life and not experienced any success. Success is a "destination", achievement is a "journey". Just like not all very demanding journeys take you to prestigious destinations, not all prestigious destinations have involved the travel of demanding journeys. There are of course cases where very demanding journeys do lead to prestigious destinations. It is the journey that requires the skill, the knowledge and is the test of character; and it is because of the journey that I have made to date and currently undertaking; which is high in altitude and made up of very steep gradients; that I consider my life to have been full of achievement that I can be very proud of. I am still alive, I have survived depression, anxiety and epilepsy; I have overcome phobia, I have developed a high level of fitness, I have become a consistent meditator, I have become assertive and outspoken, I have developed advocacy skills and can solve other peoples' life problems, I am a genuine guy with his own principles and values that have given him a huge confidence; I have had numerous character building experiences, I am an "action guy" and not just a "talk guy", I have become a positive thinker; and more, which the becoming of, as well as achieving of, have all been chapters of a very large journey that I am currently trekking.

Another example of achievement, is a guy with learning disability, who has no numeracy nor literacy skills, has required care in the community and can now can hold down a simple job. This person has experienced a greater achievement than the A-stream privately educated individual, who got 7 A's in their highers, whose teachers were forever saying good things about them, went to university to study law and became a lawyer living off a big salary, living in a big house; in a very upmarket suburb. The lawyer has experienced an incomparably greater amount of success, but the learning disabled guy has experienced greater achievement.

What have we got to learn from this? Achievement is "getting to the top", and success is "at the top"; and what we can learn from this is that the size of what is at the top is not a measure of the amount of struggle, altitude, gradient and climate that a person has had to endure and master to get to the top. Getting two-thirds up one mountain in one's life- time is very often an incomparably greater achievement than someone else getting to the top of another mountain. There are too many people in their seventies who have "only" climbed halfway up their mountain who look at people aged thirty at the top of their mountain and think the thirty something year old has made more of their life, however, the thirty something was climbing a much shorter mountain with little gradient, meaning the seventy year old has lived a life with much more achievement; where achievement always co-exists with 'living', therefore anyone whose life has abundant achievement has also had abundant living which is what life is all about.

Unless someone is prepared to start climbing other mountains once they have got to the top of their first encountered mountain then they will stagnate. Success provides the option of living the rest of your life in the comfort zone. If you are not climbing then you are not growing. Your life has already come to a conclusion. This is where we get on to the subject of "no pain, no gain". People at the top in our society tend to hold positions where they climbed and got to the top at too young an age and then stagnated meaning they stopped undergoing any further maturation which is why we live in a society that's judgemental as hell, as judgementalism is just infantile thinking that stems from a simplistic understanding of the real causes/issues/reasons behind things due to lack of exposure, desire for openness to new experience and an unwillingness to learn new things. The man who is fifty and two thirds up his mountain, or the man who is in his seventies starting his third climb will take no sides until they've heard all the facts when they see a man with a growl hit a man with a smile. The man who got to the top of his mountain at a young age and stagnated will always take the side of the man with the smile. Too many psychiatrists climbed their mountain by a young age and stagnated; and when left in front of an angry man laying into a society that the psychiatrist has always seen as being a society with a smile on its face, since it was good to him, he will always believe the angry patient to be the culprit and give him some terribly stigmatising diagnosis for doing nothing other than giving a witness account of his own life. The psychiatrist thinks "Society was good to me, therefore, this criticism of society can only be imagination, which means his interpretation of events must be down to paranoia".

This has been an excellent example of how transparent the world has become to me due to my meditation practice. It's lifted all that fog that society has filled my head with since being a child making me see the things I was not seeing.

CHAPTER 40

I am now back to living in Glasgow, after living four continued years in isolation living in Helensburgh. The move to Helensburgh from Glasgow was about moving to a town, as it was believed that living in a town of 15,000 people, as opposed to living in the centre of a city metropolitan area of 1.7 million people, would be an easier place to make social connections. Unfortunately, this did not turn out to be the case, and I spent the last two years pretty much just travelling in and out of Glasgow to Costa Coffee; working on the starting of my peer support mental health service; going back twenty five years to remaster the science of chemistry and to finish the writing of this book; conquering feelings of burnout, anxiety and depression with my meditation practice and positive thinking; where I visualise and positive affirm successful outcomes for these three projects in the same way I positive affirmed for Fairway Advocacy.

I would describe myself as someone who had "gone over the edge of the cliff, but did not fall", as a result of these cognitive techniques and aerobic exercise; without the need for anti-depressant nor tranquiliser medication. As a molecular biologist as well as a cognitive practitioner; my personal, with the aim to become professional opinion, is that psychiatry in cases like mine is a massive "stitch up", and I will not be reduced to intoxicating my body for the purpose of an industry; especially when industry is the cause in so many cases of those ending up on these drugs. What these cognitive techniques offer is not just an alternative therapy that has been proven by many studies to be more effective than years of psychiatry, but also a remedy for torpedoing an industry, that exploits others' misery, out of the water. Therefore, these cognitive techniques are consistent with my political orientation as well as ethos on human wellbeing.

I have now decided to re-join a different church after leaving a previous church that I was a member of two years ago. I have decided to join this church as I believe becoming a regular member of a local congregation will, over a number of years, provide me with an alternative to family. I believe that the church can play a BIG ROLE in bringing back together communities. The coffee session after the service is invaluable and has made me realise that there should be community lounges where isolated people can just walk into, put on the kettle, make a coffee, sit down and start talking to someone. There could be a pool table there, an urn, television with DVD's, CCTV, books, a games table for chess/card playing (security on door so no gambling)/other, and very importantly; an opportunity to share issues amongst people who can empathise and advise, as they have the necessary life experience and knowledge to do so. My local community lounge would have an advocate there for example! The square pegs of society need somewhere to meet, as it creates a habitat for those of us who live in an uninhabitable world.

I have decided to play chess and join my local chess club as it is an intuitive game played by intuitive people. I must meet intuitive people since I find myself living in an unintuitive world. This planet as a whole in my opinion shows symptoms of a learning disability. It lacks insight, initiative and intuition. The difference is though the lack of these faculties does not come from a learning disability. It instead comes from an obsession with POWER, GREED and STATUS; pulling the strings of people who just CONFORM, and pushes those who don't have these obsessions nor choose to conform; as they are principled, into going over the edge of the cliff, and unfortunately in many cases fall either through stress related illness i.e. Stroke, Heart Disease, Excessive Alcohol Consumption or through a voluntary way out i.e. suicide. It will be interesting to see how many mental health charities bother to reply to my letters requesting the opportunities to provide my peer support service to their clients; or just like the neurological charities with my advocacy charity, snub my letters as a result of, guess what; GREED, POWER and STATUS!!!! I already have not heard back from two of them and have only yet sent two of them letters with this request. Is losing faith in the world and people really a symptom of depression, or is it just an evidence based conclusion made from the constant unreliability and non-genuine behaviour of others that is forever re-occurring; where psychiatrists, if it becomes too problematic for you, will say that you have difficulties settling into society as a result of being at odds with it in terms of your views, beliefs and values, which "evidences" Personality Disorder. Then they will publish a research paper saying that suicide is much more prevalent amongst those with personality disorder, and use this as evidence of those having had personality disorder. Two psychologists, from the **Diagnostic Statistical manual (DSM) 5 Personality Disorder Evidence Taskforce,** resigned from the Taskforce back in 2012; as the new classification of personality disorders was too flawed and ignored evidence.

As part of my universal credit application, which I claim purely because people don't allow me to work; I have been referred to psychiatry, and have now been officially diagnosed with 'Paranoid Personality Disorder', because I think everybody is out to get me! I would say that my "Suspicion" is pretty evidence based. They are ignoring all the evidence I shared with them. There is no one way in which we should behave. How I behave is not how you should behave. That's what's wrong with conformity. I came into this world a number of "to be determined variables", just like you did. We are all a unique "padlock code". Some of us have more digits in our code than others. The more digits, the more complex your life has been. My digits are made up of family score; susceptibility to being discriminated/bullied score; extroversion score; outspoken score; temperament score; seizure threshold score!!; people confidence score; performance confidence score; principled score; intuition/insight/initiative score; life experience and knowledge score etc; and some of these scores have already been determined before birth e.g. seizure threshold score; and others have developed during our lifetime, such as performance confidence score; and how we behave will be determined by our scores for these different variables, and therefore, if you subtract 'pressure to conform' from the world, there would be no two people alike. That's why conformity makes people mentally ill, and so does non-conformity, as society creates this ideal way in behaving and being for everyone, which if you do not behave and be like, you are called a "social-reject", in the case of those who have not been diagnosed with a mental health problem; or if you have been diagnosed with a mental health problem, you are called "MAD", which drives you mad. It's true, psychiatry labels people as a way in covering up the realities of the world that we live in, and I am being labelled with Personality Disorder in the same way socialists who stood up against far right authorities used to be thrown in cells and labelled criminals. Meditation has made me so much more mentally transparent as well as the world and people around me. It's amazing what you learn from just focussing on your breathing, and you realise that you are a bag of strengths and not a bag of weaknesses that society portrays you as being. It's right that I look over my shoulder more than the psychiatrist, as my susceptibility to being discriminated and bullied scores are much higher than his!!!

In chapter 30, it was mentioned that I have an IQ of 120, and have high ability to apply intellect to practice. It was mentioned that scoring high on these two variables causes you to see many more shades of grey than most people; meaning you develop views, beliefs and opinions that are at odds with society's; as the views, beliefs and opinions of society; are the views, beliefs and opinions of people who see fewer shades of grey than you, as well as, those who also score high on these two variables i.e. IQ & ATIP but score low on morality. My IQ score of 120, is an IQ score that falls within a zone that 1 in 7 of the population fall within. This equates to 14% of the population having an IQ of 125 or above. I also mentioned that I believe those with high IQ and high ability to apply intellect to practice make up 5% of the population. I find it interesting that according to an article in the Guardian Newspaper in 2004; the number of people who are affected by personality disorder in the UK comes to 13%. This figure is very close to the 1 in 7 who have an IQ of or above 125. The BBC in 2011 reported that studies have recorded 4% of the population as having a personality disorder. This figure of 4%, is not far off my figure of 5% that I believe to represent people who have both high IQ and ability to apply intellect to practice. What the Guardian's figures suggest, in combination with the prevalence of IQ above 125, is that there may be a relationship between high IQ and personality disorder. What the BBC's figure, in combination with my observations and theories I've constructed through my meditation practice, point towards is that there is a relationship between having high IQ, high ability to apply intellect to practice and having personality disorder. These figures and observations would suggest that personality disorder is nothing more than having a greater knowledge and understanding of the world and its people, as well as seeing more shades of grey than most; therefore, making you a more informed as well as principled person than most, therefore, personality disorder is a term designated to those whose functionality is so high that they are seen as posing a threat to the status quo of society, since society is managed in the most illogical as well as dishonest ways to benefit the few, at the expense of the many. Personality disorder, in other words, could be described as a condition that prevents people making a mug of you i.e. the very type of person an exploitative society will not like. People who see few shades of grey judge a person using wealth, status and power as variables when making their judgements about people; however, those that see many shades of grey judge a person using the following variables: assertiveness, honesty, outspokenness, experience, authenticity, confidence, discipline, susceptibility to peer pressure, susceptibility to conform, political orientation, values and beliefs, discomfort threshold, love for the comfort zone, and any other variables missed that determine one's honourability and character worthiness. In a world full of "low lives" you would expect society to wish for everyone to use wealth, status and power as a means in determining one's character worthiness. It's a way in brainwashing people into believing cheats are saints. Some of us are more brainwashable than others. Those of us that can't be and refuse to be brainwashed are labelled as having paranoid personality disorder. It's society's way in saying, "You see everyone! There he is again, thinking all of us are up to no good!!", and in my case followed by, "Typical of someone with a brain condition".

CHAPTER 41

Chess will be a great game to play, as like I said; it's intuitive and I score high on this trait, which is why I pull my hair out over the behaviour of this world. I see a guy speeding the other night to prove himself to pedestrians as a result of another guy who was speeding. One guy just puts his foot down going full speed ahead in 5th gear in a 30mph zone, and the other guy does an immediate right turn at full speed into 5th Gear over a bridge; and I think "Crashes, kills husband; wife has nervous breakdown, daughter/son taken into care by social work as mother deemed too mentally unfit to be looking after child, child grows up delinquent due to feeling unloved and forgotten about; child ends up suffering from drug addiction resulting in the taking of loans that they can't pay back to fund drug habit, child ends up at the bottom of the River Clyde twenty years later". I further thought to myself "The majority of the most intuitive of our road's drivers can only see a bent bonnet in their minds when they think of a collision with another car". I then thought to myself: "Someone is constructively dismissed over their epilepsy/diabetes/recovered stroke/recovered heart attack etc, can't feed and clothe a family, house re-possessed, can't get another job due to "reasons for leaving", goes back into former workplace and murders the boss". The car driver who killed the husband gets three years in prison; and a driving ban for a further three years when he gets out. The former constructively dismissed worker gets 25 years. The former employee kills because someone destroyed his employability, deliberately causing family mayhem; the driver chose to make a reckless selfish egocentric decision to put his foot down. Who committed the worst of the two crimes: THE DRIVER, by a long way!!! If you ask me, there is a reason to give reckless drivers without causing damage, the death sentence. This is because their intuition and initiative score is so low that they are very probably going to kill someone. This would be living in a preventative society, and give the person who murdered their boss the three years as they did what they did because their temperament and pain threshold had been met as a result of someone else's morality score being very low. Are we not better off without the person whose morality score is very low? And are we not better off without the person whose intuitive score is very low, who kills people in car crashes; especially when the victim of the car crash has a very high morality score? Yes, we are in my opinion. Would you not agree that two very flawed personalities resulted in tragedies for two other personalities, which one could say if had not been at the mercy of the two flawed personalities, would to this day still be functioning members of society? Again, my answer to this is "Yes", but guess what: Neither the reckless driver, nor the discriminative boss, meet the diagnostic criteria for any of the different personality disorders!!!!!

Now, take a look at me: I walk 20 miles a week and do a little over two half marathons of calorie expenditure per week in the gym for the purpose of longevity; I eat a diet high in anti-oxidants for the same purposes of longevity; I eat fruit as well as oily fish and wholegrain for both longevity purposes as well as anti-depressant purposes, as these foods increase my dopamine and serotonin levels; I positive think and don't allow negativity into my mind when it comes to any self-evaluation; I know what I'm eating for lunch today as well as dinner tonight so I can stick to my 3,000 calories per day allowance e.g. 4 pieces of battered haddock and chips for lunch (1500 cals) -400 cals walking + tortollenis and tomato for dinner (1300 cals) + King size Snickers (426cals) + 2 apples (120cals) = 2,826 cals for the day. I also limit my alcohol consumption to way beneath the weekly allowance; I walk every round trip journey that comes to less than five miles; I meditate twice daily to combat anxiety and depressive disorders; I do two half marathons a week in gym for mental health purposes; I prioritise my spending, I have high discipline evidenced by diet/ gym/ walking over driving/alcohol consumption; I don't engage in any habit known to be bad for health; I recognise my weaknesses and go about remedying them e.g. recognising my rage and anger and addressing this through the use of meditation and thought blocking; I can apply intellect to practice allowing me to make well informed decisions; I am assertive, evidenced by my advocacy charity; I have not been floored by any set back I've had in life i.e. despite the issues in this book; I am still standing with aims and goals that I am determined to succeed at achieving; I have had the life skills and personality to survive such a rough ride as well as survive and adapt to family abandonment; I am a person who someone talking to could have a life transforming conversation with, such as a person suffering from depression on anti-depressant medication or someone wanting to have a lot more confidence than they have at present etc. This list could go on so I will stop adding to this list, but I have added enough to demonstrate that no one could say I am a bad role model; no one could say that I am a bad or reckless person, and instead could only be described as insightful, responsible, disciplined, high morality, having principles that are of an ethos that advocates a fairer world where life is a level playing field for everyone, believing in mutuality where people should treat others the way they wish to be treated themselves; has healthy moral and self-esteem through the use of alternative remedies as well as through achievements made i.e. advocacy charity etc. Despite the listing of many of my behaviours ,and the reasons behind them and what they say about me as a person; I am diagnosed as having a personality disorder, which I find farcical when the credentials I have listed in this paragraph are all evidenced from the decisions that I make which have been shaped by my personality type. When I look at the lifestyle choices of many and am aware that their choices are determined by personality type, it makes the diagnosis of personality disorder very unscientific indeed, and nothing more than a name calling exercise. Just like when we were all little children aged six in the playground, we called the classmate who was different in some way a "Spastic"; adult society calls the person with any form of individuality that makes them different to the rest as being someone with a personality disorder. The logic behind calling someone a "Spastic" at age six, is the same logic behind calling someone a "Personality Disordered Person" at the age of 44.

I am diagnosed as having paranoid personality disorder'. You will have your own opinion, but as a meditator and as a molecular biologist I have to disagree, as this term "Paranoid Personality Disorder" in my opinion, is just a way in sweeping under the carpet the following:

Social work training, Thelmer Turner Homes, Epilepsy Connections (not just your employer but also your friend of fourteen years), Richmond Fellowship, Loughborough University teacher training, Epilepsy Society, ASA support work agency, nurse training, neglectful treatment by the police, family abandonment.

Paranoid personality disorder just allows for the politicians to sweep under the rug the failings of the Equality Act 2010, and deny that there is a discrimination problem concerning those living with disability as well as deny that social exclusion is the reason for why I am living off the benefits system. My reports of discrimination are just put down to me having a paranoid interpretation of others treatment of me and allows for the social exclusion of people like me especially when employers want "reasons for leaving" and "explained gaps in employment" listed on their application forms.

This book could go on and on. The difficulties of living in an intolerable society, intolerant of anyone whose either a good person or a disadvantaged person, are so great. It is for this reason that people like myself "Walk this path alone" through this world that is foreign to the idea of friendship or family, and too familiar with hatred, intolerance and persecution. I am; however, surviving it; where each day has made me a stronger person despite a more abused as well as neglected person. Time has proven me to be larger than the abuse and the neglect that I have been on the receiving end of which in a perverse way has been a massive confidence booster that is transferable to entrepreneurship where I invent my own world (maybe universe) since this world has proven to be cut out for one purpose in my life and that is to reject me. Some of us are too honourable to be here and an honourable man's world is a "self- made world". People like me create our own world by selecting our own populace i.e. networking; using our own self- taught life skills and knowledge i.e. life experience; marketing ourselves e.g. giving talks and engaging on social media; using our own resources e.g. fundraising or inherited wealth and most importantly our high sense of self and not just being another one of the others!!

CHAPTER 42 - WHY BEING A FIT HUMAN BEING, WHO BELONGS TO THE MAJORITY, IS THE MOST STIGMATISING THING ONE COULD BE!!

One of the purposes of this book has been to open the eyes of the reader and put into perspective how irrational the stigma of those living with epilepsy and mental health problems is. One thing I have drawn attention to is how most people living in our society are brought up with a self-loathing that comes from belittlement and put down by our friends, family, industry, media, societal expectation, teachers, employers, neighbours and any other I have missed out. I have also drawn attention to the fact that this self-loathing causes people to want to "fit-in" and be like one of the others, therefore, resulting in a love to be a member of the majority and a major disliking towards being a member of any minority; unless superior amounts of money, fame, skill or power are the defining feature of that minority. This love for being a member of the majority causes everyone to dress the same way, talk the same way, behave the same way, think the same way, spend their money the same way; thus, causing people to refuse to be the people they are and instead be the person they believe others want them to be. They therefore see their "true selves" as being inferior to the rest which fills them with great insecurity about who they are. They spend their lives running away from themselves and instead running towards the identity shared by the many. It is this mentality that fuels conformity. It is also this mentality that fuels judgemental behaviours towards anyone seen to have a weakness, dysfunction or anything out of the ordinary that makes them different to the majority thus causing them to become a member of a minority.

As the majority spend their lives with the front of their minds saying: "I am a member of the majority", but the back of their minds thinking: "You portray yourself as a member of the majority, so you will like yourself, and be liked by others", they live in a state of denial over what they truly think of themselves, which is "not much". As they do not like themselves, they get defensive when they are told by someone that they are not very good looking, or when they are told that they are not as good at something as someone else is. It is also why they get jealous when they hear that someone has more money than they, or when someone has more status or power than they. It is why, very often, when they see someone doing really well at something, they at the back of their minds are hoping that that someone will suddenly hit some bad luck and fail at what they were achieving. I reckon this was a major reason as to why when I was running my advocacy organisation, where I was winning cases for those with disability against social work, housing, employers and many other as a one man band with no training; just learning on the job, the only thing that the Scottish Independent Advocacy Alliance would say was that I was giving advocacy a bad name. This I dare say was the same reason no other neurological charity would refer clients to my advocacy charity when they had issues needing resolved.

It is because of this not thinking very much about oneself, that people don't question logic, nor, challenge opinions and decisions that are about to be; or have been made by others, which is why most work colleagues would participate in a constructive dismissal of someone or do anything under the orders of anyone above them (which they see as being almost everyone else around them). The request to participate in such a dishonest and damaging action against someone who is a member of a minority is further encouraged by the conformist's views on people who belong to that minority, which as already mentioned are formed from their own insecurities about not being a member of the majority as well as their self-loathing induced aversion to minorities.

This self- loathing experienced by the majority is also why people are painfully self-conscious when they meet new people. They fear the evaluation, others give them. They believe everyone to think very little of them because how can you think others think highly of you, if you don't think highly of yourself. This is why when people come across a person who they give a poorer evaluation of, than the one they believe others would give of them, they get a joy knowing that someone is in a worse position as they when that someone meets new people; therefore, to celebrate this, they want to both see this person receive negative evaluation as well as enjoy imagining themselves in that person's shoes momentarily, to then put themselves back in their own shoes and be very grateful that that person is not them, which for once in their lives gives them a feeling of security. People also love to put themselves in others shoes and imagine the pain that person must be feeling since they know what pain they would be feeling, and jump back into their own shoes and feel a strong sadistic satisfaction. This is therefore the reason why everyone loves to pick on the D-stream boy; the boy with the birthmark; the new start on first day of new job; the guy with social anxiety disorder; the autistic guy with poor social skills; the shy person; the clinically obese person and so on.

The reasons for the majority targeting the vulnerable person are exactly the same reasons behind those in high socio-economic positions being all high on their inflated moral and self-esteem, and appearing as well as feeling super confident amongst others. It is because of this feeling of super confidence that many will also take a jibe at people they see as being of less worth than them which in their case is the majority. Imagine that! You are brought up feeling the need to fit in as you saw the majority being above you and now you see the majority below you. That must make you feel like something that was once less than bronze, turned into something made of gold. The thing is though, this "super confidence" is not real confidence as the minute that person loses that socio-economic position, they suddenly lose that super confidence. Someone with "real confidence" does not require anything to separate him from the rest that equates to some kind of superiority over the others. A person with real confidence feels confident because of their lifetime achievements, and what they say about themselves to themselves, which no one can take away. These people have proven themselves to themselves; therefore, they do not need the approval of others; therefore, do not feel the need to conform, which encourages them to live outside their comfort zone living new experiences, acquiring new skills and knowledge; further growing in character and personality, making them much more life educated and wiser people. These people don't need to get drunk to enjoy a night out on the town because they have so much knowledge, experience and a passion for so many things that they would rather spend all night talking about these things than talking the drunk garbage that you hear going on around you. Look at me, come and stand beside me at the bar and look at what you would learn if you hadn't read this book, and what life transforming information could be departed to that person if they had epilepsy, depression or anxiety; and can you imagine if I got standing beside someone who had as equally as much to talk about but on another subject such as real life politics and war. To experience such an encounter, which provides a huge learning opportunity, requires one to speak to strangers; which unfortunately involves them coming out of their comfort zone.

Having discussed the self-loathing induced thoughts and behavioural outcomes of the majority of human beings, it would be fair to say that if they want to treat me disrespectfully because of the stigma that is associated with epilepsy, depression and anxiety; then I could do exactly the same with them, as there are grounds for saying being "typically human" carries as much stigma if not a lot more.

There is sound evidence for saying that the Diagnostic Statistical Manual, that has the diagnostic criteria for mental health conditions in it, should have a medical condition called "Typical Human Personality", that could be described as having the following diagnostic criteria:

Feelings of Self-loathing

Feelings of inferiority

Feelings of grandeur when in high socio-economic position

Defensiveness and hostility towards others due to feelings of inferiority

Intolerantly impatient of others

A tendency to contribute towards the mental scarring of others

Seeks sadistic gratification through watching of soap operas, making jibes of others, spectating distress of others but not offering to help, playing of inappropriate practical jokes, treating some people less favourably than others and other sadistically gratifying behaviour

Will behave in needy ways and make needy choices for the purpose of approval by others

Does not behave in a way that is navigated by values, opinions and beliefs thus making them inconsistent in what they say and do as well as making them easily exploitable and manipulatable

May fail to develop principles as a result of conforming to a capitalist/exploitative/very far right wing society, explaining a tendency to behave in an unprincipled way

Totally lacking in initiative, intuition and insight creating a very simplistic understanding of a very complex world resulting in very unwise decision making, very often to the detriment of others

Lacking in ability to think outside the box

Believes anything they are told due to never questioning logic

Extremely unpragmatic

Low adaptability

Feelings of Jealousy

Inability to say "No" due to pressure to be Mr/Mrs Kind

Obsession with Power, Greed and Status

Tendency to declare war for the purpose of Power, Greed and Status

Tendency to kill innocents through erratic behaviour e.g. reckless car driving, war, conflicts caused by pride and ego

Dishonesty

A tendency to let others walk over them

A tendency to cause collateral damage in the lives of others through lack of initiative, intuition and insight e.g. family breakdown, damaged careers, reduced employability, acquisition of disability and ill health Impaired Social Skills- a) have a tendency to only be able to form conversation with people they are very familiar with i.e. acquaintances, colleagues, family members and friends. Will demonstrate clique behaviour towards any person who does not fall within one of these categories. This is due to inability to construct and maintain conversation with strangers and an inability to find a common ground that they can form a short- lived temporary relationship from. b) Have low confidence stemming from self-loathing which creates paranoid delusions that others are negatively evaluating them which also impairs social functioning causing avoidant behaviour e.g. will need a friend to take them to a party where they will not know anyone

A tendency to overindulge with intoxicating compounds to compensate for low confidence

Ambiguity between views and actions taken e.g. campaigning for a living wage on the Monday, as they are left wing, but at same time accepting a

disproportionately large pay rise as part of a promotional package on the Tuesday

Fear of the discomfort zone and an aversion to new experience

Judgemental due to a requirement to live in the comfort zone, where only source of education on minority groups and sensitive issues/subjects i.e. disability, race, sexuality etc is media

Persistent negative thoughts and tendency towards always predicting worst outcomes

A taking of things for granted, creating impatient, demanding and intolerant behaviour that causes symptoms of burnout and nervous breakdown in others

There is no doubt about it and that is the more hardship you have had in your life the fewer of these typical human personality traits you will have. Hardship makes you a better person. It gives you empathy and a "treat others the way you wish to be treated yourself" mentality, as never in a million years would you ever wish to be as bad as the people who have treated you badly. You will therefore find many people with disability, people from the LGBT community and people who belong to racial minorities possessing a much fewer number of these traits.

If you were to ask me what is the most stigmatising condition one could live with i.e. "Typical Human Personality" or being epileptic, I would overwhelmingly believe "Typical Human Personality" to be much more stigmatising. I would also have to say that the stigma of "Typical Human Personality" would be justified, as all these symptoms say "STAY WELL CLEAR!!!". These personality traits have put me off ever wanting to marry someone, have a family, work for someone or with others, have friends and have as little to do with others on a peer-peer basis or superior-subordinate basis where I am the subordinate. I have become judgemental of the human race and it is this that psychiatrists refer to as "paranoid personality disorder" when in fact my judgementalism is down to a stigma towards people who are typically human that is well earned. It is the case that psychiatry takes it out on me, the well- earned stigma of being a typical human being.

If psychiatry has it down in its books that I should be like all the above in order for me to be defined as being of fit mind as well as personality, then I am afraid to say it but psychiatry is very much a flawed science. I also have to say that if having paranoid personality disorder means that your personality traits are at odds with the above "symptoms of normal personality" then it is "normal personality" that should carry the greater stigma as my personality ticks all the following traits, which I would expect you to agree with having read this book:

Empathetic towards anyone with a vulnerability- evidenced by voluntary and paid work as well as my experiences in this book

A great amount of initiative, intuition and insight-evidenced by the lifestyle choices that I make and why I make them, such as the diet I follow and exercise regime I keep to. This is also evidenced by the being at odds with an illogical society that creates non-sensical boundaries and hurdles, thus, causing me a lot of frustration. In other words, my "Non-conformity" evidences me to score high on these traits.

High problem- solving skills- evidenced by resolving 120 cases when running Fairway Advocacy as well as the fact that I have self- treated my depression and anxiety and found ways in curbing seizures that I have felt coming on

Highly adaptable- evidenced by the fact that I can speak to an academically educated person as an advocate, and then meet with a moderately learning disabled former client for a coffee and a two hour chat

Highly assertive- evidenced by my advocacy work as well as my ability to deal with antisocial neighbours that this book has not touched on the subject of

No interest in social position- evidenced by the chapter where the difference between achievement and success was discussed. I judge a person by the amount of "climbing mountains with steep gradients" they have done in their life, as well as judge someone on the amount conformity plays in their views and behaviours

Does not get jealous- evidenced by the fact that "Achievement" is what gives me my pride and neither position, possessions nor wealth

Questions logic and highly pragmatic- evidenced by the fact that one of the things that has frustrated me over the years is the lack of logic that has been present in our education establishments and employment settings e.g. why does it take three years to train a nurse at university, and why should a guy with a tendency to run off to London on a skateboard be allowed a bike.

High trait confidence – evidenced by my confidence score at any one time of day, which is high due to the amount of achievement there has been in my life e.g. conquering depression, anxiety and not letting epilepsy defeat me, winning 120 advocacy cases, proving teachers wrong by achieving my degree

Non-needy- evidenced by my ability to have coped in this world without a single friend or family member without it compromising my confidence, moral or self esteem

Scores very high on discipline- I walk 20 miles per week as well as do two half marathons in the gym; I follow a 3,000 calories per day diet; I can say "No" to a fifth pint; I meditate for 50 minutes morning and night,

No fear of the discomfort zone- evidenced by overcoming my crippling fear of public speaking the day I threw away my beta blockers; sat in lectures where there was a risk of seizures; got through every morning and night time awakening as a child where there was either a seizure or risk of seizure; walk 20 miles a week and do two half marathons in the gym; have started to do card tricks in public with people sitting on park benches; and I am sure you can work out other not mentioned.

Little trust of others- justified by the list of personality traits found under the diagnostic criteria for "Typical Human Personality" that has been evidenced by my life experience.

My lack of trust in others is because of the following traits found in the first list of traits that could be described as being symptoms of "Typical Human Personality". These traits are:

"Ambiguity between views and actions"

"Does not behave in a way that is navigated by values, opinions and beliefs thus making them inconsistent in what they say and do as well as making them easily exploitable and manipulatable"

"May fail to develop principles as a result of conforming to a capitalist/exploitative/very far right wing society explaining a tendency to behave in an unprincipled way"

"Inability to say "No" due to pressure to be Mr/Mrs Kind"

"Will behave in needy ways and make needy choices for the purpose of approval by others"

"Judgemental due to a requirement to live in the comfort zone where only source of education on minority groups i.e. disability, race, sexuality is media due to an aversion to learning from new experience"

"Totally lacking in initiative, intuition and insight creating a very simplistic understanding of a very complex world resulting in very unwise decision making, very often to the detriment of others"

"A taking of things for granted, creating impatient, demanding and intolerant behaviour that causes symptoms of burnout and nervous breakdown in others"

We all live different lives, and some of us will be exposed to these traits in others, more often than most, depending on our life circumstances. There are two types of leader: The "moral leader" and the "immoral leader". If there is an immoral leader in charge, and the staff below them are easily exploitable and manipulatable, then anyone who is at risk of immoral treatment has a right to fear the immoral leader and have little faith and confidence in their colleagues behaving honourably since they will just carry out any orders that are given to them from above. It is the case, therefore, that if you have difficulties with learning or you live with a condition that has a lot of stigma attached to it, and you have an immoral leader, you should be conscious of how the stigma combined with the immorality of the leader could result in you becoming majorly compromised, especially living in a world where you can be so easily disposed of and replaced by someone else the next day. It happens! It's been evidenced by this book! In a world where you are so easily got rid off and replaced in no time, it is correct for you to not trust anyone in a workplace with an immoral boss who would not care about the collateral damage sacking you would have on other areas of your life and the lives of those closely reliant on your income if you live with a vulnerability. It's okay for a psychiatrist who has only ever known professional colleagues; living in a world where people are favourably judgemental towards him as he is a doctor and, therefore, create the impression to him that the world is a friendly, tolerant place where everyone behaves professionally at all times; to believe that the complaints of people like me are just down to paranoia. If anyone is suffering from delusions of reality, it is the science of psychiatry. The diagnosis people like me find ourselves labelled with have been created by people to sweep under the carpet the abusive, exploitative and manipulative nature of our society to prevent a revolution. It is also a diagnosis that today's psychiatrist does not question the logic behind the creating of and just accepts as a medical diagnosis. Remember that list about typical human personality where one of the traits in humans is that they don't question logic? Labelling someone with "personality disorder" is irrational when you look at the list of traits that define normal personality and so is any stigma associated with any vulnerable minority when you look at the personality traits that define the majority. Paranoid personality disorder is nothing more than saying "You are unlike the majority, which means you are more honourable, bolder, smarter, more outspoken, not easily walked over, more logical, better at seeing through peoples' true incentives and therefore a risk to a society that gets away with exploiting and manipulating less life educated people. You have an honourable ethos and therefore are a threat to capitalism, hierarchies, bosses' egos, continued inequality of wealth and poor workers' rights. You will end up socially excluded for having these traits as they are traits that allow people advocates (Remember Fairway Advocacy), who stick up for others' human rights. We will find a name for you that will make everyone look at you and say "Yuck!!" and stay clear off you". Therefore, the labelling of people as "personality disordered" is nothing more than name calling, which is what stigma is all about. If stigma is about "shame", then I must say, there is much more stigma in being of normal personality and very much a pride to be taken in being Personality Disordered!!! And what this world fears is that the "Personality Disordered" make more people "Personality Disordered" through their good influence and spreading of the word, making the world a kinder place with greater equality and regard for human rights.

So, what does paranoid personality disorder really mean? Looking at the traits that cause me to not trust the human race, it basically means I am someone who has seen a mountain of evidence throughout my life to date that is supportive of humans being of these already listed seven personality traits, meaning I would not trust a human as far as I could throw one. That sounds a logical, evidence based, non-judgemental, experienced, well-informed thinking that is evidence of being of sound mind. Did I not previously say that personality disorder is being an upright guy in an upside- down world!!!

The Milgram experiment is a classic example of behaviour seen by humans that evidences that you should not trust a human unconditionally as this experiment demonstrates that so long as the order to harm comes from a person in a position of authority then other peoples' attitudes are "Don't look at me. I'm only doing my job". It's the classic "I have a wife and family to feed and clothe". How often did we hear this being said when you were being brought up in the eighties. Others used this statement as though it was in fashion. A good example of this can be found in an article titled "Branding a soldier with Personality Disorder" that was published in the New York Times on the 24th February 2012. This article tells the story of a woman called Captain Susan Carlson who was a counsellor in the US army who was deployed to Afghanistan with the Colorado National Guard where we are told that everything fell apart for her. During her deployment she had been accused by a soldier of making sexually inappropriate remarks which resulted in her suspension from her counselling duties and referred to an army psychiatrist. The psychiatrist diagnosed her as having a personality disorder which was a diagnosis that the military had been using to discharge thousands of troops. As a result of this diagnosis, Captain Susan Carlson was sent home. It was months later that she found in her medical file evidence of her command specifically asking the psychiatrist to diagnose her with personality disorder. Veterans' advocates said that Captain Carlson had stumbled across evidence of something that they had been struggling to prove and that was military commanders had been pressuring psychiatrists to issue unwarranted psychiatric diagnoses to get rid of troops. Since 2001 the military had discharged 31,000 service members because of personality disorder. Veterans' advocates have been saying for years that the Pentagon uses the diagnosis of personality disorder to discharge troops that they see as being troublesome or wants to avoid giving benefits to as a result of service- connected injuries. It is believed that the psychiatrists have been diagnosing military troops, who are no longer medically fit to be soldiers, with personality disorder to avoid having to diagnose them with Post Traumatic Stress Disorder (PTSD), for the purpose of not having to give these discharged troops benefits that a diagnosis of PTSD would entitle them to. According to this newspaper article a diagnosis of post traumatic stress disorder can cost the US army 1.5 million dollars in benefits over a soldier's lifetime. As you would expect there is denial by the authorities that such manipulating of psychiatrists occurs. If this story is true then it would be right to say that these psychiatrists would keep increasing the voltage, thus, killing other people under the orders of authority; whereas I would not, if I and them were to participate in a Milgram experiment. I would say "No" to further increases of trauma and report the abuse because of these personality traits of mine that psychiatrists would say are evidence of personality disorder. This evidences that personality disorder was invented to label people who are prepared to go against the grain of an abusive/negligent/incompetent authority which is a prerequisite of rebellion. As has already been mentioned, the US army were using this diagnosis to discharge trouble makers.

CHAPTER 43

I am going to share with you a present day issue in my life that is an example of the human behaviour of others that results in a person like myself being diagnosed with paranoid personality disorder, and that is an experience that I had this morning with my factors who are the Govanhill Housing Association. Just a few days ago on the 2nd September 2020 my factors came to my building to do maintenance work on my close entrance. As Billy Connolly says, "The close, is the entrance from the street, followed by the staircase that takes you up to your flat" for those reading who are not aware of the term "Close". Billy said this as part of a joke, taking a jibe at the typical English having no understanding of Scottish Patter. All said in Good humour!

When the contractor came out to the block of flats, he started making lots of hammering noise that disturbed my ability to enjoy my own top floor home on that morning and would certainly have caused me to have cancelled any appointments or meetings I may have had if I worked from home. The fact that no notice of this was given in advance so that residents could rearrange prior arrangements to accommodate this work was in my view unforgiveable. It was inconsiderate and short sighted. I therefore wrote to the factors and told them that they should give me notice in advance whenever they are planning on doing loud work so that their work does not collide with my interests. What I got as a reply was that their remit does not require them to give me advance notice, and therefore, they will be giving me no notice in the future of any work. The factor said, as part of their defence, that according to the contract they only have to tell the tenants about work that comes to a certain amount that is above £200 in costs, and that the cost of this work was below that threshold. My immediate reaction to this was to think to myself that there will of course be a policy where we as residents have to give our permission for our money to be spent in large quantities for work to be done as part of their maintenance work. I, however, also recognised that telling people about work to be done because of disturbance made by noise; and telling people about work for the purpose of being given the go-ahead as a result of cost, are two completely different matters.

A few days later on the 3rd October I received a letter from the factor telling me that there had been a report made about how the back close area was untidy with litter and broken toys and that they did not provide maintenance for this area but they could do if we paid an extra £68.00 per year. What surprises me is that first of all I know that none of the neighbours in my close would have reported this mess as it is their children that create it, and as well as this they live their lives in the most reckless ways such as drilling holes in walls at 10.30pm in the evening while I am in bed reading my kindle. They have no respect for one another. I have lived there a year and see their gardens on the ground floor overgrown and unkept with litter in them, the two on the middle landing do unannounced DIY work that is so loud at the most anti-social times, and the flat across the landing from me is vacant as it keeps getting broken into.

I know from my experiences as an advocate, as I have in the past written to this housing association on behalf of clients with disability, as well as from the letter that I wrote the previous week, that if this housing association don't see the dealing of someone's complaint as being a part of their remit, then they would give as a reply "Not interested" to anyone making a complaint about the unkept conditions of the back close area. I therefore find it hard to believe that anyone who reports me and my neighbours for keeping the backyard untidy would get, as a response, the housing association sending a letter to us telling us to keep the back yard tidy. I would definitely say from past dealings that the complainer would get something similar to the following quoted reaction: *"We do not advocate for residents who have complaints concerning the behaviours of residents living in other closes. You can speak to your neighbours with the intention of resolving matters or you can contact the Glasgow City Council Environmental Protection Services."* Such a response would certainly be consistent with the response I got from them to my letter complaining about the excess noise, that told them that I had enough issues with problem behaviour from my neighbours and didn't need them acting as bad examples; instead, what I got was a letter saying that they don't get involved in neighbour disputes of the kind I was describing i.e. disputes where they have no power to intervene and that I could always approach the environmental protection services. This housing association most likely saw an opportunity to start charging for a service that we were not asking for and tried to create a demand by saying there had been a complaint.

I also had a letter sent from this housing association back in August saying "It seems that you have not paid a bill owed to us that covers the period between January and March of 2020". When I wrote to the housing association, I informed them that as they had not behaved professionally over the unannounced noise, I was not paying this bill until I got that guarantee that I would always be informed of loud work prior to the day such work would take place on. In the reply there was no demand for that payment to be made. Just a very blurred explanation for why I had been sent that bill. On the day I receive the letter about the back yard there is again no letter requesting that money be paid that I was refusing to pay. I noticed that the letter about the money owed sent to me in August uses the words "It seems". It is pretty black or white if you have paid a bill or not, and therefore, I would expect the letter to have used the words "You have not". The usage of the word "seems"; the lack of request for payment in their response e-mail to me concerning my letter of complaint over noise made on the 2nd September; the fact that they said in their e-mail reply regarding my complaint that I would be sent the content of that e-mail in a letter as well, which I have still not received; the fact that they are telling us of a complaint that their remit does not involve the addressing of (when they have a culture of saying "not interested" to anything they do not see as their responsibility) and the fact that they are now offering to provide a service that costs £68 per annum in response to "this complaint" they received, gives me every reason to believe that they are just saying that there has been a complaint to try and get us to buy a service that none of us are interested in. What gives rise to this suspicion is the inconsistency between what they say they are not prepared to do for me, as it is not a part of their remit, but what they are prepared to do for someone else that is as equally not a part of their remit. The typical human personality trait of others that gives rise to this suspicion in me is listed above as being "Ambiguity between views and actions". I am also more educated than everyone else in my close as I have been a disability advocate and I know that if the back yard does not fall under their jurisdiction then it is the city council environment protection services that the person's complaint should be reported to. The fact that there is no reference to the environmental protection services in this letter also gives rise to suspicion. Surely if someone had reported this complaint to them, then the housing association would have instructed them to phone the environmental protection team, and the housing association would have had to have told us they had done this in the letter they sent to me and my neighbours. It therefore can be said that my suspicions are not just down to a behaviour that I observe that is consistent with "typical human personality" but also because of a breaking of ranks within proper policy and procedure. I obviously detect these things and question them as well which others do not, and therefore, I would say that another term for paranoid personality disorder is "Streetwise Personality". This "personality disorder" is a strength and not a weakness and is something that people who are more informed about the world, as a result of greater life experience through living outside the comfort zone, have.

It is also my belief that my reaction to this letter offering this new service is evidence of myself coming from the high functioning end of the functionality continuum. My querying of logic, as well as being able to join the dots up between letter demanding we keep the back area clean and the following:

1. previous reactions of housing associations to correspondence sent to them over professional matters when I was an advocate;
2. the fact that I had mentioned in my letter of complaint over the noise that the neighbours do not talk to anyone as there is a loss of community, therefore, they could so easily send a letter to all of us saying that the other five had all said "yes" to this new service, and that our bills would be going up by £68.00 per annum without any of us checking with one another that we had agreed to this;
3. the purpose of the environmental protection services;

and come to the conclusion that we as tenants should not give the housing association unconditional trust, and instead, query the offering of this service further, tells you that I have high IQ and high ability to apply intellect to practice, thus, making me high functioning, therefore, not easily fooled or conned, nor, walked over as a result of having more "people confidence" due to having this neurocognitive advantage over others. This makes me unpopular with authority in a world where it   is the individual's word against the authority's, making me prone to name calling by a system that was previously invented for the purpose of reducing the "leadership effect" someone like me is capable of having, thus, preventing socialist uprisings and the giving of more power to the people. If psychiatry was around in the 14th century, King Edward I of England would probably have had his English Psychiatric Association label William Wallace as having paranoid personality disorder to put off Scottish civilians following his leadership, especially when he was making claims like "Today we beat the English, but they will be back!!".

This area of psychology that was very likely a creation of psychiatry protecting the interests of an industrialised world that makes money and gets away with wealth inequality through the use of abuse and exploitation of others, is one that needs to be challenged in the name of democracy.

When I wrote my letter of complaint to the housing association, I had memories of the psychiatrist at the Jeanie Deans in 2019 asking me as part of his diagnostic questions "Do you complain a lot?" and I thought to myself, this fits my belief on how personality disorder came to be, which is very similar in context and identical in principle to the theory that the American Psychiatry Association invented personality disorder under the instruction of President Nixon according to philosopher Olivia Goldhill. It could be said that the people living in my close are like the workforce and my demanding prior notice of loud noise and querying of other matters is evidence of me being the trouble maker who gets in the way of the employer abusing and exploiting, and fortunately for me my flat belongs to myself therefore they cannot have me gone, like they could in a workplace, however, if my flat did belong to the housing association, which is the case with most of their tenants, they probably would find a reason to have me evicted and thrown out into the street and made homeless. When I wander the streets of Glasgow I sometimes wonder if any of these people sleeping rough were the ones that stuck up for the rights of the other tenants by raising complaints and objecting to future plans and procedure, bringing in third parties such as advocates, local councillors, Member of the Scottish Parliament, media etc.

Just before Fairway Advocacy closed, one of my clients with high functioning autism made many complaints about the living conditions to his social landlord. He spoke his mind. He complained at his social work meetings about the social injustice that the system was guilty of and how the social workers were just judgemental and didn't like the way he had been given a community payback order and liked to wind him up at his supervision meetings so he would lose his temper. I had to attend the meetings with him as he did lean across the table while telling the social workers what he thought of them. I had to put my arm across at these meetings to keep him from going too far over the table and the social workers tried to spin it, that I was aggressive. I knew that if my client lost his temper and did something impulsive he would end up in prison. The social worker shouted at me and said at one of the meetings "Do you think there's nothing wrong with a man doing a community payback order going to gay nightclubs". I couldn't believe the judgementalism I was hearing.

I had resolved a number of this client's complaints, however, it was the case that just a few days after our closure I learned from a cry for help message from this client, left on an answer machine, that he had been evicted and now made homeless. They had actually thrown him out of his accommodation. I've been teaching you about the world of epilepsy, welcome to the world of autism. Social exclusion never gets talked about by our politicians and it is by far the biggest killer in people living with epilepsy as well as those living with other disability, especially the hidden disabilities. The lives of many are way too complex to be living in, and have the needs met by, a very simplistic construction called "society". The real definition of social exclusion is where your life is so affected by a number of complexities that your needs outsmart society, resulting in society and its people exhibiting avoidant behaviour towards you. You will either adapt to this abandonment by society and grow knowledge and skills that will enhance you, or you will not survive the turbulent storm caused by society's avoidance and it will break you. I am glad to say that therapies like Meditation, Visualisation, Distraction, Cardiovascular Exercise, Diet, Positive Thinking and Cognitive Behaviour Therapy go about making sure social exclusion makes you.

This book started with me at age three running around with a toy hoover in the city of Leeds in a lounge, where I was suddenly overcome by a simple partial epileptic seizure that was to become complex partial epilepsy at the age of ten when I started to have seizures happening at a frequency of one every 36 hours. It was for the next thirteen years that I would experience one seizure every 36 hours, where my seizures for the vast majority of the time either occurred upon awakening in the middle of the night or within the first two hours of being out of bed in the morning. The mornings required a great deal of concentration in the trying to prevent myself from having a seizure. I therefore know that there will be children/adolescents/young adults throughout Glasgow and beyond, who every morning need to waken up naturally and avoid sudden awakenings before getting out of bed, and also need quiet environments so that concentration is not affected in carrying out the mental activities that I used to carry out that helped prevent morning seizures. It was the case that noise such as the dog suddenly running into my room and barking loudly at a passing train could bring on a seizure.

The possibility of lost earnings, of someone working from home, was one potential outcome of the housing association refusing to give prior notice of any maintenance/repair work due to be carried out, however, there is a potential second outcome that could have much more catastrophic consequences than lost earnings. This potential second outcome could be a person with epilepsy who is vulnerable to morning seizures being suddenly woken up by loud hammering in the close bringing on a seizure. Depending on the type of seizure the consequences of having such a seizure in the bed could be suffocation or being left too mentally fatigued for the rest of the day to be able to go to work, go to a job interview, catch a plane etc. The potential consequences of having a seizure when up out of bed, depending on the type of seizure, could be burns; lost teeth; head injury; back injury; broken bones; emotional/mental trauma of having a seizure; bad disfiguring bruising/scarring; leaving the house without locking up; leaving a child unsupervised; home being burned down; having an injury in the shower; drowning in the bath etc.

As already mentioned I had sent a letter a to Govanhill Housing Association dated 13th September 2020, and in it I said that that they really should give people advanced notice of maintenance/repair work as many people with depression are fed up with the self-centred nature of this world and that they would see such unannounced noise being made as being nothing other than both a housing association and a contractor only being interested in making money even if it is at the expense of their own client's health and wellbeing. This is particularly hard for a depressed person whose politics is left wing. I said in the letter that there was a recognised symptom of depression called "Noise annoyance" and that this can make a depressed person very irritable and impulsive and cause a depressed person to attack a workman. I said that people like the housing association as well as the contractor criminalise people. I actually told the workman, on the day of his unannounced work, that he was lucky that my depression was symptom controlled as he could have been attacked if I wasn't a meditator. The law too often criminalises the good guy and puts its arm around the greedy, selfish, non-insightful, reckless, disrespectful of others' needs person. Depressed people tend to be principled people living in an unprincipled world. That will be partly why I am the only one who complains, and also why I say depression is probably a rare condition, and that what most people who say they suffer from depression really suffer from is low morale and self-esteem. In other words, they suffer from insecurity as a result of not believing themselves to fit in as well as they feel they should, in order for them to be seen as a credible excuse for a human being.

Even if the threshold in the contract says that they do not need to inform you of any work to be done on the close that is less than £200 at the time of signing; peoples' needs change and they do go on to develop neurological, learning or mental health disabilities that they did not have at the time of signing the contract. If someone's mother with dementia moves in with them, then the mother could start becoming hysterical with anxiety. These people who we give the responsibility of looking after our every day needs to are so uneducated!!!!!!!!!!!!

I have sent e-mails to a S***Y T*****n who is a member of the Factoring Team at Govanhill Housing Association, and on the 1st October 2020 I responded to her e-mail that she had sent on the 29th September, in response to my letter sent the 13th September, that basically said that Govanhill Housing Association (GHA) (Must not be confused with Glasgow Housing Association who are also referred to as GHA) would not give me any prior notice of any future maintenance/repair work that had been arranged with the contractor. I put in my e-mail that if there was someone with learning disability like autism living in my home, they could become very distressed due to sound sensitivity and start displaying challenging behaviour if workmen were to just suddenly start hammering and drilling. This is especially the case when walking down the stairs of the close.

The next few pages give you a chronology of the e-mails sent to S***Y T*****n between the 29th September and the 9th October. In bold are the most relevant parts of the body of the text in the e-mails sent concerning the complaint I was making about the total disregard shown towards those with sudden noise induced symptoms of disability and the need for prior notice of noisy work.

The below e-mail is S***Y T*****n's response to my letter sent to the factoring team on the 13th September:

Complaint - Ascog Street 2/1 Inbox

S***Y T*****n @g*********a.org>

Tue, Sep 29, 5:09 PM

to me

Dear Mr Bone

Further to your letter of 11th September, a copy of my response to your letter was posted out today. I am also emailing the contents of my letter below.

Kind regards.

++

Dear Mr Bone

I refer to your letter of 13th September, received by us on 21st September. Given the contents of the letter, we have logged this a Stage 1 complaint.

You mention receiving a reminder letter and you state that "when one pays for a service they should only do so if th e service has bee n professional". As the one of the Managers, I absolutely agree with you that our services should be professional. However, I am not aware of any issues raised by you relating to services provided in the quarter to 31st March 2020. That quarter's charges were invoiced on 10th July and due for payment within fourteen days. This was well in advance of the events of 2nd September. We invoice retrospectively so everything included in that invoice was already paid on your behalf by the Association a number of months ago. If there are any issues relating to the items included in that invoice please let me know.

I note that you intend to refer the noise made by Mears on 2nd September to your local councillor. You also mention noise made by some of your neighbours on occasion. If you have any issues with noise made by others we would encourage you to contact Glasgow City Council (**www.glasgow.gov.uk**) for their advice on the matter. You should, however, bear in mind that there will always be "living noise" in multi-occupancy buildings.

With regards to common repairs being carried out, you will appreciate that it is unavoidable for many repairs to involve noise being made. The repair carried out by Mears on 2nd September involved reglazing the rear close door. I am sorry to hear that our contractor did not provide you with details of the approximate length of time required to carry out this sort of work. I note what you say about different people having different lifestyles. We instruct approximately 1,000 repairs every month. This means that it is not feasible for us to programme in times for common repairs to be carried out at a time to suit a number of owners.

In your letter you quoted a section of the Property Factors (Scotland) Act 2011 regarding repairs As per Section 6.1 in our Written Statement of Services we do have a threshold in place under which we do not need to seek authority from owners for common repairs. The value of the repair

carried out on 2nd September was under the threshold. Please see below the relevant section of our Written Statement of Services:

"The Association has the delegated authority of the owners within the block to instruct and have carried out repairs and maintenance to the common parts of the block being factored provided that the anticipated cost to each owner of any one item at the time when it is instructed will not exceed £200 or such other sum as may be agreed with a majority of owners of the block or set out in the Deed of Conditions for the property."

I am sorry but I am unable to give you any guarantee as per your request that there will not be any unannounced common repairs taking place in your close. Even if a repair is in excess of the threshold we would notify owners that work was going to take place but we would not be able to confirm a specific date when repairs would be carried out. With the number of repairs that are carried out on our behalf and ever changing priorities as and when emergencies happen this is just not possible.

If you have any queries regarding the above please let me know and I would be happy to discuss. We have a two stage complaints process and my response concludes Stage 1. If you wish to escalate your complaint to Stage 2 please let me know.

Yours sincerely

S***Y T*****n

Manager

On the 1st October I replied to the e-mail S***Y T*****n sent to me on the 29th September. My 1st October 2020 e-mail can be seen below:

Re: Complaint - Ascog Street 2/1

Tim Bone @*****.com>
Thu, Oct 1, 5:11 PM

To: S***Y

Dear Mrs/Miss T*****n,

First point I would like to raise in response to your letter is:

1. You completely disregard the complaint that I make about my neighbours.
You make reference to "Living noise" in your letter and that I should learn to
accept this living in a multi-occupancy
building. This response does not recognise my complaint which was not about
"living noise" but about people not knocking on your door just
to let you know that they are about to carry out loud intrusive work for the
purpose of ensuring that they will not be compromising you with their noise
and if so for the second purpose of scheduling an agreed time so that there are
no clashes when the work is eventually carried out. To not give advance notice
that requires nothing more than a knock on a door and the asking of a simple
question is
inconsiderate considering their noise could make things like hosting a dinner
party or entertaining guests impossible as well as do things such as take very
important phone calls and conduct skype meetings.

2. You mention the following in your letter "We instruct approximately 1,000
repairs every month. This means that it is not feasible for us
to programme in times for common repairs to be carried out at a time   to
suit a number of owners". My letter never asked you to arrange a time for
work and repairs to be carried out at a time that was   convenient with me.
What my letter asked for was that you tell me when repairs will be carried
out so that I can arrange to be elsewhere that   day if the noise from work is
going to stop me from being able to work from home on that day or so I can
cancel appointments and have them re-arranged for another day so client
time is not wasted nor does professional image become compromised nor do
I lose earnings.
3. You mention in your letter the following "We instruct approximately 1,000
repairs every month. This means that it is not feasible for us to programme
in times for common repairs to be carried out at a time to suit a number of
owners." I struggle to believe that your human resources facilities cannot
arrange nor keep a record of times, dates, addresses, jobs to be done,
contractor's name. That is very simple basic information. What you are
telling me is that you do not know who is coming into your clients closes, on

what days, to do what jobs. Not very impressive and certainly not good for
security.

4. You are saying that you do not give people advance notice of work
to be done and all work makes noise. I would have expected you to have
known this and that is this is in breach with the Equality Act. If
someone has a disability that makes them prone to reacting to loud noises
that could compromise mental wellbeing and physical health then they need
to know in advance of such work being carried out and when   it will be
carried out so that they can make arrangements not to be at home on the
day of the noise. If someone has nocturnal seizures and is suddenly awoken
by very loud noise in the morning then they can could have a seizure. This
could be very dangerous if the seizure is in bed
as it could result in suffocation. If a person has autism and suddenly
experiences very loud noise they could suddenly exhibit challenging
behaviour which could seriously compromise them and anyone living with
them. Unannounced noise can also be a risk factor for anyone who   suffers
from Noise annoyance as a symptom of their depression or an anxiety
disorder. If I become compromised by someone with learning disability or
mental health problems as a result of unannounced noise
I think it would be fair to say that with you having received this
e-mail, and you having a knowledge of my predicament my injuries could
have been avoided with a simple three line letter telling me work will
be done, what will be done, when it will be done and who it will be done by.
To not be able to provide such a simple communication can only be
described as incompetence. To say that the word to use is "impractical",
which your letter claims the sending of such a communication to be, is
laughable.

I now need to ask myself "Am I dealing with incompetent people and should
therefore expect nothing more than this incompetence" or should I further
pursue this. I better watch what I say here as I know that
too often pride and ego of the authority are bigger determinants than what is
right and wrong in determining the outcome of a complaint. Pride and ego
determining the outcome of a complaint is defensiveness
which is symptomatic of being in agreement with the claims made by the other
party. What you say you can't do creates a whole load of questions regarding
human rights issues that will need answering from an independent source.

This is a decision that you are quite right in saying I will make and as part of that decision I am currently seeking advice from a lawyer over earnings as well as equality law. My decision has therefore not yet been made and you will hear back in the next few days.

Regards,

Tim Bone

S***Y T*****n's e-mail reply to the above e-mail from myself can be seen below:

RE: Complaint - Ascog Street 2/1 Inbox

S***Y T*****n

Tue, Oct 6, 12:22 PM

to me

Dear Mr Bone

Thanks for your email.

1. Residents have a right to carry out activities in their own home which may make a noise within the parameters of regulations about noise and wider legislation. I wasn't disregarding your complaint about your neighbours. However, we wouldn't expect residents to confer with others in their building before they did anything that makes a noise or, as you suggest, negotiate alternative times with their neighbours. If residents wish to arrange to do this amongst themselves they can do so but that's a matter between residents. Glasgow City Council may be able to offer you guidance on what would be considered acceptable / unacceptable in terms of noise depending on specific circumstances.

2. I'm afraid that we can't give you advance notice of repairs being carried out. We look after a number of buildings and this isn't a service that we can

practically offer. What I would also say is that some repairs inevitably arise at very short notice. I can see that to date we've carried out 2 common repairs at your close in 2020, one internal and one external repair. We also carried out 2 common repairs in 2019 so our attendance at the close has been minimal.

3. Anyone carrying out a common repair on our behalf is one of our approved contractors.

4. I note that you're taking advice and look forward to hearing from you.

Regards.

S***Y

S***Y T*****n
Govanhill Housing Association

On the 9th October I responded to S***Y T*****n's e-mail. It can be noticed in point 4 of my e-mail that I had informed her that I had a fictional friend called Alistair, who visits once every two weeks as a means of coping with social isolation; who has epilepsy and has seizures first thing in the morning, where he relies on using cognitive techniques to prevent seizures that involve great concentration, which can be impeded upon by sudden loud noises. I informed her that sudden loud noise could therefore cause Alistair to have a seizure, and if Govanhill Housing Association were to just post a three sentence length letter through my door, telling me about any maintenance/repair work scheduled for a particular day, I could arrange for Alistair to not visit the night before such work is due to begin. I attached a model letter for S***Y T*****n to read, letting her know what minimal work I was expecting from her in the writing of such a letter. This e-mail sent to her on the 9th October can be seen below, and the content of the model letter that I had attached to my e-mail is quoted below the e-mail:

Re: Complaint - Ascog Street 2/1

Tim Bone @*****.com>Fri, Oct 9, 11:27 AM (13 days ago)

to S***Y

Dear Mrs/Miss T*****n,

Many Thanks for your response.

1. First point is that my letter never asked you to involve yourself
or give your opinion on the legitimacy of what my neighbours on the second
landing have been doing. I was making reference to my neighbour's behaviour
as I had made progress with them and that there was the possibility that what
happened on the 2nd September might have opened old wounds that were
healing. I had already told you I was
going to my councillor therefore that should have been enough for us
to never discuss the issue again. That was now business between me and my
councillor who I plan on seeing after the lockdown. To ask you to address and
resolve this matter requires nothing more than what I have attached. I have
therefore done your job for you even though I pay
you.
The neighbours' previous behaviour was mentioned as a reference to example
what I have already been up against and would have expected something
more professional from yourselves. I think there has been a failure of
yourselves to think "outside the box". The consensus
amongst the public would be that to give me such notice is COURTESY which
any person in receipt of a paid service from a service provider should expect
from their service provider.
2. You have to recognise that a one size fits all system is impractical. It takes
nothing to have a record of who lives in what house and what special
requirements they may have that can be easily accommodated by Govanhill
Housing Association. If I asked 100 people if Govanhill Housing Association
could provide a letter like the one attached to those who require it then I
believe that 100 people would
all say "Yes". I'm sure at one of your in-house training days you
could have a freethinking exercise on "Why would a resident need to be told in
advance that loud intrusive noise was going to be done"
3. I also find it very poor customer service for you to say "Tough
luck, if you have to lose earnings and have to unexpectedly cancel an
appointment with a client who maybe very distressed". I think you forget that

the residents are your bosses. We employ you. That close is jointly owned property that Govanhill Housing Association do not
own. We are not residents of one of your Govanhill Housing Association homes. Just like the Part 3 of the Environmental Protection Act says, we have a right to enjoy our own homes and that no one behaves in a way that stops you from enjoying your own home or behaves in a way that compromises health.

**4. I will finish of by informing you that I have a friend called   Alistair who stays the night, maybe once a fortnight, as a means of coping with social isolation. Alistair has learning disability and
epilepsy. Alistair has morning seizures and has to try some cognitive techniques in the morning to prevent such seizures from occurring. The usage of the cognitive technique requires great concentration of Alistair's. Any unannounced disturbing repair and maintenance noise can act as a distraction thus impairing Alistair's concentration that can bring on a seizure. People with learning disability also have a heightened sensitivity to sound which in Alistair's case could cause him to become anxious thus also bringing on a seizure.**

I therefore ask you to reconsider your refusal to provide such prior notice of when work will be occurring so that alternative arrangements can be made to prevent clashes that are both compromising to wellbeing and health.

Regards,

Tim Bone

CONTENT OF ATTACHED SAMPLE LETTER; EXAMPLING THE NOTICE OF WORK TO BE DONE THAT I WAS DEMANDING, CAN BE SEEN BELOW:

"Dear Mr Bone,

I write to you to inform you that there will be maintenance/repair/renovation work being carried out on the following day ………………… at the following time………….

The work to be carried out will be:…………………………………………..

We do hope that this will not inconvenience you.

Yours Sincerely,

On the 16th October I sent a reminder e-mail to S***Y T*****n as she had not replied to my e-mail sent the 9th October asking for an advance notice letter to be sent to me prior to any maintenance/repair work so that seizures in Alistair could be prevented. The response I got was basically that the Govanhill Housing Association were not going to send me a letter and that a guest such as Alistair would therefore just have to run the risk of having a seizure. The e-mail reply can be seen below:

Complaint - Ascog Street 2/1 Inbox

S***Y T*****n
Fri, Oct 16, 2:33 PM

to me

Dear Mr Bone

Thanks for your email below.

We don't usually inform owners of impending repairs and have no intention of starting to do so. The repair that prompted you to contact us was the reglazing of a door. This was noted during the lockdown and was instructed after the restrictions on the type of repairs that we were able to carry out were eased. The contractor attended on 2nd September and was on site for one hour. Should you feel that the Association is contravening environmental legislation by carrying out repairs you are welcome to take advice on this.

You included a comment in inverted commas in your paragraph 3 – this is certainly not something I said. The properties at Ascog Street are residential, so as factor we would expect that these are normally used for residential purposes.

If you've any queries regarding the above please let me know.

Regards.

S***Y

I sent an e-mail on the 19th October to S***Y T*****n in response to the above e-mail she sent me. This e-mail can be seen below:

Re: Complaint - Ascog Street 2/1

Tim Bone @*****.com>

Mon, Oct 19, 8:38 AM (3 days ago)

to S***Y

Dear Mrs/Miss T*****n,

Thank you for the quick reply to my reminder e-mail sent to you on the Friday 16th October. This e-mail was reminding you of an e-mail sent to you on the 9th October which I had not yet received a reply for.
In response to my e-mail it is evident that if I paraphrase your previous comments and answers to my requests in previous e-mails between you and myself, you are quite simply saying:
"Govanhill Housing Association will not send a letter to your home informing you of work to be done that will create noise that could give your friend Alistair a seizure even though this letter would prevent Alistair from having a seizure triggered by this noise". You are effectively saying that you are prepared to be the cause of guests
in my own home have seizures that could cause head injury, burns, lost teeth, suffocation and other potential outcomes of having a seizure because of excess noise caused by building and maintenance work that Govanhill Housing Association could have given advance notice of in the form of a letter or a phone call which would have allowed the avoidance of having a guest like Alistair round at mine on the morning that the work was taking place.

I find the above staggering, especially when this request made by me requires minimal work from you, and if you imagine it was you living with the burn or the head injury and you learned that the only thing Govanhill Housing Association had been asked to do to prevent this from happening was send a letter like the one attached; I think you would be living with a rage for the rest of your life that would lead
to the development of anxiety disorders and potentially suicide. I would say that the ordeal that you would be prepared to put my friend through to fulfil your aim and objective on the day of a repair or maintenance job is on a par with the ordeal that the Japanese were prepared to put their prisoners of war through to fulfil their aim and objective. That is not an exaggeration. I am sure you would find some section, subsection in the Human Rights Act that would cover this.

I will simply ask you this one question that only expects a one word answer. There is no need to write back to me with paragraphs of explanation and argument. You have made it quite simply obvious to me how prepared you are to contribute towards the creating of an unsafe environment within my home for someone with epilepsy. I hate to think how you treat your own Govanhill Housing Association Clients living in your own homes that have disability. The question I therefore have to ask you is this:

*"If it were me with the epilepsy who could have seizures upon sudden awakening or sudden impaired concentration when using cognitive exercises to prevent seizures from coming on due to unexpected loud noise caused by maintenance and repair work, would you be prepared to give me advance notice so that I could stay at a friend's the night
before such work was due to begin in my close?"*

This question is a closed question and quite simply asks for a "yes" or "no" answer.

I will finish off by explaining why in paragraph 3 of the e-mail sent
on the 9th October I had put in what appeared to be quotation marks, something that you had not said but you believed I was claiming you had said in the exact words that appeared to be "quoted" . These words were:

 "Tough luck, if you have to lose earnings and have to unexpectedly cancel an appointment with a client who maybe very distressed".

I would like to say that never did I say that these were your "Exact words". What I was doing was something called "PARAPHRASING" you. I was taking your words from previous e-mails and putting into other words for the purpose of condensing the conclusion from everything discussed in all previous e-mails between you and myself over this matter; and also for the sake of providing greater clarity. I have also paraphrased you at the beginning of this e-mail when claiming what you have effectively said in your last e-mail about Alistair..
Quotation marks can also be used as inverted commas. Inverted commas are used when you wish to put emphasis on a word or phrase. I used inverted commas to put emphasis on the paraphrased words. There was no corruption of truth in the paraphrasing of your words. It is the case that you have said that I am not going to get a letter giving me advance notice of maintenance/repair work after me telling you that this letter is needed to prevent such work from causing me to have to cancel appointments either last minute or during such appointments where by the nature of the appointments i.e. mental health, these clients will often be distressed. This will inevitably cause loss of earnings and I would find that "Tough luck" and .I am sure your IQ is high enough to know that I would find that "Tough luck". Therefore, the words:
"Tough luck, if you have to lose earnings and have to unexpectedly cancel an appointment with a client who maybe very distressed", I think you would have to agree, is an honest accurate record that concludes what you have been saying to me. I have this as evidence in all the e-mails you have been sending to me.

Now if you could just get back in touch with a "Yes" or "No" answer to the beneath question:

"If it were me with the epilepsy who could have seizures upon unexpected sudden awakening or impaired concentration when using cognitive exercises to prevent seizures from coming on due to
unexpected loud noise caused by maintenance and repair work, would you be prepared to give me advance notice so that I could stay at a

friend's the night before such work was due to begin in my close?"

Yours Sincerely,

Tim Bone

On the evening of the 19th October I arrived back at my home and thought to myself that I would have mixed emotions if the Govanhill Housing Association replied to my e-mail with an answer of "No" to my closed question I had sent earlier. I did think to myself "Imagine that, a closed question being sent at 8.45am in the morning and it being 4pm and this S***Y T*****n hasn't yet been in contact. How long does it take to answer a simple [Yes/No] question?" I then thought "Checkmate!" It was when I started to browse the internet on my phone that I saw the name S***Y T*****n come up on my notifications. I didn't know whether to look at this now or in the cafe I write this book in. I was put off looking as I was on my own, in a flat, with it dark outside; having recently woken up with night time anxiety provoked by not knowing anyone in the world combined with thoughts of not having had any good experience with a human being since I had left my friends at school. The others had just been a bunch of walkovers, disappointments and betrayers. I thought to myself "Do I want to be on my own tonight with no one to share this next punch of social exclusion with". I thought, "Do I want to risk experiencing a fit of rage that will go round and round in my mind amplifying in amount and intensity with each cycle, or do I want to leave it to tomorrow where I am out in public in a café where I won't feel as alone when experiencing this punch". I then thought to myself "On the other hand, if these people say 'No' as their answer to my question, then it is evidence of them being a cold, uncaring, very right wing, shameful organisation whose name I could expose badly, thus, damaging their professional image". I thought that maybe such an e-mail giving "No" as an answer would allow me to pursue action that might give me closure on all the other injustices that authorities as well as people in positions of responsibility have got away with over the years.

After having these thoughts I decided to open the e-mail and as I had expected the answer was "No" but worded in a cowardly way. The e-mail sent on the evening of the 19th October by S***Y T*****n answering my question on whether or not Govanhill Housing Association would give me prior notice of maintenance/repair work in the knowledge that I have epilepsy and that excess unannounced noise can cause me to have seizures can be seen below:

RE: Complaint - Ascog Street 2/1 Inbox

S***Y T*****n

Mon, Oct 19, 4:41 PM (3 days ago)

to me

Dear Mr Bone

Thanks for your email.

As far as we are concerned we have already answered the question and we will not be responding further on the issue.

Regards.

S***Y

S***Y T*****n Manager

It is clear from this e-mail that they would not care about someone having an upon awakening tonic clonic seizure and suffocating in their bed as a result of their hired workman coming round and making unannounced loud excessive noise, and they are even prepared to admit to it.

As this housing association are not short of tenants and income, due to being providers of social housing; as well as, the Scottish Government relying on their existence due to the introducing of subcontracting of social housing from local government to third parties called Housing Associations; which happened under New Labour during the Tony Blair era, this Housing Association believes itself to be above the law. As they believe themselves to be above the law they have now moved into the private sector and started providing factoring services to private home owners, and now believe that they can get away with providing their customers with the minimum service. They know neighbours don't talk anymore and therefore, they take advantage of the fact that there will never be a consensus agreement amongst disgruntled clients to get rid of them and replace them with other factors, especially when the rest of your neighbours don't have an ounce of common sense and behave in ways that cross boundaries that results in neighbour conflicts and fallouts. In a close where we all have relatively high IQ and relative high ability to apply Intellect to Practice, these neighbours would be my allies instead of my enemies. It is because of their low ability to apply intellect to practice that they keep annoying me, causing me to fall out with them; which only gives psychiatrists more ammunition to say I have a personality disorder, as I fall out with everyone simply because they stand on my toes. Remember the Functionality Continuum!! If you are high functioning trying to play a role in society where you are subordinate to someone else, then you are the "owner being walked by the dog". The only way you will be the "owner taking the dog for a walk" is if you turn to entrepreneurship and become your own boss. It is obvious from my experiences that I have become very misanthropic, where my misanthropy is at a level where I hate society and its people, but I can still meet someone for the first time where I see them as a blank canvass; where I allow them to paint a picture of themselves, as I am aware that I belong to a population of people who feel the same way as I, and that stops me from thinking that all people are the same every time I meet someone new. I give everyone an opportunity to prove themselves on a one to one basis, but I'm afraid to say it on a seven billion to one basis the former party has painted its picture and its left me with a feeling of disgust.

There are square peg people who have been far worse affected than I have been, who are misanthropic at a one to one level, and I believe that these people hate people so much that they can take a life without feeling regret, and will carry out the most immoral behaviour as a way in "get back" towards a society that has treated them with such immorality. I reckon that many of these people are found in organised crime and don't care whose lives they ruin with drugs and arms dealing as well as protection money racketeering. Misanthropy will either make you either recluse yourself, refuse to be like others by choosing to help others or unlearn everything you were taught about morality and become society's worst enemy. I have become quite religious since taking up meditation, and believe that those who recluse themselves; as well as those who help others, will go to heaven, and those who fight an evil by becoming an evil will come back to this hell.

It's a difficult life being SMART, "DISABLED", OPEN MINDED, PRINCIPILED and BRAVE; living in a STUPID, PHYSICALLY UNFIT, JUDGEMENTAL, UNPRINCIPLED and VERY COWARDLY world!!!!!!!!!!!!!!!!!!!!!!!!

CHAPTER 44

SO WHAT DOES THE FUTURE HOLD?

It is now the 11th November 2020 and I have been without any friends, acquaintances or supportive family, and have had no conversation with anyone but my father and mother since March 2020 due to the "Lockdown" resulting from the Covid 19 pandemic. I have met with my father a number of times that could be counted on three hands, and my mother that can be counted on one hand; however, we do not have a good relationship, and meetings with my mother have been upsetting as having her in my home or just being in her company makes me reflect on what a cold mother she has been that only fills me with a rage and strong feelings of isolation for the next 48-72 hours. I therefore decided that I could no longer meet with this woman and therefore I have not seen her in the last three months. I have continued to meet with my father approximately every three weeks; however, we do not have a good relationship, and I don't enjoy his company as we just let differences in opinion over his paternal skills, and the grudge I hold towards him for sweeping issues under the carpet, get between us as they have caused major incompatibilities that result in clashes that have the same effect as meeting with my mother had i.e. feeling rage and isolation for the next few days. As a result of this I have decided that meeting with him is not in my interests and that I should just come to terms with the fact that I do not have a family, and let go of all rage towards family and anxiety caused by the isolation, so that I can move on and make the most of the present and give myself a future I truly deserve. I have therefore completed a course that has awarded me with a Cognitive Behaviour Practitioner certificate and I am now waiting for the end of lockdown so that I can start networking and teach courses to people with anxiety and depressive disorders where I teach those attending the same cognitive tools that I have used to control some mental health conditions and conquer others. I also plan on teaching these skills I have used, to people with anxiety and/or depression, on a one to one basis as a person who has 'walked the walk' and can therefore 'talk the talk'.

Despite choosing to come to terms with being a man living in isolation, walking an isolated path through isolated terrain; as well as feeling positive about being able to use the skills, knowledge and experience acquired from walking this path, it was the case that on the 8th and 9th November 2020 I had two lazy days in my home, as over the previous six days I had accumulated a total of two marathons of exercise in the form of 26 miles walking; and two half marathon visits to the gym. Over these six days I was symptom free of depression and anxiety and spent the whole week experiencing a feel good factor. It didn't bother me that I was socially isolated and that I was alone in this world. This knowledge instead filled me with dopamine and gave me a buzz as I looked forward to the challenge of navigating the world entirely on my own. It was the case, however, that the quietness and lifelessness of the flat, over these two days, just made me reflect on the reasons behind my isolation. This caused me to develop depressive symptoms and in the early hours of the 10th November 2020 I woke up with the room feeling like it was spinning caused by strong feelings of burnout with thoughts that were generating huge amounts of panic and rage as a result of prolonged social isolation. I felt like I was being pushed into a really tight corner with feelings of anxiety going through the roof as well as anger and rage; which also causes anxiety as you think "Am I going to lose my mind and go out to Helensburgh and shoot dead all members of my family when they next meet with one another?" As I was feeling this, the meditator in me immediately told me to "LET GO". The meditator was saying, "As convincing as this anxiety and rage is, if you just let go of the thoughts they will eventually subside and so will the emotions". In response to this I just let go of all thoughts. It was as though a major storm was going on in my head and while I let go of the thoughts, I imagined the thoughts being clouds just flying through the "sky" in my mind, and as much as I felt I should be engaging with them, I instead just chose not to engage with any of them. I did this for about twenty minutes and suddenly the thoughts switched off and I was calm and relaxed and the mental storm had subsided. It was now mental peace and tranquillity, and I felt that I had survived a storm which if I had not known about "letting go", would have blown me over causing me to lose all sanity; however, as I let go, I instead remained "standing". I then managed to get back to sleep for the remaining three hours and had no seizure.

I woke up two nights later on "the edge" between strong mental discomfort, that was mixed with intense feelings of helplessness and hopelessness, and giving up on all living; where if I had gone over the edge, I would have had no interest in taking another breath and would have called it a day on living as a result of being completely burned out to the point of needing a hoist to get me of the floor, and a carer to put a set of clothes on me. I felt myself on the verge of going over the edge and at the same time being pulled away from the edge through voluntarily making the effort to keep myself mentally present. When this happens, you have to make sure the depression doesn't make the cynic in you choose to stop you from voluntarily choosing to keep yourself present and instead have you engage with thoughts such as "My life has been a disaster"; or "I live in an ecosystem that makes people like me extinct"; or "I am experiencing extinction"; or "I hate every man, woman and child on this planet"; therefore, you have to let go of the depressive thoughts as well as the anxiety inducing thoughts which by doing will make you increasingly more present. By remaining present I could get through the night in one piece, falling asleep for a couple of hours at a time, wakening up with very strong feelings of burnout and feeling like I was not going to be able to get through the next two minutes of life; to feeling the burnout subside as I made myself present, where I felt myself calming down and experiencing a resurrecting effect. I would have described the night as being a night full of "close shaves" where none of them managed to "sever me". I kept myself present by eliminating from my mind all thoughts to do with the past or future as well as keeping out of my mind, any knowledge of their being such a thing as past or future; simply by letting go, and focusing on the lamp that sat beside my bed, telling myself that the only thing that defined existence was that lamp. I told myself that nothing had come before, nor, will there be anything come after that lamp, and that there had only ever been that lamp. There were no planets, no countries, no people, and   no such thing as anything that had come before or after it. This made me increasingly aware of the present moment by giving the present moment much more focus, thus, increasing its presence. I was basically doing a meditation like the one I do sitting on the couch, but instead of using my breathing to allow me to let go, I was instead using "100% focussed pre-occupation" with an inanimate object to let go of the disturbing thoughts. Feelings of burnout were being caused by thinking about the isolation in the past as well as thoughts of anticipating 24/7 isolation in the future. Feelings of anger and rage were brought on by thoughts about what people, especially family, had done to me in the past as well as thoughts about what I would like to do to these people in the future. Feelings of hopelessness and helplessness were brought on by thoughts of all the efforts I had made in the past to resolve my isolation, and how these attempts had failed, and how no other way could be tried in the future; and therefore the future was going to be full of failed attempt, after failed attempt etc causing more burnout and depression as well as frustration and feelings of hatred and rage increasing with each cycle to the point of me losing all control and going mad by shooting dead every member of my family. It was therefore the letting go of all future and past thinking and only leaving space for present moment thinking that put out the flames that past and future thinking were causing, thus, freeing me of all cruel emotions caused by both past and future thinking.

It was the next day that I went to the gym and did my four miles walk, 40 minutes on the bike and did my hour on the cross trainer, thus, burning off 1,800 calories, which is equivalent to eighteen miles of aerobic exercise. After this workout I then came back home and did a 30 minute very deep meditation where the depth of the meditation was likely encouraged by the meditative effect of the exercise, and I slept like a log with a couple of awakenings where I woke up with strong feelings of confidence and euphoria. I felt a million miles away from where I was the night before.

It is because of the experiences mentioned in the last few paragraphs as well as other similar experiences over the years that I would like the first classes that I teach these alternative remedies to, to be classes for those with panic disorder, anger management and major depressive disorder. I have thought about teaching those with epilepsy about the benefits of meditation, but there is a lot of paranoia amongst neurologists and other related disciplines that meditation might worsen epilepsy. I am of the opinion that it does not. I believe that it can reduce seizure frequency. Evidence of this is that when I have forgotten a dose of medication or have been sleep deprived and had a seizure in the gym I have never had a seizure while exercising. The experiencing of seizures in the gym have instead been while resting between exercises or in the shower room. I have never had a seizure on an exercise bike, cross trainer, treadmill or swimming pool. They say that when you do intense exercise you are in the meditative zone as you remain in the present moment as you counter the temptation to rest and instead keep going. The discomfort from the exercise keeps you in the present moment. People say they get bored of their exercise routine as they are doing the same exercises over and over again. It is impossible to get bored of a challenging exercise routine. If you become bored of an exercise routine then it means your workout is too easy and is no longer challenging enough; which in that case you need to increase the exercise intensity. Your exercise no longer has a focus i.e. the discomfort that keeps you present. You can't become bored when in the present moment. When I sit on a couch and do my meditation; letting thoughts pass through my mind as well as not engaging with them while focussing on my breathing, I am not thinking "How much time have I done", nor am I thinking "How much time have I to do" as my mind is in the present moment and not thinking 'past' or 'future'. I therefore do not become bored, as boredom is thinking "How much time have we done?" and "How much time have we to do?" combined with "How unrewarding and unchallenging has this activity been since starting and now?" and "How unrewarding can we expect this activity to continue to be from now to end?". People in boring, repetitive, unrewarding jobs will relate with this. You are looking at the watch, constantly asking these two lots of questions, which brings on boredom. It is, therefore, interesting how boredom can bring on a seizure, and how meditation prevents boredom. This fact, therefore, may make the claim that meditation is good for epilepsy, more credible than the claim those saying the opposite make.

It was after the attack of panic and rage during the early hours of the 10th November that I woke up that same morning at 7.30 am and during my meditation session it came to me that I should get the symptoms caused by family abandonment officially recognised. I thought it was wrong that I suffer from these torturous symptoms that would have killed me if it were not for me teaching the expert patient programme where I learned about meditation.

I have decided that I am going to go to my General Practitioner and tell him that I fit the definition of having been abused. According to the National Health Service website psychological abuse is defined as "an unreasonable and unjustified withdrawal of services or support". All my cries for help have just fallen on deaf ears over the last five years. I just suddenly found myself with no family support without any justification. Despite me giving my family plenty descriptions of my symptoms and how isolation and abandonment were the causes of them, my family still showed no interest. As I can say for sure that their deaf ears would have killed me if it were not for the meditation, I could never seek repatriation, therefore, I now find myself not just without family but also without prospective family. I will never be able to forgive them for how they have treated me; and as a result of that, their deaf ears have created for me an irreversible set of living conditions that without the meditation would be too mentally torturous to endure. It is for this reason that I want these mentally torturous symptoms recognised as being symptoms of abuse. I therefore seek a mental health diagnosis that is recognised as being caused by abuse. I certainly wish to seek an official diagnosis of 'Social Anxiety Disorder' as this would at least recognise the abuse that I received from my mother when I was a boy i.e. the overly critical childhood. A diagnosis that recognises that I have been abused would give me closure as when I have been angry with my family for not helping me, they have said that they don't help me because I am angry and make them feel threatened. They evidence their claims by making reference to the anger that I am experiencing over the phone. I tell them that they dress up my symptoms of neglect by them as being the reasons for neglecting me. They say that my anger is the precursor to the neglect when it is the neglect that is the precursor to the anger. I feel that this is as big an injustice and cover up as the experience in social work training where they denied ever being on the phone to me and that I had imagined voices over the phone. I want a doctor to tell my family, "No, it was the neglect that came first and the anger is a symptom of the neglect". This would give me a lot of closure. I also wish these symptoms that have held me back throughout life, and would have caused me to take my life, to be recognised as being symptomatic of a trauma related mental health condition, as at present the diagnosis of 'Paranoid Personality Disorder' does not recognise any of the abuse as well as breaches of trust that those who held positions of responsibility over my personal development were guilty of during my formative years and beyond. This protects the abusers from me making a litigation claim or taking any other legal action against my school, universities attended, family, past employers and others guilty of my mistreatment throughout my life. I therefore want psychiatry to recognise that I do not have a paranoid personality disorder and what I am instead is someone who has a rational dislike and distrust of the human race as it has abused me all of my life due to its judgemental attitudes, fear of difference, failure to develop views/beliefs/values of their own; making them easily manipulatable and exploitable, and a failure of them to develop outside the box thinking causing them to behave in ways as well as make reckless decisions that "stand on my toes", creating an incredible number of relationship difficulties. The correct diagnosis is 'Misanthropist'. According to the Merriam-Webster dictionary, the definition of Misanthropy is:

"A hatred or distrust of humankind"

I now need to get this book on the market as I need the money, therefore I am going to stop here. I am feeling good about my future projects as I know that I have the skills and abilities to make a success of my peer support mental health service evidenced by my ability to run Fairway Advocacy, winning 120 cases between the years 2014-2017, as well as from the self-management of my mental health conditions that goes back as far as 1993. I also have training experience from the days when I delivered the Expert Patient Programme, where I was always given good praise in my course delivery evaluations, as well as when I delivered self-management courses to those with disability when I worked at Disability Information Greater Glasgow, despite it possibly being a charity that was nothing more than a front; and when I delivered mental health management courses at Epilepsy Connections where they constructively dismissed me very possibly because of their own deep rooted insecurities preventing them from wanting anyone who knew more than they entering their patch.

I will continue to be using meditation, exercise and the power of positive thought to control the mental health symptoms that I will have to continue to contend to during the growing of my projects. Despite having night time awakenings where I have strong anxious and depressive thinking that makes me feel that I am going to break down and not be able to find the energy nor motivation to take my next breath in a world I have no support from friends or family in, I am glad to say that my meditation practice and what it has taught me about the workings of the mind has prevented these awakenings from happening every evening and instead one every five evenings when you average it out, where that one in five night is down to lots of mind wandering during my meditation sessions. I can also defuse these attacks when they happen by doing an on the spot eyes open meditation where I focus on a lamp when I feel really burned out by isolation or let go of thoughts remaining present. The letting go of thoughts defuses the burnout but takes longer than the focussed concentration on the lamp. The letting go of thoughts during such intense emotions is better left to 50 minutes meditation sessions on the couch that play much more of a preventative role.

I am glad to say that never have these nocturnal attacks of anxiety and depression stopped me from being able to get up the next day and work towards my goals and never have I had such nauseating symptoms during the day.

I have found that when I incorporate two aerobic workouts per week into the equation, on top of the meditation, I am having no nocturnal attacks of anxiety and depression as the gym makes the meditations deeper as well as increasing neurotransmitters concentrations such as dopamine and serotonin. It is the case that these nocturnal attacks start to become one every five nights when either my attendance at the gym drops from twice a week to once or when for some reason, I have to go a stretch of time without attending the gym e.g. injury.

CHAPTER 45

In a nutshell, meditation has provided me with the following benefits which have been:

The rehabilitating of my ability to concentrate when reading and listening

The rehabilitating of my ability to process information when reading and listening

Large reductions in rage and trait anger levels

Huge reduction in time spent thinking about past events that have traumatised me; and huge increase in ability to make myself present when past or future thinking is exacerbating anger, rage, depression and anxiety

A large reduction in intrusive thinking; continuing towards the total elimination of intrusive thinking

Much improved memory

Reduced seizures

It is also the case that aerobic exercise has successfully controlled symptoms of obsessive compulsive disorder between the years 1999-2012 where I destroyed all obsessive thinking that had me constantly experience mental distress caused by tormenting thoughts telling me to give up things, turn down things or bring an end to things that were very meaningful to me. Aerobic exercise also gave me the determination and confidence to keep bouncing back from all set backs experienced during these years and beyond

I have used 'thought blocking' to reduce existing anger, rage and irritability during 2008-2012. With thought blocking, if I caught the strap of rucksack on a door handle or got a cable caught on the corner of a table, I was no longer feeling the need to shout out loud "You bastard!" and instead felt impartial and unbothered.

I have used Visualisation to prevent Performance Anxiety (subtype of Social Anxiety Disorder) from getting in the way of me driving a car after passing my driving test.

I have used positive thinking in the form of visualisations, positive affirmations and thought blocking to pass my driving test back in 2012 as well as win 120 cases when I ran Fairway advocacy between the years 2014-2017.

I resorted to slow breathing to prevent myself from experiencing symptoms of anxiety that crippled my ability to vocalise and had me trembling like mad when giving presentations to audiences of any size between the years 2001-2012. This has unleashed a career path for me that is a road that leads to being your own boss.

I used mental arithmetic in the preventing of daytime seizures where anxiety or sleep deprivation could bring them on between the years 1994-present

I have used distraction during the years 1993-1997 to control symptoms of obsessive compulsive disorder where I constantly worried about HIV infection

I now use positive thinking, meditation as well as aerobic exercise to make a success of working towards my future aims and goals. My only frustration is that I did not know about the power of visualisations and positive affirmations when I was an undergraduate student at Glasgow University. If I had known about these tools back in 1993-1997 I do believe that I would have got a much better degree than I did. I got a third class honours degree in molecular biology at a time in my life where I was having a seizure every 36 hours as well as being on strong anti-convulsant medication. I was also during these years living with an anxiety disorder i.e. symptoms of obsessive compulsive disorder as well as living with the scars of school that had me believe I was the thickest student and that a guy like me could only ever expect a pass at best. I do believe that if I had known about visualisation and positive affirmations as well as thought blocking during my honours degree, I would have left university with a much better degree avoiding 23 years of mayhem. I am therefore so glad that I now know about these tools of positive thinking, and have evidence that they work due to what was achieved at Fairway Advocacy; and how I passed my driving test first time round, and look forward to using them with the successful setting up of my peer support mental health service.

I therefore wish to share these experiences, and what I have learned with others; and therefore, would hope others reading may have learned something from this book that they can take away with them and use to make improvements in their character as well as in their lives.

I am glad to say that there is such a "destination" that the journey I am on is capable of taking me to where I see myself being happy, and that is in the success of this book; the establishing of professional contacts; the meeting of honourable people through the church; the creating of my peer support mental health service; and an amount of success that allows me to enjoy life, as up until now it's just been about fighting and surviving in a very judgemental and right- wing world. What's the worse of two crimes: The person who is dragged out of a cell and shot through the back of their head as a result of campaigning for a fairer more democratic electoral system in a dictatorship society; or an education system that discriminates and excludes a sense of purpose person because of a condition like epilepsy, causing major depression combined with a loathing of the human race as a result of a lifetime of abuse and neglect; resulting in feelings of anger and rage, causing relationship difficulties; making it impossible to hold down a job; resulting in being diagnosed with paranoid personality disorder by a judgemental psychiatrist for the purpose of denying that society has a discrimination and prejudice culture; resulting in a life on the benefits system combined with loss of purpose; resulting in the picking up of a gun and then shooting himself in the side of the head? I leave that question for you to answer.

www.ingramcontent.com/pod-product-compliance
Lightning Source LLC
Chambersburg PA
CBHW070106260726
48658CB00001B/6